CYCLE OF LIES

THE FALL OF LANCE ARMSTRONG

JULIET MACUR

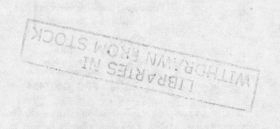

WILLIAM
COLLINS

William Collins
An imprint of HarperCollins*Publishers*
77–85 Fulham Palace Road
London W6 8JB
WilliamCollinsBooks.com

This William Collins paperback edition published 2014

1

First published in Great Britain by William Collins in 2014

A catalogue record for this book is available from the British Library.

ISBN 978-0-00-752063-3

Printed and bound in Great Britain by
Clays Ltd, St Ives plc

MIX
Paper from
responsible sources
FSC **FSC® C007454**
www.fsc.org

FSC™ is a non-profit international organisation established to promote the
responsible management of the world's forests. Products carrying the FSC label
are independently certified to assure consumers that they come from forests that
are managed to meet the social, economic and ecological needs of present or
future generations, and other controlled sources.

Find out more about HarperCollins and the environment at
www.harpercollins.co.uk/green

To my two greatest loves, Dave and Allegra

To my heroes, Mama and Tata

This is my body. And I can do whatever I want to it. I can push it, study it, tweak it, listen to it. Everybody wants to know what I'm on. What am I on? I'm on my bike, busting my ass six hours a day. What are you on?

—LANCE ARMSTRONG

CONTENTS

CYCLE OF LIES

PROLOGUE

The $10 million estate of Lance Armstrong's dreams is hidden behind a tall, cream-colored wall of Texas limestone and a solid steel gate. Visitors pull into a circular driveway beneath a grand oak tree whose branches stretch toward a 7,806-square-foot Spanish colonial mansion.

The tree itself speaks of Armstrong's famous will. It once was on the other side of the property, fifty yards west of this house. Armstrong wanted it at the front steps. The transplantation cost $200,000. His close friends joke that Armstrong, who is agnostic, engineered the project to prove he didn't need God to move heaven and earth.

For nearly a decade, Lance Armstrong and I have had a contentious relationship. Seven years have passed since his agent, Bill Stapleton, first threatened to sue me. Back then, I was just one of the many reporters Armstrong had tried to manipulate, charm or bully. Filing lawsuits against writers who dared challenge his fairy-tale story was his quick-and-easy way of convincing people that writing critically about him wasn't worth it. Over the years, he came to consider me an enemy, one of the many he and his handlers had to keep an eye on.

Only now, after he has fallen, have we agreed to something approaching a truce. Though he'd deny it, I know that he has chosen to sit down with me because he thinks he might be able to control the direction of my book. No chance, I've told him. After multiple criminal and civil investigations into whether Armstrong orchestrated a sophisticated doping regime to win seven Tour de France titles; after all the testimonies from riders who knew him better than anyone else, and who contradicted under oath every public defense Armstrong had ever given; after he lied, lied and lied some more, the most notorious athlete of our generation realizes I'm suddenly holding a lot of rope. And *I* realize that, even now, he imagines himself to occupy a position of almost absolute power.

"You can write what you want," he tells me in one of our many conversations. "But your book is called *Cycle of Lies*? That has to change."

I've interviewed him one-on-one in five different countries; on team buses that smelled of sweat-soaked Lycra at the Tour de France, in swanky New York City hotel rooms, in the backs of limos, in soulless conference rooms; and for hours by telephone.

Now, in the spring of 2013, after his whole world has come crashing down and moving trucks are en route to dismantle his beloved estate, I've come to visit him at home in Austin, Texas, for the first time.

Yes, fine, come on out, he said. Beset by endless obituaries of his celebrated (and now fraudulent) career, he wanted to ensure that I wrote "the true story."

So here I am parking beneath the grand oak that Armstrong had moved because, why not? I look at the house and think of his yellow jerseys. A month after the United States Anti-Doping Agency released 1,000 pages of evidence against Armstrong and stripped him of his Tour titles, he had Tweeted a photo of himself lounging, arrogance itself, on an L-shaped couch in this house, his seven yellow jerseys hanging ceremoniously behind him: "Back in Austin and just layin' around." That was November 2012. Seven months later, will I find him still defiant?

Before I can pull the keys from my car's ignition, a cherubic face under tousled, curly brown hair appears at my window and two small preschooler hands slap the glass. It's Lance's youngest son, Max.

Armstrong stands behind him in flip-flops, wearing a black T-shirt over black basketball shorts that brush his scarred knees. His eyes are hidden by dark sunglasses.

"Say hi to Juliet, Max," Armstrong says.

"Hi, Joo-leee-ette!" Max says. Then he turns to his dad and asks for ice cream, a request that makes his father giggle, something I'd never seen him do before.

"Yes, you get ice cream," Armstrong says. "You've been good, buddy, really good."

We walk up the front steps until Armstrong stops at the door. He moves his eyes to the tree, the house, the life he has enjoyed.

"Great place, right?" he says.

"Yes," I say, "are you going to miss it?"

Armstrong doesn't want to move, he has to. His sponsors have abandoned him, taking away an estimated $75 million in future earnings. He would owe more than $135 million if he were to lose every lawsuit in which he is a defendant. To "slow the burn rate," as he calls it, he has stopped renting a penthouse apartment on Central Park in Manhattan and a house in Marfa, Texas. Next to go is this Austin estate, traded in for a much more modest abode near downtown.

His former sponsors—including Oakley, Trek Bicycle Corporation, RadioShack and Nike—have left him scrambling for money. He considers them traitors. He says Trek's revenue was $100 million when he signed with the company and reached $1 billion in 2013. "Who's responsible for that?" he asks. "Fucking right here." He pokes himself in the chest with his right index finger. "I'm sorry, but that is true. Without me, none of that happens."

After his sponsors cast him aside, he tossed their gear. There's a chance you could catch a glimpse of one of his Dallas friends wearing Armstrong's custom-made yellow Nike sneakers, with "Lance" embroidered in small yellow block letters on the shoes' black tongues. A Goodwill outlet in Austin is replete with his former Nike clothes and Oakley sunglasses. The movers, who packed up his guesthouse a week before I visited, will have to contend with whatever brand-name gear is left in his garage: black Livestrong Nike caps, black Nike duffel bags with bright yellow swooshes, Oakley lenses and frames and a box of caps suggesting "Yes on Prop 15," a 2007 Texas bond plan for cancer research, prevention and education supported by Armstrong.

It was 1989 when Armstrong moved to Austin from Plano, a suburb of Dallas, showing up in this progressive town as a rough, combative and pimply-faced teenager, with frosted wavy brown hair, a gold hoop in his pierced left ear, a silver chain around his neck with a dangling pendant in the shape of Texas, and a fake ID.

On an income of $12,000 a year, and with the help of a local benefactor named J.T. Neal who had taken Armstrong in, he lived in a studio apartment for $200 a month. He dressed it up with an oversized black leather couch, a matching chair and, above the fireplace, a red-white-and-blue colored skull of a Texas longhorn.

From a cramped studio to a sprawling estate: a reflection of

Armstrong's ascension into modern American sainthood—a cancer survivor who beat the world's best cyclists in a grueling race, dated anyone he wanted and made millions in the process.

Armstrong loves this house. He loves its open spaces and floor-to-ceiling windows. He loves the lush, landscaped yard where his kids play soccer, and the crystalline pool (a "*negative-edge* pool, *not* an infinity pool, get it right"). Behind the house are rows of towering Italian cypresses.

He moved here in 2006 after winning a record seventh Tour de France. He once said the place was his safe house—inside it, "nobody's going to mess with me." Having eluded near-constant attempts to expose his doping, he could take a left down the main hallway, then a quick right, and disappear into his walk-in wine closet to grab a bottle of Tignanello and toast his good luck.

On a table next to a couch is a 36-inch model of the Gulfstream jet that had been Armstrong's favored means of long-distance flight. It's white with black and yellow racing stripes. He and his buddies often stood up when the plane took off, "surfing" as it rocketed into the sky. Armstrong had sold the plane for $8 million in December 2012, as he braced himself for the inevitable legal fees that would follow USADA's exposé of his cheating.

Just as we settle into his media room on the big house's second floor, his twin daughters, Grace and Isabelle, burst in. The preteen girls are replicas of their mother, Kristin: beautiful and blonde. Their open smiles reveal gleaming silver braces.

"Hi, Dad! Did you buy those skirts for us off the Internet?" Isabelle asks as she and her sister use the couch as a trampoline.

"Yeah, Dad, did you buy the skirts?" Grace seconds.

"No, not yet," Amstrong says. "It's almost time I had a beer. It would be nice if one of you ladies got me a beer. Shiner Bock."

Grace shouts, "Shiner Bock! Don'tcha know, it's a beer—that's B-O-C-K. It's not a twist-off."

Once he has the beer in hand, Armstrong looks at me and says, "So this is my awful life. Just so awful."

He says how much he likes having kids in the house—children are transparent and pure, too young to con him. I ask if he feels like people have taken advantage of him, if he feels used.

"Uh, yeah," he says.

"Who?"

"Everybody. Get in line."

The kid who once decorated his living room with a steer head has become a collector of sophisticated, expensive art. His sensibilities are apparent, if perplexing. Upon entering his house you see a panel of stained glass eleven feet tall and five feet wide that, upon closer inspection, is actually a panel comprised of hundreds of colored butterflies—a Damien Hirst piece called *The Tree of Life*. Hirst is known for his provocative installations (e.g., a severed cow's head being feasted on by maggots in a glass case). In 2009, when he decorated an Armstrong racing bike with butterflies, the animal rights group People for the Ethical Treatment of Animals called the work "horrific barbarity."

The more I see of Armstrong's art throughout the house, the odder his curatorial eye seems. To call his choices dark is to be kind, to call them controversial is too simple. All Armstrong will say of any of them is that they are "fucking cool."

Look, though: Above the fireplace in the expansive formal dining room, flanked by marble bowls made to contain a church's holy water, is a photograph of urine and blood called *Piss and Blood No. VII*. It is by Andres Serrano, the photographer made infamous for his 1987 photo of a plastic crucifix in the artist's urine. There is something harmonic in being in the same room as both the photograph and an athlete who claims to have passed hundreds of urine and blood drug tests.

On the far side of the room is Armstrong's office, dimly lit, built of dark shades of wood: a spot to brood. Sitting at his desk in a corner, Armstrong has a direct view of his Tour de France trophies—seven deep purple porcelain cups with delicate gold designs—perched high on the wall atop bookshelves, each in its own spotlight, each luminescent.

To the left of his desk is artwork that may speak to his broken relationships with family, friends, lovers, teammates. A sepia-hued photograph by Luis González Palma shows a man and a woman in an embrace, dancing. Or are they really? A second look and I see spikes protruding from their backs. Armstrong would admit only that the piece is gloomy.

And then there is the Jesus art.

To the right of his desk is a seventeenth-century Spanish painting of the crucifixion that takes up nearly the entire wall. Four women pray at the feet of Christ, his head slung and crowned by a glowing gold halo. Years ago, the painting hung inside the chapel Armstrong had built for his ex-wife, a Catholic, inside their home in Girona, Spain. He himself is not a religious man. He says he considers organized religion to be gatherings of hypocrites.

Around the corner from his office, overlooking a stairwell, there is another vision of the crucifixion. The piece's full effect is apparent only from certain angles, where an image of Christ nailed to the cross comes into view.

"One man has taken the blame for a thousand sins," Armstrong says. But even in the presence of these crucifixes, he is talking about himself. Like he wants me to write that he has been made a martyr for cycling's century of dopers and this is the way to make sure I do.

He walks over to a coffee table in his office and picks up a sculpture—an arm from hand to elbow. The sculpture, by Japanese artist Haroshi, is made with many layers of pressed skateboards. The sculpture's middle finger is sticking up.

"This is pretty much the story of my life," he says. Then he shoves the sculpture in my face. I notice Armstrong's hands. On each palm, there is a small wound where he'll tell me a doctor burned away a couple of cysts. I think of the stigmata.

"Fuck you," he says, laughing.

Seven years ago, he told his three oldest children from his failed marriage—Luke, Grace and Isabelle—that they would graduate from high school while living in the house by the big oak tree. He owed them that. They had followed him from Texas to France to Spain countless times. At last they could plant some roots. "I promise," he said. "Dad's not moving again." They would live six minutes from their mother, Kristin, and could count on the familiarities of the giant kitchen table surrounded by black-and-white photos of their family. They knew where Dad would be on most weeknights—on a couch in front of the TV, watching CNN's *Anderson Cooper 360°*. In the summer of 2012, Armstrong built an addition onto the first floor so his growing family would have a seventh bedroom. Already, the house was his headquarters. He lived there with his girlfriend, the willowy blonde Anna Hansen, and their two children, four-year-old Max and two-year-old Olivia, a Shirley Temple lookalike. Armstrong and his clan had planned to stay here, safe and happy, for a long time.

But now the movers are coming. It's June 6, 2013, five years before Luke's expected graduation. In the morning, a line of black trucks will pull into his driveway and out will spill workers in black short-sleeved shirts. Already, the atmosphere is funereal. The movers have already emptied out the 1,633-square-foot guesthouse, a mini-mansion, with its matching tan façade and burnt orange roof.

On June 7, I return to see those workers clear the main house. They take Armstrong's Tour trophies from their illuminated shelves, cover them with green bubble wrap and place them in blue boxes. In a moving box marked #64, one mover places a silver frame containing a 5x7 photograph of Armstrong's 2005 Discovery Channel team sitting at a dinner table after his seventh and final Tour victory. He, his teammates and longtime team manager Johan Bruyneel are holding up seven fingers. A yellow rubber Livestrong bracelet hangs from each man's wrist. A table is littered with half-empty wineglasses. A former life.

Box #64 goes onto the truck with the rest. I follow the movers into the media room. Wearing white cotton gloves, they take down the seven yellow Tour leader's jerseys framed above the couch. The day before, as Armstrong and I sat in this room, he had an idea. He asked if I wanted to lie on the couch, if I wanted to pose for a photograph under the jerseys that were still left.

"It'll be funny," he said.

I didn't get the joke.

In the dark before dawn, Armstrong left the big house for good. At 4:15 a.m. on June 7, 2013, with Hansen and his five children, he drove to Austin/Bergstrom International Airport for a commercial flight to the Big Island in Hawaii, where they would remain for the first part of the summer.

Armstrong tells me he didn't look back at the house he had built. He says sentiment has never been his thing. The move means only that part of his life has ended and another will begin. That's all it is, he says. Maybe he believes the words coming out of his mouth. Maybe he doesn't.

Several days later, only two of his possessions remained on his estate. One couldn't fit in the moving truck: a 1970 black Pontiac GTO convertible given him by the singer Sheryl Crow, with whom he had a very public romance that ended when he pedaled away just before she got cancer. The car, with its evocations of another Armstrong failure, carries a price tag of $70,000.

And, finally, left over in the living room of the guesthouse was a fully assembled drum kit. Just another piece of the man's discarded life. *Oh beat the drum slowly and play the fife lowly*, I thought while I looked at the set, words of a song I know from my time working in Texas,

> *Take me to the valley, and lay the sod o'er me,*
> *For I'm a young cowboy and I know I've done wrong.*

PART ONE

LIES OF THE FAMILY

CHAPTER 1

L ance Armstrong's mother, Linda, is always the hero of her own story. As she tells it, the two of them—she and Lance—struggled to survive in Dallas's Oak Cliff neighborhood in the hardscrabble projects on the wrong side of the Trinity River. They had only each other. The boy never met his father; she raised him alone. She said she taught him to ride a bike, encouraged him as an athlete, paid for his equipment, bought their home, traveled to all his races, secured his sponsorships and was out the door with him at 7 a.m. every Saturday so he could administer a beating to yet another set of, say, prepubescent middle-distance runners.

In her autobiography, *No Mountain High Enough: Raising Lance, Raising Me*, she revels in the constant question, "How did a single teenage mom manage to raise a real live superhero?" In the author's note, before the story unfolds, she warns of her "totally biased, subjective, slanted, rationalized, and confabulated" account. She even says, "Someone else might have a different perspective." She dared those people to write their own book.

She used pseudonyms for her three ex-husbands: Eddie Gunderson, Terry Armstrong and John Walling. She calls Lance's father "Eddie Haskell" after the sweet, conniving character in the 1950–'60s television show *Leave It to Beaver*. The Gundersons were Lance Armstrong's first family. Eddie Gunderson and Linda

Mooneyham married while they were in high school. The baby came seven months later.

The shotgun wedding united two troubled families. Both of Armstrong's grandfathers had been heavy drinkers whose wives fled with their children after one sodden mishap or another. His paternal grandfather was so mean that he would put kittens in fruit jars to smother them. Armstrong's father was an alcoholic with as many wives as his mother would have husbands—four.

By the age of twenty, Armstrong had had three different fathers: one biological, one adoptive and one step. (In her book, Linda Armstrong writes of the failures of her love life as having been the result of "stupid, self-undermining, counterintuitive and utterly stinko" choices.) After that, Lance was tossed about in the tumult of a dozen stand-in fathers of his choosing.

As a motivational speaker, Linda has made a living off bromides of her struggles to raise the greatest cyclist the world has ever seen, telling her audience, "We had everything against us," and "It was about survival." She talks about how Lance once showed up at a race in the mountains of New Mexico without a long-sleeve shirt and how, while the other racers had fancy gear, he had to borrow her tiny pink windbreaker to stay warm. He broke the course record.

She talks about going "from poverty with no money to personal success" and emphasizes that she played an integral role in her son's accomplishments. "I really believe that your children are a product of you."

By her telling, she has been the single constant presence in his life. Early on, she made it clear that she, and only she, would shape her son. The first step in that process began when she removed him from the Gunderson family. Armstrong's mother has told her side of that story for years. It's a story that a lifetime later brings Willine Gunderson Harroff, Eddie's mother, and his sister, Micki Rawlings, to tears.

Linda Armstrong has said she was alone in raising Lance, that others in Lance's life played only bit parts no matter what they contributed or how long they were involved. She called herself a single mother though she was only without a husband for a year before Lance was sixteen and a half—and even then her first husband's family said they helped her get by, babysitting while she worked. Over time, the media played up the tragedy and triumph of it all: that one of the greatest athletes in history was a product of a teenage mother who had struggled for survival with no one to lean on but her young son.

Linda's mythmaking didn't sit right with the rest of Lance's family, according to Willine Gunderson.

The Gundersons had their own version of Lance's childhood to tell. For one thing, they called Lance's father Sonny. He was a handsome, blue-eyed rebel with shiny brown hair, a mischievous grin and a willingness to help friends steal tape decks from parked cars. He once rode his motorcycle through the back door and into the kitchen of a high school girlfriend's house, causing her parents to call the police.

In their neighborhood of Wynnewood, a middle-class area of the city—nothing like "the projects of Dallas" proclaimed by the promotional videos for Linda's public speaking—the Gundersons were neighbors with another family, the Mooneyhams.

Linda Mooneyham was a high school homecoming princess and a star on the school's drill team. Sonny asked her for a date. Soon enough, they were going steady and cruising around town in his souped-up Pontiac GTO. He had a bad-boy charm that caused him, one night in the winter of 1970, to whisper to Linda, "Make love, not war." That evening, she got pregnant. When a sixteen-year-old Linda refused to get an abortion, her mother told her to leave the house. Far from being left on her own—with "everything against us"—she found a family that took her in. She lived in Sonny's house. She became, in effect, an adopted daughter of Willine Gunderson, whom family members called "Mom-o."

Willine was a single mother with an ex-husband always late on child support payments, when he sent them at all. For forty-three years, she worked at Dallas's First National Bank. Her sense of family was so strong, she says, that she insisted her two daughters and Sonny go to church together three times a week. She never criticized her absent ex-husband because she wanted her children to make up their own minds about him. She and Linda became as close as best friends during Linda's pregnancy.

On Linda's seventeenth birthday, she and seventeen-year-old Sonny were married in a Baptist church packed with fellow high schoolers, some no doubt noticing the bride's baby bump beneath her flowing, pleated white dress. That was February 1971. The boy arrived in September.

He was named after Lance Rentzel, the Dallas Cowboys star wide receiver who the year before was arrested for exposing himself to a ten-year-old girl. At the window of the maternity ward, his father saw that the newborn's head was misshapen: too long, too narrow. His mother, a petite woman, delivered him at 9 pounds, 12 ounces.

"What's wrong with his head?" his father asked, as tears rolled down his cheeks.

"It'll get better," one of his sisters said. "It'll be fine, I know it will."

Linda took a part-time job at a grocery store. Sonny worked at a bakery and delivered newspapers, but fatherhood didn't bring with it a sudden maturity. As a minor, he had made frequent appearances in juvenile court. In 1974, when his son was two and a half, and he and Linda had already divorced, Sonny Gunderson spent his first night in jail as an adult. He had been arrested for breaking into a car.

Their marriage lasted for just over two years. Linda would claim in her book that Sonny had been so rough with her that her neck and arms were bruised. Years later, the ex-husband admitted that he had slapped her, but only once.

Gunderson told his family that he spent months after the divorce in a zombie-like state. He wanted to fix what he had broken, but had no idea how. He often sat across the street from his son's day care center and watched the boy play on the playground. He couldn't pay the child support, or wouldn't. He ignored the demand notes as they piled up in his mailbox, accusingly.

To his father's family, Armstrong was Lance Edward Gunderson. They still saw him at Christmases and other family gatherings, where he played with his cousins. They still have photos of him, yellowed and fading. His grandmother has a 4x4-inch photo album made for her by Armstrong's mother. Linda signed the album with her boy's name, "To Mom-o Willine. Love, Lance."

Willine "Mom-o" Gunderson is Armstrong's paternal grandmother. In nearly every photo of her with the infant Lance, she is kissing him, her eyes closed, the kind of moment a grandmother wants to last forever. Her son is partly to blame for how short-lived it really was.

Whenever he saw Lance, Gunderson acted like a kid himself. While his mother and two sisters watched, he gave the boy rides on his ten-speed bike and motorcycle. Inevitably, some outings ended with acrimony. Lance once came home with a quarter-sized burn on his calf where it had rubbed against the motorcycle's exhaust pipe. Another time, he suffered a bloody toe when his foot became tangled in the spokes of a bicycle. Linda blamed Sonny for his neglect and chastised Willine for allowing the boy to get hurt while in her care.

Willine told the young mother, "You can't keep him in a golden cage his whole life."

Linda snapped back, "I'm the one that knows what's best for him."

"She was maternal," Willine says, "but she was so young, she didn't understand that babies love more than one person in their life. She didn't want him to love anybody but her. But babies love anybody that will love them. That doesn't take from the love that they have for their mother."

When Linda filed for divorce—on February 15, 1973—she just couldn't stand Sonny anymore. She married Terry Armstrong, a salesman, in May 1974, a year after her divorce papers were signed. Though Sonny couldn't know it at the time, his life with Lance would soon be over.

The Armstrongs would eventually move away, ending any contact with the Gundersons, and Terry officially adopted Lance as his son. Linda said in her autobiography that Willine agreed it was best for Lance to never see the Gundersons again. But whenever someone suggests as much to Willine her mouth drops open. "Ooh, no, no," she says.

Willine last had direct contact with Linda and her family

when Lance was five or six. She had gone to his maternal grand-mother's house with Christmas gifts for him. "Linda told me not to take anything more from you," the grandmother told Willine. "What little stuff you give him is not worth the trouble Linda has with Lance after he has had some contact with you."

Shaking with distress, Willine quietly said, almost to herself, "You've got no right to tear a family apart," and walked away with the presents in her hands and tears in her eyes.

For years after Lance was gone, Willine and Micki kept his picture inside oval gold lockets that hung around their necks. In his grandmother's locket, he is an infant, maybe ten months old, wearing a fire-engine-red romper. In his aunt's, a toddler with a goofy smile.

To this day, Willine is haunted by the last time she saw Lance. She was babysitting him, and he was about four. His mother swung by to pick him up, and found him under the Gunder-sons' dining room table. The grandmother remembers the boy saying, happily, "I'm just going to live under here. I won't take up too much room. I'm just going to live under this table." But his mother grabbed Lance by the arm and led him through the front door, the boy crying as they went. She slammed the door. The grandmother never saw the boy again.

The Gundersons had no idea that the Armstrongs were living in Richardson, a northern suburb of Dallas, and had no money to hire a lawyer or investigator to find him. The Gundersons held out hope that Armstrong would come looking for them someday, maybe when he had children of his own. At their church—Four Mile Lutheran, which his relatives helped found and build east of Dallas 165 years ago—the congregation for years had prayed for Armstrong every Sunday.

The Gundersons wrote to Armstrong occasionally, but he never answered. They rarely called Linda's family, and when they tried they heard only the click of a phone being put back into its cradle.

Linda's brother, Alan, felt sorry for Sonny and was the Gundersons' only source of information about the boy. He once came over to Sonny's place and gave him a school picture of Armstrong, a color 8x10. The Gundersons inspected Lance's face closely, the first time they had seen it in more than five years.

He had the same deep blue eyes as his father, and the same high cheekbones. They wondered if he possessed other family traits: Would Lance be hard and stubborn? Did he have problems with authority? Did he see the world in extremes? Did he hold grudges?

Armstrong's grandmother is now nearly ninety. When she turned eighty, she moved in with Micki, who resides in one of Dallas's most exclusive neighborhoods, among mansions and estates with guardhouses. Her husband, Mike Rawlings, was elected mayor in 2011.

Willine's thick brown hair has turned snowy white. Her once rod-straight posture has become permanently bent. She uses a walker and needs thick glasses and bright lights to see. Her hearing is going, too, but her mind is sharp. Next to her bed she has photos of six of her seven grandchildren and six of her eleven great-grandchildren—but not a single photo of Lance Armstrong at any age, nor photos of any of his five children. It's as if Lance Armstrong had never existed in her family.

CHAPTER 2

The last name is all that remains of Terry Armstrong. Just as she had erased Eddie Gunderson, Linda removed Terry. Divorce records show they were married fourteen years, until Lance was nearly seventeen. Linda, meanwhile, continues to represent herself as a single mother who raised her son alone.

In her career as a motivational speaker –that pays her as much as $20,000 a pop—there is hardly a word about Terry's involvement in Lance's life. (Some newspapers have quoted her saying the marriage lasted only until Lance was thirteen. She declined to be interviewed for this book.) In her autobiography, she never uses Terry's name. She calls him "the Salesman" or "Sales." The best allowance she makes for him is that "Sales coached Lance's Little League team, he did do that. He gets some credit for effort there, but I'm not sure how much he enjoyed it. Lance wasn't the budding baseball star Sales would have liked him to be."

In truth, Terry Armstrong could not have been more different from Eddie Gunderson. One had been the cool bad boy in the Pontiac GTO spending late nights at R&B clubs rather than with his wife and newborn child. The other was the twenty-two-year-old son of a minister, a churchgoer with a steady job and an eagerness to be a father.

A wholesale food salesman who hawked barbecued meats and

corn dogs to schools and businesses, he had met Linda Mooney-ham Gunderson at a car dealership and was smitten with the cute, spunky brunette. He looked like the kind of guy who could buy a car with cash, which was its own sort of handsome. They started going steady and it fast-tracked into a marriage proposal. With Linda, Terry married into the role he had always wanted: father to a son. With Terry, Linda had found a solid, stable provider.

According to divorce records, and Terry himself, the two were married for most of the boy's formative years—ages two through sixteen. In that time, Lance learned how to compete in his trade-mark way: as an irritable, cocky bruiser.

Both father and son were driven by an intensity that often turned to ruthlessness. Lance saw it when Terry coached his foot-ball teams and advised him in his early efforts in bike racing. Terry could be demanding, especially when his son didn't meet his expectations.

At the boy's first BMX bike race, Lance fell and started cry-ing. Terry marched over to the fallen child and said, "That's it, we're going." Then he grabbed Lance's bike. "We're done. No kid with my name's gonna quit." Properly admonished, or frightened, Lance got back on his bike and competed in another race. Terry thought it was proof of his son's toughness.

When Lance was seven and then eight, he played for the Oil-ers, a team in a YMCA tackle football league in Garland, Texas. Terry Armstrong was one of the coaches. At the team's first prac-tice, Terry gathered the players and the fathers around him.

"Let me tell y'all about this football team we're gonna have here," he said. "If your kid's not any good, he ain't playing. This is not just a show-up-and-run-around situation. We're going to win."

Against the league's rules, he videotaped other teams' work-outs and held after-school practices in the privacy of his backyard to gain an edge. His idea of a bedtime story for Lance was an old copy of a Vince Lombardi fire-and-brimstone speech about win-ners and losers. Once, when he believed Lance had loafed through a football game's fourth quarter, he didn't talk to him for a week. Lance would come to the dinner table, and he'd say, "You're just a loser—you didn't put the effort out." Meanwhile, his team of eight-year-olds went undefeated through eleven games.

Terry and Linda never were a perfect match. Neither claims to have ever been madly in love, or even that love was the founda-tion for their union. Neither Linda Armstrong in her book, nor Terry Armstrong in interviews, can remember any details of their wedding.

Several of Lance's pals say that his mother was more of a friend to him than a parent. They remember Lance once asking her to get dolled up so she could ride around in the limo he had rented for his prom, making it quite an uncomfortable trio—Lance, his prom date and his mother. Lance's friends and some of his for-mer coaches say Linda was a permissive parent who indulged her son's every wish. (Example: He drove himself alone to his driver's license test.)

So, according to Terry Armstrong, he became the disciplinar-ian by default. When Lance disobeyed or mouthed off—both frequent occurrences—Terry had a routine. He waited for Linda to come home. He armed himself with his fraternity paddle be-fore telling Lance, "Grab your ankles!" Then he used the paddle against the growing young man's rear end.

If Lance didn't clean his room—not so much as a sock out

of place, per the protocol of Kemper Military School in Boonville, Missouri, where Terry had been wrapped in a blanket and viciously beaten by other cadets—Terry administered two licks. Talk back? Two licks. Years later, Lance described those spankings as traumatic, saying that the pain was more emotional than physical.

Terry and Linda often fought about Lance's schoolwork. Terry remembers, "I would say, 'You can't go outside until you get your homework done,' and she would say, 'Well, he's my son and I make the rules.' I would ask for his report card, and she would say, 'I'll handle it, he's my son.'"

One perhaps inevitable result of the parental disagreements was that Lance became an angry, aggressive child. Classmates from middle school said he was a classic bully, "picking on people that were vulnerable and harassing them on a daily basis." He always seemed to be fighting something or someone.

As he entered high school, Armstrong remained an outsider, a short, slight kid with Brillo Pad hair and a cowlick that could not be conquered by comb or brush. He was arrogant in sports, but less confident socially—at least partly because he had stopped playing football. It was Texas, after all, where football sopped up everyone's attention.

Terry Armstrong said his son quit football in middle school because he became furious when teammates failed. He gravitated toward individual sports like running and swimming, where he alone could control the outcome. He was a natural there and his father pushed him because he didn't think Lance would get to college based on his academics. "One thing I'll always say about my son, and I still love him to death, but he's not the brightest tool in the shop," Terry says. "He did not have the discipline to go to school. That's the one reason I pushed him so hard in athletics. I knew athletics was going to be his way to school. He was lazy. He didn't want to study. He wanted to go run. He wanted to go ride his bike. He wanted to go play."

Terry made sure Lance had all the advantages in sports and other extracurricular activities. The best catcher's mitt. A brand-new drum set. Top-of-the-line bikes. A red Fiat convertible. "What Lance wanted, Lance got," said Armstrong's neighbor and close friend Adam Wilk.

Lance worked out with a small coterie of pals that included several future high-level athletes like Chann McRae, who became a cyclist on the Postal Service team with Armstrong. Though the young athletes mostly delighted in pushing each other to perform better, Lance's joy did not come in winning competitions by an inch. He needed to humiliate his opponents. Wilk recalls him saying, "Did you wear your panties today? You are a weak pussy. You suck—why did you even show up?"

Although Lance did poorly in school, Linda was proud of his athletic accomplishments. Wilk said, "If it wasn't for sports, you would look back and say Linda did a crappy job raising Lance." Wilk didn't know what Armstrong would have done with his life if it hadn't been for his athletic gifts. "A juvenile delinquent, maybe in jail?" he said. "I can't remember him having any other interests. He was focused on winning, and to me, he's still fixated on it."

Lance Armstrong was fourteen when he learned about Terry's secret life. They were traveling to a swim meet in San Antonio. He saw Terry writing, then tossing away pieces of crumpled paper. The boy picked up a sheet of the paper and saw the beginnings of his father's love letter to a mistress. To spare her the pain, he didn't tell his mother. But Terry became an enemy to be crushed— another lost father.

Right away, Armstrong found a replacement: Rick Crawford, a professional triathlete. Crawford didn't know what was in store when he met the fourteen-year-old Armstrong at a Dallas pool. They were swimming laps in adjacent lanes. Armstrong went all out to beat him. Crawford was impressed.

He's not sure how it happened exactly, but Crawford—twelve years older, never a coach—helped Armstrong launch his triathlon career. Armstrong promptly became a star in the niche sport, someone race directors wanted at their event. They marketed him as a prodigy, a boy threatening to challenge the sport's best athletes. Crawford was astonished at how quickly Armstrong excelled. His national triathlon ranking improved by the day, Crawford says, the number dropping "like shit through a goose." They trained together for eighteen months.

Crawford says he was taken aback by Armstrong's combativeness. He heard him at races tell competitors, "I'm going to kill you. You are pathetic." He would say those things at the starting line *and* the finish. Crawford remembers telling him, "Lance, no. Not cool. Buddy, let your legs do the talking."

On training rides, Crawford had to keep an eye on Armstrong, who saw every motorist as a threat. In a kind of bike rage, he would chase down cars that had come too close to him in order to curse and threaten the driver. He wouldn't temper his emotions for anybody. Crawford noticed that was especially true when it came to the way Armstrong treated his father.

At first, nothing stood out to Crawford as unusual at the Armstrong residence in the Los Rios neighborhood, a solidly middle-class section of Plano. The Armstrongs lived in a simple brick ranch-style house: three bedrooms, 1,500 square feet, a patch of lawn, a couple green shrubs.

Then Crawford began to hear Armstrong's stories of his family's problems. He heard about Armstrong and his father taking swings at each other and landing on a glass coffee table, smashing it. "He was encouraged to be bad," Crawford says. Family friends saw a teenager out of control.

While Linda and Terry Armstrong argued at home, Crawford spent more time with their son, training and traveling to events where they both were treated to free airfare and fancy hotel rooms because of their athletic abilities. That, too, was a learning experience. The night before a triathlon in Bermuda, Armstrong "borrowed" a scooter that Crawford had rented and returned it to the rental company hours late. Later, in a bungalow that housed several other professional triathletes, Armstrong broke glasses and bottles when he took a cricket bat and smacked a ball into the place's wet bar.

Crawford had had enough. He was tired of doing the job of this kid's parents who, in his view, were lousy. He pinned Armstrong against a wall and growled, "You're done, dude."

"Screw off," Armstrong said, "you're not my dad! Don't ever talk to me again."

As he had with his biological father and Terry Armstrong, he left Crawford behind.

"I guess you couldn't blame him," Crawford says. "He was already staying in five-star hotels and having people adore him."

Crawford remembers Armstrong's behavior as Oedipal. He says most of the father figures in Lance's life have ended up as villains and that every girl he has ever dated looks exactly like his mother.

In turn, Armstrong calls Crawford a bitter, "crazy and angry" guy. He also points out that Crawford went on to help athletes dope. In 2012, years after he split from Armstrong, Crawford admitted to helping pro cyclists Levi Leipheimer and Kirk O'Bee of the United States Postal Service squad use performance-enhancing drugs. Crawford said he did it only because Armstrong had set the team's standard of doping. He said those riders were neophytes who heard that Armstrong and other elite riders on the team were taking part in a sophisticated drug program. They only wanted to keep up. Still, Crawford later was fired from his coaching job at Colorado Mesa University for allegedly doping an athlete there, a charge he denies. As for the matter of Armstrong's doping—might Crawford have ever helped a young triathlete bend the rules?

"No," he said. "I would never put drugs into a young kid."

Linda Armstrong always looked for people who could help Lance—and along came Scott Eder, a local sports promoter working for the sneaker company Avia. He crossed paths with Armstrong in 1986 at a biathlon in Dallas. After Armstrong won the event, Eder delivered a free pair of Avias to his house, and—one imagines—walked away with exactly what he was after.

Linda asked Eder, "Can you watch over my son, kind of act like his agent?"

Eder became, as Lance said later, "a coach meets agent meets big brother."

Armstrong had already proven himself to be an amazing athlete. He was only thirteen when he won his first triathlon, an IronKids event, and was second in that year's IronKids national championship. At fourteen, he was sneaking into races for adults, with Terry Armstrong changing the date on his birth certificate to make him eligible. The next year, he competed for the second time in the President's Triathlon in Dallas, an event featuring many of the sport's stars, like Mark Allen, an eventual six-time Ironman world champion.

A fifteen-year-old Armstrong wasn't far behind the top competitors. He beat Allen in the swim. In the bike portion of that 1987 race, he pedaled alongside Allen and got his attention. "Are you Mark Allen?" Armstrong said. When Allen said yes, Armstrong remained by his side for nearly the rest of the event. Armstrong finished sixth, but made a name for himself as the next big thing in the sport.

Allen later told the President's Triathlon race director, Jim Woodman, that the young Armstrong's abilities were uncanny. "He couldn't shake him, and that freaked him out," Woodman said. The next year, Armstrong won the triathlon. He also won the Texas state championship, beating his own former mentor, Crawford, for the title. *Triathlete* magazine claimed that he would be one of the greatest athletes in the history of the sport.

By the time he was sixteen, he was making $20,000 a year and had turned pro. Eder was acting as his traveling secretary, event negotiator, marketing director and road manager. He compiled triathlon schedules, secured sponsors and budgeted for their races. Eder also arranged for Armstrong to spend two summers training in California with top triathletes.

In all, Eder told me, he traveled with Armstrong to more than twenty-five out-of-town races. He showed me the itineraries he had typed up on his typewriter. The travel—which included stays in expensive hotels like Bermuda's Princess—was often paid for by the event sponsors. Armstrong was only a kid, and he already was being treated like a superstar. The Armstrongs didn't need to spend a penny.

Linda has claimed to have been by her son's side at most of those competitions. Eder differs. "She went to about three," he says.

He saw the kid as a brawler with a touch of paranoia. If you glanced at him the wrong way, he might say, "What the hell are you looking at?" He'd sneak into a bar, get into a fight, and this underage boy would go back home with a bloodied nose and raw knuckles.

He once threw a Kestrel racing bike—one of the first generations of all-carbon-fiber racing bikes—across several lanes of road after his tire went flat during a Miami triathlon. Kestrel dropped its sponsorship of him. The tantrum had hurt Armstrong's marketing appeal, especially since it was captured by television cameras.

This reputation preceded him, yet people in the sports world still wanted to glom on. They sensed that he had a great future. But the better Armstrong fared as an athlete, the more of his humility he lost. Already, no one was brave enough to stand up to him. He would get into fights at school. He would drink. He would drive too fast. His coaches and sponsors around town heard all about it, and couldn't or wouldn't stop it.

Eder said Armstrong's relationships with father figures would always go bad for one reason or another. Once, Eder had to convince Jim Hoyt, the owner of the Richardson Bike Mart, that he should continue to sponsor Armstrong despite the teenager's off-the-bike antics. Hoyt was another early benefactor, one who had been there nearly from the start. Armstrong was kicked out of the store at age twelve because he took gear he never returned, Hoyt told me. Then he was kicked out again at seventeen because Hoyt had co-signed a loan on Armstrong's new white Chevy Camaro IROC Z28 and Armstrong had abused his generosity. Trying to outrun the police one night, Armstrong abandoned the car at an intersection before sprinting away on foot. Police impounded the car and showed up at Hoyt's door because his name was on the vehicle's registration.

"A week later, that little prick came to my house with his friends to actually get the car back," recalls Hoyt, a Vietnam veteran who earned a Silver Star in combat. "I rolled up my sleeves and said go ahead, just try to get it back from me." Hoyt reported back to Eder: "Your boy screwed me again."

It was another ten years before Hoyt spoke to Armstrong again.

By Lance's senior year of high school, Terry Armstrong was gone. Linda Armstrong had tracked down a mistress. (Terry told me there were so many he didn't remember this one's name.) When Terry came home from work one day he found his wife and the other woman sitting together on a couch.

"Who are you?" he asked the mistress.

Terry Armstrong lost both his wife and his son. In the divorce decree, Linda Armstrong was awarded her husband's Cadillac as well as all the money and retirement accounts in his name. The house was to be sold, with the proceeds divided equally. But Terry Armstrong insisted that his wife and son live there until Lance graduated high school. According to divorce records, he also assumed all the family's debt, including monthly payments on his wife's 1986 Buick Skylark and $8,265.78 on credit cards.

Scott Eder said Terry Armstrong would often call and ask

about Lance. Many days, Eder saw Terry hiding behind bushes to watch his son train in an outdoor pool. Lance saw him once and told Eder to deliver a warning: If Terry Armstrong keeps stalking him, he'll kick the crap out of him.

Lance viewed life as increasingly unfair. His senior year, he felt that all of Plano East High School was out to get him. The school wouldn't let him graduate with his class because he had too many absences: days he took off for triathlons and for training in his specialty, cycling, at the United States Olympic Training Center. He was preparing for the cycling junior world road championships in Moscow, where he amazed everyone by leading the race so forcefully that some of the sport's top names still remember how his amazing performance caused them goose bumps. (He exhausted himself way too fast, though, and finished back in the pack.)

He and his mother didn't think he should have to follow a state law that mandated a minimum number of days a student had to attend class. Lance was "that guy with the mom who was always making a stink about him getting out of school," according to one of his classmates. His mother argued that he should graduate, but school officials wouldn't budge.

That led them to Bending Oaks in Dallas, a nontraditional school with about a dozen students per class. As a private school, it didn't have to follow public school rules and wouldn't have the same problem with Armstrong's absences that his last school had. He'd be able to graduate on time, so long as his tuition was paid. And Terry Armstrong, the man whom Armstrong's mother would call an absentee father, was the one who wrote the check.

In his airy three-bedroom ranch straight out of a Pottery Barn catalog, Terry Armstrong lays a box on the kitchen table. He pulls out card after card, photo after photo. A Father's Day card: "I didn't get to pick my dad, but I'm glad my mom picked you." Inside, in a child's writing: "Love, Lance." A photo shows Lance driving Terry's father's golf cart. There's a photo of Lance at the organ in a church where his grandfather preached.

Terry Armstrong shows off a smiling Lance on his grandparents' couch, and then another with a smiling Linda in the same spot on the same couch. The photos have writing on the back: Christmas 1983. Lance was twelve, a few years from becoming a triathlon star. Though he had lost touch with his son soon after Lance's cycling career took off, Terry followed him in the newspapers and on television. On his office wall, he kept photos that showed the evolution of Lance from boy to man. The most recent shot is of Lance and Lance's children that Terry had printed from the Internet and framed. He said Lance's achievements thrilled him and that his son's troubles caused him heartache, though not nearly as bad as in 1996, when Lance was diagnosed with cancer, and Terry was not allowed to enter his son's hospital room in Indianapolis.

After Lance won his first Tour de France, Terry Armstrong was astounded to hear Linda's claims about their years as a family. He wondered, "Linda was a single mom? Her first two marriages were quick ones? Lance and his mom always had their backs against the wall?" He was sensitive about mistakenly being called Lance's stepfather, not adoptive father, by news outlets, including CNN.

Terry tried to fight back by writing those outlets to say that they had the story wrong. He sent copies of his marriage certificate and divorce decree, showing that he had been married to Armstrong's mother for fourteen years. He wanted to set the record straight, but a lawyer discouraged him because Terry "didn't have the ink," meaning Lance had the power of the press. Reporters, especially in the United States, were in love with the Lance Armstrong story. Then came Lance's autobiography, *It's Not About the Bike*, which cast Terry as a terrible father, and then Linda's book piled on. Terry called the stories "a constant battery of mistruths."

He had planned to confront his ex-wife at one of her book readings in 2005. He said he waited until the last minute before walking down the center aisle to take a seat in the front row.

Tami, Terry's new wife, who had never met Linda, sat apart from her husband so she could ask, "Did you or did you not raise Lance yourself?" Linda said, well, you just need to read the book.

Terry Armstrong said he held his hand up that day, waving it like a kid trying to get the teacher's attention. But the author ignored him. Only after the reading, as Linda sat at an autograph table, did the former partners in marriage come face-to-face.

"I really enjoyed the book," Terry told her.

"Really?" Linda said.

"Yes," he said. "I love fantasy."

CHAPTER 3

John Thomas Neal was an independently wealthy real estate investor and massage therapist, a forty-eight-year-old husband and father, who worked as a *soigneur* in elite cycling. *Soigneur* is a French term meaning "one who cares for others." In cycling, it is a person who gives the riders massages, prepares their lunches and water bottles, cleans uniforms and transports their baggage to and from hotels. A fixer, nurturer and wise counselor, Neal had worked with professional athletes on the beach volleyball tour and swimmers at the University of Texas. But his passion was cycling because he loved the sport and the travel.

He had fled Montgomery, Alabama, after growing up amid the race riots of the '60s. In Austin, his open mind and eclectic tastes matched the city's liberal attitude. He once hosted a gay wedding at his home, originally a church on a hilltop overlooking the city's skyline. Though he had a law degree, legal work didn't satisfy him and he didn't stick with it. Anyway, he could afford to quit because he married into money.

Neal, who was maybe 5 foot 8 and had a very slight build, was a huge sports fan—University of Texas football, swimming and volleyball, professional tennis, cycling, you name it—and wanted to find a way he could work in the sports business. He couldn't coach because he wasn't the aggressive type, nor had he ever been an athlete. Massage therapy was the answer. The clinical aspects of it fascinated him. He also loved the idea of being trained to cure people's ills.

Neal was so serious about his new vocation that he traveled to China and spent several months learning Eastern healing techniques, including how to perform acupuncture on the inner ear.

Back in Austin, he volunteered to work with the athletes at the University of Texas. In time, he had made enough connections and had cultivated a reputation in the Olympic sports world for being so good at his job that he was hired to work as a *soigneur* for the Subaru-Montgomery professional cycling team. Former United States Olympic cycling coach Eddie Borysewicz was in charge of it. Thomas Weisel, an investment banker who was a legend in financial circles, was the owner.

When he first signed on, Neal worked races only in the United States and hadn't heard much about doping in the sport, except that performance-enhancing drug use among cyclists was prevalent in Europe.

He met Lance Armstrong in 1989 at a Texas triathlon after Borysewicz told him to look out for the budding cycling star. Armstrong's all-out effort at the 1989 junior worlds in Moscow had caught Borysewicz's eye. The coach convinced him to switch to cycling from triathlon because cycling was an Olympic sport, while triathlon wasn't.

Armstrong, arguably the hottest up-and-coming cyclist in the world, later landed a spot with the Subaru-Montgomery team. By then, Neal and Armstrong knew each other well.

Nearly a dozen athletes in Austin—both men and women—still say they were closer to Neal than to their own fathers. He brought them into his family and gave them some stability. Lance Armstrong was just the latest athlete in need.

Armstrong was relocating to hilly Austin from flat Plano because the area's terrain was perfect for training. At a steeply discounted rate, Armstrong moved into an apartment complex owned by Neal. Near downtown—among tall trees, twenty paces from Neal's office—it was a comfortable, safe place that Armstrong could call home. Later, Armstrong told the *Dallas Morning News* his apartment was "killer . . . s-o-o-o nice!" He and Neal met every day, sometimes several times a day, for massage treatments and meals. It gave Neal satisfaction to know that he could make a positive impact on the life of a teenager who needed some guidance.

Neal's first impression was that the kid's ego exceeded his talent. Armstrong was brash and ill-mannered, in desperate need of refinement. But the more he learned of Lance's home life, the sorrier Neal began to feel for him. He was a kid without a reliable father. Linda Armstrong was pleased that her son now had a responsible male role model in his life, and Neal lent a sympathetic ear to her as well while she dealt with the rocky transition between marriages.

Neal soon recognized that Armstrong's insecurities and anger were products of his broken family—he felt abandoned by his biological father and mistreated by his adoptive one. Armstrong didn't like to be alone, so Neal often met him for breakfast at the Upper Crust Café, just down the street from Neal's house, and for lunch at a sports bar called The Tavern. Armstrong ate dinner with the Neals three or four times a week. The Neals' three children would be there, along with the occasional Armstrong friend or a student Neal was mentoring. It was nothing fancy—sometimes just slow-cooked beans eaten with plastic utensils out of mismatched mugs, as if they were on a camping trip. But they were a family.

Frances, Neal's wife, and Armstrong were the group's jokers. They might chase each other around the dinner table. They might sing parts of the song "Ice Ice Baby," by the Dallas rap star Vanilla Ice, a song that then sat atop the music charts. One would sing, "Ice ice baby!" and the other would reply, "Too cold, too cold!" On some days, they would bring their show to the Neals' motorboat, where they would spend the day swimming or water-skiing.

It was arguably the happiest, most uncomplicated time in Armstrong's life. He no longer had to worry about Terry Armstrong, and his mother's current marital woes were 215 miles north on Interstate 35, back in Plano. His world centered on Austin and Neal, who gladly opened up his home or apartments to national team cyclists—like future Postal Service teammates George Hincapie, Frankie Andreu, Chann McRae and Kevin Livingston—who wanted to train with Armstrong in the Texas Hill Country.

The day after Armstrong moved into his new apartment, the Neals saw him ride in Lago Vista, thirty-five miles from Austin. Armstrong did poorly and admitted to Neal that he'd been up late the night before, drinking at an Austin strip club named the Yellow Rose. Neal passed it off as Lance's being just another rambunctious teenager testing his newfound freedom.

The call from Armstrong to J.T. Neal came before dawn on an August morning, 1991. Could Neal come to San Marcos and pick him up? Armstrong wasn't stranded on the side of the road in the Texas outback. He had not blown out a tire on his bike in a marathon training ride. He was in jail.

The night before, thirty miles from Austin, Armstrong had partied with some coeds from Southwest Texas State University. As they frolicked in an outdoor Jacuzzi at one coed's apartment complex, they made so much noise that the police came to quiet them down. But that was only Armstrong's first meeting with cops that night. The second was the big one. Pulled over for driving erratically, he thought he could talk his way out of trouble. So what if he had appeared drunk and refused to take a Breathalyzer test? He was sure the officer would be impressed when he told them who he was—the best young cyclist in the entire country.

Had he been a quarterback, maybe the ploy would have worked. But a Texas police officer could not care less about a guy boasting about his prowess on a bike. No, it was off to the county lockup.

Neal, always concerned about Armstrong's drinking and driving, came and got him from the San Marcos jail the next day. Months later, upon receiving a notice informing him that his driver's license could be suspended, Armstrong forwarded the letter to Neal. On the envelope, he wrote, "J.T.—This came today?? Have a great Xmas! Lance." Now acting as his lawyer as well as his friend, Neal helped Armstrong beat the charges and keep his license.

In turn, Neal received from Armstrong something rare and precious: Armstrong's trust. Armstrong sent him postcards from training trips and races—such as a note dated August 16, 1991, from Wein-und Ferienort Bischoffingen, Germany:

J.T.—Hows it going? Well, Germany is very nice. As you probably know the worlds are a little over a week away and Im [*sic*] nervous as hell. At least I'm riding good now! Wish you were here! The boys say "hello." Lance

Neal was an admitted cycling groupie. He was never athletic enough in any sport to be a hotshot jock—he rode a bike, but only recreationally—but now he could walk among those jocks and be accepted and respected by them. He had the job of a cycling fan's dreams.

Neal loved that the national team riders and American pro cyclists knew who he was. Some even called him for advice. In Hincapie's case: *I was stopped by customs with a suitcase filled with EPO and other drugs, what should I do?* Some of them, like Armstrong and Hincapie, were open with him about their drug use. Whether Neal was complicit in any of that drug use is unclear. He said, though, that a *soigneur*'s job in the United States was different from that of one in Europe, where the job had long required an intimate knowledge of pharmaceuticals. He had learned that from his fellow *soigneurs* who had done work overseas. Only once did Neal inject Armstrong, Neal said: a vitamin shot in the rear end.

In those early days, Armstrong didn't hide the fact that he received regular injections. Neal always said that Armstrong never liked to do things for himself, that he felt entitled to have someone wash his car for free or make restaurant reservations. At first, he didn't like injecting himself, either. A coed named Nancy Geisler, Neal's office assistant who was close with both men, said that Neal once asked her to give Armstrong a vitamin shot because he'd be out of town and couldn't do it. She presumed that it was just a part of Armstrong's training regimen.

Armstrong was nonchalant about it when she filled in. She saw no label on the vial from which the syringe had drawn its liquid. She assumed that Armstrong had been doping and that Neal knew it. Only years later did she think, "Had I been a part of something illegal?"

According to Neal, Armstrong relied on shots and IVs for recovery and a pre-race boost of energy. On the eve of the road race at the 1992 Olympics, fellow Olympian Timm Peddie walked into Armstrong's hotel room and saw Neal and a gaggle of USA Cycling officials standing around Armstrong as he lay on a bed, hooked to an IV. Peddie was astonished at the openness of the procedure. Everyone there stared at the unexpected guest until Peddie left as quickly as he had come in. He hadn't been sure what he had seen. Maybe a blood transfusion? An infusion of electrolytes or proteins? He only knew that he himself had never received an IV of anything before a race. Armstrong was, evidently, special.

In the early 1990s, U.S. cycling had a single star, Greg LeMond, who in 1986 became the first American to win the Tour de France, a feat he would repeat in 1989 and 1990. But his victories had little impact on the sport in the United States. LeMond had ridden for a European team and his success came primarily in Europe, out of sight of America's sports fans.

Armstrong, however, came into the sport with the dramatic backstory—the struggling single mother who had dropped out of high school to raise him—and he raced for an American team,

Motorola, starting in 1992. Young and charismatic, he was set to be a star, and he wanted fame badly.

He insisted that Steve Penny, the managing director for USA Cycling, sell the hell out of him to raise awareness of the sport. News about cycling had rarely gotten much past the sports pages' agate section.

Penny persuaded Descente, the federation's new clothing sponsor, to produce a poster of four top athletes on the national team: Armstrong, Hincapie, Bobby Julich and the 1991 junior road cycling world champion, Jeff Evanshine. In the years to come, all would admit doping or serve a suspension for breaking anti-doping rules. The poster featured a dramatic photo of Pikes Peak behind the riders, each of whom carried a look of grim determination on his face. In the lower left-hand corner of the poster was a list of the "U.S. Team Rules."

RULE #1:   Don't mess with Lance, Bobby, George and Jeff.
RULE #2:   No Whining.
RULE #3:   It doesn't count unless you do it under pressure.
RULE #4:   There is no "Back Door."
RULE #5:   There are no rules: Winning the Gold in
           Barcelona is the only thing that counts.

As much as Armstrong loved being a star, his devotion to celebrity may have run a distant second to his hunger for money. J.T. Neal sensed that early on.

He saw Armstrong driven by money—how to get it, how to keep it and what he had to do, ethically or unethically, to get more of it.

* * *

In 1993, Armstrong chased a million-dollar bonus. The pharmacy Thrift Drug offered the prize to a rider who won three big American races—the Thrift Drug Classic in Pittsburgh, the Kmart Classic in West Virginia, and the CoreStates USPRO national championship in Philadelphia. Each required a different strength: Pittsburgh's was a demanding one-day race, West Virginia's a grueling six-stager that rewarded the best climbers and Philadelphia's an event geared toward sprinters.

Armstrong, only twenty-one, won the first race and surprised everyone. Five stages through the second race, he was among the favorites to win. So, with the possibility of a million-dollar payout dangling in front of them, several riders on the Motorola team allegedly devised a plan to guarantee victory.

They allegedly offered to pay some riders on the Coors Light team a flat fee of $50,000 to help Armstrong win the million-dollar prize by not challenging him for the victory in the rest of that second race and the entire final race. Coors Light was a strong team with riders who also were among the top contenders.

Later that night, several riders from each team discussed the deal in Armstrong's hotel room.

If Armstrong won the million, both teams would benefit. Armstrong would receive the prize money—$600,000 taken in a lump sum—and would walk away with $200,000 while the balance would be distributed to his team and other cyclists who had helped him win. Each rider on Coors Light would be given $3,000 to $5,000, according to Stephen Swart, a Coors Light rider who claimed to be in on the discussions.

As long as America had no idea how it happened, Armstrong's $1 million jackpot would also give cycling the positive publicity it needed to grow. It was a win-win all around.

The practice of throwing races had existed for decades, and was as much a part of the sport as doping. Joe Parkin, an American who raced in Europe, said so in his book, *A Dog in a Hat*. He wrote that selling victories was a common and accepted practice in Europe in the late 1980s. A rider racing in his hometown might shell out several thousand dollars to win. The losers would get guaranteed, easy money. Everybody left happy, pockets stuffed with cash.

Parkin wrote, "My experience as a pro cyclist in Europe has left me with a somewhat altered moral code, such that many of the things that bother normal people are invisible to me."

Armstrong won the second race in the million-dollar race series. Then, in the last moments of the Philadelphia race—the final race in the series—Armstrong was in a breakaway of six riders when he took off toward an impossibly steep climb called the Manayunk Wall. None of the other riders in the breakaway chased him, leaving him to win the race in what seemed like a heroic solo effort.

Before the race, Neal thought Armstrong would win because he was the strongest rider. Only after the event did he learn that Armstrong had paid his way onto the top of the winner's podium.

Armstrong told Neal that in the race's waning miles he bribed Italian rider Roberto Gaggioli, so Gaggioli would let him win. He offered Gaggioli, one of Armstrong's top opponents, $10,000 to hold back when Armstrong took off on his solo breakaway, and the Italian agreed to the bribe. Gaggioli later said Armstrong had given him $100,000 in the deal, though that amount seems improbable.

Neal, uncomfortable with the apparent shameless dishonesty, said that he chastised Armstrong for cheating.

"For God's sake," he told Armstrong, "stop bragging about it."

Neal also was upset with Ochowicz, who he suspected was in on the deal. He didn't like Ochowicz very much anyway. He complained that the team manager knew little about cycling tactics and that the only thing he did was gorge himself on the peanut-butter-and-jelly sandwiches that were kept for him in the team car. He felt that Ochowicz was a bad influence on Armstrong, a kid who didn't need much prodding to break the rules. It was now evident to Neal that Armstrong's moral code would be forever altered. Armstrong, according to a person with direct knowledge of the situation, would later win the Clásica de San Sebastián race in 1995 only after bribing another rider in the final few miles, but that he was just following the sport's well-established customs.

If Armstrong ever had a conscience, the sport's established customs helped convince him that it didn't matter.

In the television broadcast of the prize ceremony, Armstrong summed up the victory with an ironic hint at the fact of the race: "Everybody won today."

That year, 1993, Armstrong's star rose sharply. Not only did he win the million, he also won his first stage of the Tour de France. In August, at twenty-one, he became the second youngest world road racing champion ever. With Motorola planning to leave cycling, Armstrong's brilliant season gave his team reason to believe it would gain a new sponsor, probably one with much deeper pockets.

All of a sudden cycling mattered. Reporters from around the world descended upon Austin. ABC News interviewed Armstrong and his mother, calling him a "boy wonder" and playing up Linda Armstrong's role as a teenage mom.

"Well, being young and pregnant, I was scared," she said.

Lance said: "We had to overcome a lot of obstacles and a lot of resistance in our lives. And I mean, all these people, they counted her out, counted me out."

Newspaper stories said he had never met his father and that Linda's second marriage ended after ten years. Those lies somehow made Armstrong's story even more attractive to the media.

"Lance is just what our country needs to get excited about cycling," the USA Cycling marketer, Steve Penny, said in one news report. "If someone is looking for a hero to back, Lance fits the mold."

Team manager Ochowicz said he was ecstatic about Armstrong's $1 million victory. "It's a great day for U.S. cycling." By year's end, Armstrong and the cycling team were so good that Motorola signed on for another year. The team did not have to fold after all. Armstrong had a new name for Penny: "Dime."

Back in Austin, Armstrong paid $70,000 for a new sports car, a black Acura NSX. He then asked Neal to build a garage at the apartment complex. Neal resisted, but only for a moment. For about $50,000, he built the garage. Whatever Armstrong asked, it seemed, J.T. Neal was there to say yes.

At Christmas that year, Armstrong thanked him with several gifts. One was an autographed world champion's rainbow jersey. In black marker, he wrote, "J.T. I'm very fortunate that our paths have crossed. You're truly my righthand man! Not to mention my best friend! Lance Armstrong."

He gave Neal a Rolex watch inscribed with the words "To J.T. From LANCE ARMSTRONG." Neal accepted the watch as a symbol of Armstrong's gratitude, even his love. For a number of years, Neal wore it with pride—until the day came that he decided to never put it on his wrist again.

PART TWO

LIES OF THE SPORT

CHAPTER 4

I n 1992, someone opening the Motorola team's medicine cabinet would have come across the usual items—Band-Aids, diarrhea medicine and antiseptics for "road rash"—as well as the banned stuff, like cortisone and testosterone alongside household Tylenol. Most riders didn't consider them to be real doping products. Using those drugs just meant the riders were minding their health in a grueling sport.

Cortisone, which could be injected or swallowed, reduces muscle soreness and is an anti-inflammatory for stiff, aching joints. It remains a staple for cyclists because it alleviates leg pain. Riders liken it to taking an aspirin if you have a headache, and many team doctors write bogus prescriptions for the drug.

Testosterone is a steroid, but isn't used to help riders bulk up with muscle. Rather, it allows them to recover more efficiently from a workout, so they can rise the next day and train just as hard. Riders treat the drug the way they do getting a massage or staying hydrated.

Those drugs were common in the European *peloton*. Everyone serious about the Tour looked for an edge, whether it was steroids or injectable vitamins like B12, B complex or folic acid.

Performance-enhancing drug use is bound with the history of cycling, especially the Tour de France, a three-week,

51

2,000-plus-mile race. The event, held every July, is almost impossibly hard, and has been that way since its debut in 1903.

Riders have always found ways to make the race easier. In 1904, cyclists left their bikes and hitched rides in cars, trains or buses to cut miles off the route. Every stage winner and the first four finishers were among twenty-nine riders punished for cheating that year, ushering in the Tour's dance with dishonesty.

Through the early 1900s, riders relied on substances like ether, cocaine and strychnine to blunt the pain. Some stopped at bars to chug wine and other numbing spirits. They used cocaine-based mixtures to convince their bodies they could go on when their brains said they couldn't. Riders believed they could breathe easier if first they had taken some strychnine (so highly toxic it is used as rat poison) and/or nitroglycerine (given to heart attack patients to stimulate the heart).

The abuse of those drugs was affirmed by Henri Pélissier and his brother, Francis, French riders who abandoned the 1924 Tour and then gave a blockbuster interview to a journalist, Albert Londres, of *Le Petit Parisien*. The story was titled, "Les Forçats de la Route"—"The Prisoners of the Road."

Henri Pélissier told Londres, "You have no idea what the Tour de France is like. It's like martyrdom. And even the Stations of the Cross had only fourteen stations, while we have fifteen stages. We suffer from start to finish." Pélissier showed the journalist the contents of the bag he had carried throughout the race: cocaine for the eyes, chloroform for the gums, horse ointment for the knees. Pills he called "dynamite."

Amphetamines became popular in the mid-1940s, and would lead to dangerous accidents. French rider Jean Malléjac collapsed with his bike at the 1955 Tour, six miles from the summit of

Mont Ventoux, the famous bald mountain that towers more than 6,200 feet above the Provence region of France, and fell onto boulders at the roadside, with one foot attached to a pedal and the other pawing frantically through the air. He remained unconscious for fifteen minutes in what the Tour doctor deemed an amphetamine-fueled breakdown.

Another French cyclist, Roger Rivière, landed in a tangle of metal at the bottom of a steep slope after crashing over a wall during the 1960 Tour. He broke his back. Doctors found pain-killers in his pocket, which could have distorted his judgment and slowed his reflexes so much that he had been unable to apply his brakes. He never regained use of his lower limbs. Just two years later, fourteen Tour riders left the race because they had been sickened by morphine.

The Tour and drugs went hand in hand, despite a growing public concern. Five-time Tour winner Jacques Anquetil was famously open about his own regimen. He once said, "You can't win the Tour de France on mineral water alone . . . Everybody dopes." Nothing was illegal.

By 1963, doping had grown so dangerous that a group of cyclists, doctors, lawyers, journalists and sports officials came together to push for drug testing. Two years later, France passed its first national antidoping laws and drug testing began at the Tour.

Led by Anquetil, riders balked. Before the Tour's first stage, they gathered and chanted, "No pissing in test tubes!" Their protest included walking their bikes for the first fifty meters of that stage. Félix Lévitan, the Tour director, called the riders "a band of drug addicts" bent on "discrediting the sport of cycling."

Then came one of the blackest days in cycling's dark history. On July 13, 1967, the British rider Tom Simpson began zigzagging across the road not far from the top of Mont Ventoux. He finally toppled over, then told a British team mechanic, "Get me up, get me up. I want to go on. I want to go straight. Get me up, get me straight." Spectators helped him back onto his bike, but just one hundred meters later, he crumpled onto the road again, still gripping his handlebars as he went into a coma.

Three hours later, he was dead. An autopsy report said he had died of heat prostration that led to a heart attack. But his jersey pockets told another story. In them were empty vials dusted with amphetamines.

Don Catlin, the man who set up the United States' first performance-enhancing drug testing laboratory, the UCLA Olympic Analytical Laboratory in Los Angeles, had been studying the drug erythropoietin, called EPO, from the start. It appeared on the market in the United States in 1989 as a drug used for kidney patients and AIDS-related anemia, but athletes long before that had learned of its magical powers. EPO is a powerful hormone that boosts endurance by increasing red blood cell production. More red blood cells mean more endurance. In the sport of road cycling, it turned out to be a miracle potion.

The drug comes in a vial less than an inch and a half tall. But it is filled with several doses. No longer would endurance athletes have to undergo the dangerous and logistically difficult process of receiving blood transfusions to boost their red blood cell count. Now enhancing one's endurance was as simple as pricking the skin with a needle. Athletes could receive what one unpublished Swedish study said was an average 8 percent boost in aerobic capacity. The study said the drug could cut 30 seconds from a 20-minute run. In cycling, using the drug could mean the difference between winning the Tour de France and not even qualifying for one's Tour team.

There was a frightening downside, though. EPO raised a rider's hematocrit level—the proportion of red blood cells in the blood and a measure of blood's thickness. A man's hematocrit is usually between 42 and 48 percent of his whole blood.

But with EPO, some cyclists were boosting their hematocrit into the 50s, or even higher. Bjarne Riis, the 1996 Tour champion, was even nicknamed "Mister 60 Percent" because EPO was rumored to have jacked up his hematocrit that high. The practice was inherently dangerous. If athletes overdosed on EPO, the drug would turn their blood to a viscous, sticky sludge that could cause a stroke or heart failure. Dehydration, which often occurs during long races, makes the blood even thicker. By the late 1980s, cyclists were buying the drug on the black market. Then they started dropping dead.

In 1987, five Dutch riders died of heart problems. On August 17, 1988, Connie Meijer, a Dutch rider, passed out and died while competing in a criterium race. Diagnosis: heart attack. She was twenty-five. One day later, Bert Oosterbosch, another Dutch rider, died in his sleep, at thirty-two. Again, a heart attack.

Doctors and blood specialists said EPO abuse might have played a role in the deaths of at least eighteen professional European cyclists in the years from 1988 to 1992. Ten deaths were attributed to heart problems. The cycling magazine *VeloNews* declared that "an atomic bomb" had gone off in the sport. News of the deaths was picked up by mainstream media outlets. The *New York Times* carried a headline: "Stamina-Building Drug Linked to Athletes' Deaths."

Catlin sounded an alarm with the International Olympic

Committee. As a member of the IOC's medical commission, he pressed for an investigation. The athletes had taken a drug for which no test had yet been developed. Catlin believed the IOC should do something about it, and right away, because lives were at stake.

He went with an IOC team to Europe on a fact-finding mission. He found no one who would talk about EPO. Family members refused to cooperate. Riders said they'd never heard of it. Basically, they told Catlin to go away. Again and again, he told them, *Don't be afraid to talk. We're trying to save the lives of other cyclists. Please help us.*

In reply, he heard nothing. He believed that some people were protecting not only the memory of friends, family and teammates—they were also protecting the sport. Doping scandal followed doping scandal. Something had to be done.

Catlin made his pitch in 1988. But the code of silence that had served cycling for so long could not be broken. Seven years later, Lance Armstrong used EPO for the first time.

When Armstrong signed with the Motorola team in 1992, he had already fallen in with coaches of dubious repute. The first was Eddie Borysewicz.

In 1985, Borysewicz was at the center of one of the biggest doping scandals in U.S. Olympic history. Borysewicz, a Pole, had honed his craft at sports academies in the Eastern bloc. While coach of the U.S. team at the 1984 Olympics, he was accused of pressuring riders to take transfusions of blood to get an increased supply of the oxygen-carrying red blood cells. If such transfusions were not done properly, or if the blood was not stored at the right temperature, blood doping could make a rider ill—or even kill him.

The practice was not expressly prohibited by the International Olympic Committee, but its rules said athletes could not take any medication or undergo any procedures that would unfairly affect the competition. Whether forbidden or not, Borysewicz and other team officials watched seven members of the 1984 Olympic cycling team line up inside a room of the Ramada Inn in Los Angeles to wait their turn to lie on a bed and receive blood from a relative or someone else with the same blood type. Two riders became sick. Four went on to win medals, including a gold.

Months later, the transfusions were made public, marring cycling's image as well as Borysewicz's reputation.

"Eddie B. introduced hard-core doping to American cycling, and it's never been the same," says Andy Bohlmann, who from 1984 through 1990 was in charge of the antidoping program for the United States Cycling Federation, then the sport's national governing body.

In 1990, Chris Carmichael, a former rider on the 7-Eleven team, was appointed head coach of the national team, with dozens of cyclists under his command—including Armstrong and three other promising riders from the junior national team system. Those three were Greg Strock, Erich Kaiter and Gerrik Latta.

Each of them would eventually claim that national team officials had doped them without their knowledge when they were teenagers. One pointed his finger at Carmichael. Those riders said they had received injections of substances that team officials claimed were merely vitamins or "extract of cortisone." They said they were given unidentified pills embedded in candy bars to eat during races, and drank from water bottles spiked with banned performance enhancers.

Years later, in medical school, Strock discovered that there is no such thing as "extract of cortisone." He realized that his coaches had probably injected him with the real thing, which likely triggered the autoimmune disease that ended his cycling career in 1991. He thought back to the nationals in 1990, when, he claims, Carmichael had arrived with a briefcase full of drugs and syringes and allegedly injected Strock in the buttocks under the supervision of another coach, René Wenzel. Strock remembers seeing Carmichael at other races carrying that briefcase, looking like a pharmaceutical company representative heading to see his clients.

Strock, Kaiter and Latta all sued USA Cycling, with Strock and Kaiter settling out of court. (The outcome of Latta's case is unknown.) Carmichael allegedly paid Strock $20,000 to keep his name out of the lawsuit.

And what did Lance Armstrong think of Carmichael? He told me they were like brothers. One of Carmichael's future training videos would feature Armstrong's photo on the box. Armstrong would write forewords for many of Carmichael's books. All this work was done on the premise that Carmichael was the brains behind Lance Armstrong's success. And you, too, could learn from the coach of the world's greatest cyclists, especially if you attended one of Carmichael's weeklong training camps. The cost: a cool $15,000.

Throughout the 1990s, J.T. Neal acted as Armstrong's main *soigneur* at some domestic races and at national team training camps. But in Europe and at the big races, the honor of rubbing down Armstrong went to a man named John Hendershot. Among *soigneurs* in the European *peloton* (another French word, one that refers to professional riders generally as well as the pack during a race), Hendershot was at once the cool kid and the calculating elder. Other *soigneurs* envied the money he made and the cachet that came with the cash. Wherever he walked—through race crowds or at home in Belgium—people turned to catch a glimpse. Teams wanted him. Armstrong wanted him. J.T. Neal said he was "like a god to me" and called him "the best *soigneur* that ever was."

Hendershot, an American, was a massage therapist, physical therapist and miracle worker. His laying-on of hands would bring an exhausted, aching rider to life. Eating at Hendershot's direction, sleeping according to his advice, a rider began each morning reborn. He came with all the secrets of a *soigneur* and an unexpected skill developed over the years. In Neal's words, Hendershot took to cycling's drug culture "like a duck to water." But his enthusiasm for and skills in chemistry would be remembered as his special talent.

For most of a decade Hendershot sat at home in Belgium in his makeshift laboratory, preparing for races. There he mixed, matched and mashed up drugs, always with one goal in mind: to make riders go faster.

The mad scientist conjured up what he called "weird concoctions" of substances like ephedrine, nicotine, highly concentrated caffeine, drugs that widen blood vessels, blood thinners and testosterone, often trying to find creative ways to give riders an extra physical boost during a race. He'd pour the mix into tiny bottles and hand them to riders at the starting line. Other times, he'd inject them with it. He wasn't alone in this endeavor. *Soigneurs* all across Europe made their own homemade blends of potentially dangerous mixes and first drank or injected those potions into themselves. They were their own lab rats.

Hendershot, who had no formal medical or scientific training, learned the art of doping riders by observing the effects on a human test subject—himself. He knew a formulation was way off when he felt his heart beating so fast and loud it sounded like a runaway freight train. That wouldn't work for riders already under extreme physical stress. He wanted "amped up," but not to the point of a heart attack.

If Hendershot was his own lab rat, it wasn't long before he tried his potions and pills on the riders, including Armstrong. When Armstrong went professional after the 1992 Olympics, he signed a contract with Motorola, one of the two major American teams. Because Armstrong wanted the best *soigneur*, he was immediately paired with Hendershot. It was a match made in doping heaven. Both *soigneur* and rider were willing to go to the brink of safety.

"What we did was tread the fine line of dropping dead on your bike and winning," Hendershot says.

Hendershot said the riders on his teams had a choice of whether to use drugs. They could "grab the ring or not." He said he didn't know a single professional cyclist who hadn't at least dabbled. The sport was simply too difficult—and was many times impossible, as at the three-week-long Tour de France—for riders who didn't rely on pharmaceutical help.

Hendershot believed cyclists had at most four years of clean riding before they could no longer remain in the sport. As a drugged-up *peloton* went faster, the clean riders could help the team leader for maybe the first week of a race, maybe by riding in front of the pack to set the pace or by delivering water bottles from the team car, but then would have to drop out from exhaustion. A career like that was short-lived.

When Armstrong arrived at Motorola in 1992, a system that facilitated riders' drug use was firmly in place on the team—and likely in the entire sport. Hendershot said he would take a list of drugs and bogus prescriptions for them to his local pharmacist in Hulste, Belgium, to get the prescriptions filled and to obtain other drugs, too.

Cycling was always big in Belgium—for generations, it has been one of the country's most popular sports—and the pharmacist didn't question Hendershot about the request for such a massive amount of drugs. In exchange, Hendershot would give the pharmacist a signed team jersey or allow him to show up at big races, where he would be a VIP with an all-access pass. Then he would leave the drugstore with bags filled with EPO, human growth hormone, blood thinners, amphetamines, cortisone, pain-killers and testosterone, a particularly popular drug he'd hand to riders "like candy."

By 1993, Armstrong was using all of those substances—like almost everyone else on the team, Hendershot said. He remembered Armstrong's attitude from the remark, "This is the stuff I take, this is part of what I do," and that Armstrong joined the team's program without hesitation because everyone was doing it.

"It was like eating team dinner," Hendershot says, adding that he had a hunch that virtually everyone involved in the team knew about the doping—"doctors, *soigneurs*, riders, team managers, mechanics—everyone." He called the drug use casual and said he never had to hide any of it. After injecting the riders at a team hotel, he'd toss a trash bag filled with syringes and empty drug vials right into the hotel's garbage can.

While Hendershot never administered EPO or growth hormone to Armstrong, he did administer them to other riders on the team and was aware that Armstrong was using those drugs. Hendershot said a stash of those two drugs was driven from Belgium to the team's 1995 training camp in southern France.

Riders like Armstrong could get drugs in several different ways—from Hendershot, from their personal doctor or a doctor that worked with the team, or by buying them over the counter themselves. Each rider would bring those drugs to Hendershot and he would administer them by injecting them into the rider, by mixing a potion of them for the rider to drink or inject, or by injecting them into IVs the rider would receive, based on the doctor's instructions. Sometimes the drugs would also come in pill form, and Hendershot would dole those out, too.

In the early 1990s, by Hendershot's estimation, less than half the teams in the pro *peloton* had a doctor on staff. Those teams were ahead of the curve. "Drugs level the playing field, but the better your doctor is, the better you are going to be," Hendershot says, adding that in his opinion he believes that almost all of the doctors had to be administering drugs to their riders considering the sport's drug culture.

Still, Hendershot was constantly worried that something he was giving the riders would hurt them—or even possibly kill them—especially when he was administering substances that riders had injected into the IV bags themselves or when the riders' personal doctors would prepare concoctions for Hendershot to give. He was concerned that he would be culpable if anything ever went wrong, but was constantly rationalizing his actions. Even as he provided drugs to riders, Hendershot said, he told himself, "You're not a drug dealer. This isn't organized. This is no big deal."

He knew he was lying.

He rationalized the lie by saying the process was overseen by Max Testa, an Italian who, as of December 2013, still works in the sport and runs a sports medicine clinic in Utah. In 2006, Testa told me that he gave his riders the instructions to use EPO, but never administered drugs to those riders. So if drug use was not mandated by the team, it was at least quasi-official. Hendershot trusted Testa to make sure the riders were staying safe, believing that Testa—unlike other doctors in cycling—actually cared for the riders' health, and cared less about winning or money. Hendershot put it this way, though: a doctor who refused to give riders drugs wouldn't last in the sport.

Armstrong liked Testa so much that he moved to Italy to be near the doctor's office in the little town of Como, north of Milan. Not long after joining Motorola, Armstrong began to live in Como during the racing season. He brought along his close friend Frankie Andreu, and in time several other riders joined them, including George Hincapie, a New Yorker, and Kevin Livingston, a Midwesterner. All became patients of Testa. All would later become riders on Armstrong's United States Postal Service Tour de France winning teams.

Hendershot said all those riders likely believed they were doing no wrong by doping. The definition of cheating was flexible in a sport so replete with pharmacology: It's not cheating if everybody is doing it. Armstrong believed that to be the dead-solid truth. For him, there was no hesitation, no second-guessing, no rationalizing. As Hendershot had done, Armstrong grabbed the ring.

April 20, 1994. Three riders from the Italy-based Gewiss-Ballan team stood atop the podium in their light blue, red and navy uniforms after dominating the Flèche Wallonne, a one-day race in Belgium's hilly Ardennes region. Two held bouquets of flowers above their heads as they waved to the crowd. Armstrong seethed. The Gewiss riders were flaunting their success at his expense. He had finished 36th, fully 2 minutes and 32 seconds behind the leaders.

About fifty kilometers from the finish of that Flèche Wallonne, the Gewiss riders had broken away from the pack and, as Armstrong put it later, "demoralized everyone." They pedaled faster as the *peloton* diminished into a tiny speck on the horizon behind them. They had raced along the narrow, dipping roads to the final climb up the Mur de Huy, a steep ascent with gradients as high as 26 percent. They rode up the Wall as if it were tabletop-flat. Moreno Argentin crossed the finish line first, while teammates Giorgio Furlan and Evgeni Berzin finished two-three.

It was there, in Belgium, in 1994, that the exhausted *peloton* realized what many people in the sport believed to be the amazing power of EPO. The winning team's doctor told them about it. In fact, he told the world. After the race, a reporter from the French sports newspaper *L'Equipe*, Jean-Michel Rouet, interviewed the doctor, Michele Ferrari, and asked him if his riders used EPO.

"I don't prescribe this stuff," Ferrari said. "But one can buy EPO in Switzerland, for example, without a prescription. And if a rider does that, don't scandalize me. EPO doesn't fundamentally change the performance of a racer."

The reporter said, "In any case, it's dangerous! Ten Dutch riders have died in the last few years."

Then Ferrari, who has long denied doping any of his athletes, said something that would haunt him for years. "EPO is not dangerous, it's the abuse that is. It's also dangerous to drink ten liters of orange juice."

In other words, it's all part of a balanced breakfast.

But to the uninitiated, confusion reigned. Armstrong, Andreu, Hincapie and Livingston—four riders who would become the core of American cycling—threw questions at their own team doctor, Testa. *What does EPO do? Is it dangerous? Do you think other teams are using it? Can you help us use it?*

Testa tried to convince them they didn't need the drug. He said the riders' natural abilities would be enough for them to succeed in the sport, and that it was just a rumor that all riders used EPO. "People are trying to make money off of this, you don't need it. Studies show that it apparently doesn't help very much."

Still, Testa felt EPO use was inevitable. So he gave up trying to keep his riders from it. One day, he handed each rider an envelope containing studies about EPO and instructions on its use. The literature he gave them told the riders how much EPO to take and when to take it, so they wouldn't take too much and hurt themselves or, perhaps, even kill themselves. "If you want to use a gun, you had better use a manual, rather than to ask a guy on the street," he told me. While he admitted to facilitating the drug use, Testa denies ever dispensing any doping products.

The training ride was a leisurely spin during which the Motorola riders cruised along for hours, loosening their legs. It was March 18, 1995. The day before, on the way home from Milan-San Remo—where he finished 73rd—Armstrong grumbled to Hincapie, a longtime friend, "This is bullshit. People are using stuff. We're getting killed."

Armstrong pushed the issue while the team pedaled alongside Lake Como the next day. He was twenty-three and already a world champion, and had won a single stage of the 1993 Tour de France. But he considered that only the beginning. Growing brasher by the day, he wasn't going to let a bunch of European pussies kick the crap out of him because they were using a wonder drug and he wasn't.

Armstrong approached rider after rider. "I'm getting my ass kicked and we've got to do something about it. We need to get on a program." They knew what he meant. They agreed it was time for EPO. The new drug was ubiquitous. Riders carried thermos jugs packed with ice and tiny EPO glass vials. Clink, clink, clink. You could hear the vials rattle against the ice. Clink, clink, clink. In this era of cycling, it was the soundtrack of the sport.

Armstrong might have chosen to use EPO on his own, but it wouldn't have done him much good. Cycling, despite appearances, is a team sport. There is usually one leader on each team who sets the agenda and whom the other riders support. On Motorola, that man was Armstrong, arguably the best all-around rider.

The rest of the squad are *domestiques*—secondary riders. *Domestique* is the French word for "servant," and those servants sacrifice themselves to help the leader win, partly with team tactics and partly with aerodynamics. They take turns with other *domestiques* and ride in front of their leader—or to the side, if there is a crosswind—to punch a hole in the air and allow the leader to tuck in behind and save energy. The leader is being swept along in their draft, and expends up to 40 percent less energy than he would riding alone.

The goal is to deliver the team leader as fresh as possible to the crucial point in the race. From there, he can take off and win the stage or take off and gain time on his competition in the overall race for the yellow leader's jersey.

Eventually, though, the *domestiques* burn themselves out and often peel off from their leader before struggling to finish the stage. So the stronger a leader's *domestiques* are, the better his chances to win because they will be able to hang on and help him as the finish line grows closer.

In 1995, Armstrong presented his *domestiques* with an ultimatum: If they wanted to be considered for the Tour team that year, they had to start using EPO. Don't want to? Well, there's the door. Armstrong was taking control. It was his success at stake. The Motorola program had been built around him. Finishing 73rd in a big race would not inspire sponsors to sign on. Motorola had already said it was ending its sponsorship at the end of the season. The pressure was on, then, to attract another sponsor to cover most of the team's bills.

When Hendershot took over as Armstrong's *soigneur*, J.T. Neal became Armstrong's personal assistant. In Como, he ran errands and generally made life easier for Armstrong while he raced or trained. When Armstrong dropped out of the Tour de France early—in 1993, 1994 and 1996—Neal picked him up for the trip to Como. He moved Armstrong from apartment to apartment between seasons. He ran the household. He once paid the bill to get the apartment's electricity turned on after Armstrong and Andreu had let a bill go unpaid. He repaired the clothes dryer.

When Armstrong arrived in Como after a Tour, Neal began massage sessions to prepare him for the fall's world championships. The men stuck together. Neal introduced Armstrong to art in Milan's museums. Sometimes, they simply sat outside Armstrong's place overlooking Lake Como, sharing low-calorie meals like tuna with balsamic vinegar and olive oil.

A visit to Testa was often on the day's to-do list. Though the *soigneur* Hendershot said he injected Armstrong with performance-enhancing drugs soon after Armstrong signed with Motorola in 1992, Armstrong himself claims he didn't start doping until the 1993 world championships. He said Testa gave him Synacthen, a drug that stimulates the adrenal glands to secrete glucocorticoids. Riders say Synacthen makes them feel stronger and takes away some of the pain of a difficult ride. The drug was available on the Motorola team even before Armstrong pushed his teammates to use EPO. Hendershot said Armstrong was "as clean as he ever was" at those worlds.

Neal figured Testa's job was to inject Armstrong with every needle within reach. Testa was constantly giving Armstrong IVs with substances the doctor called "liver cleansers," though the official names of those substances—and whether they were banned or not—are unclear. Stephen Swart, a teammate from New Zealand who had first raced in Europe in 1987, didn't live in Como and see Testa regularly like the American riders did, but had heard about Armstrong's drug use because the sport was so insular and rumors—especially pertaining to doping— traveled fast.

Swart, a stern, strapping guy, thought Armstrong was mandating what the team's directors wouldn't. Jim Ochowicz, a two-time Olympian in track cycling who is considered the godfather of American cycling, had founded the 7-Eleven team, the first American team to race in Europe, and stayed with the team when Motorola came on as its sponsor. It was Ochowicz who first imagined Americans challenging the European old guard, and it was Ochowicz who had made it happen.

In 1986, 7-Eleven became the first U.S. team to compete in

the Tour, and one of its riders, Davis Phinney, even won a stage. For years, Ochowicz was the point person in the U.S. for international cycling, the negotiator dealing with sponsors and the European race directors. With journalists, for some reason, he liked to play down his knowledge of the sport's inner workings.

Often when Ochowicz was asked about Armstrong and EPO, or other performance-enhancing drugs, he took on a look as if to say, How could you even think such a thing? He would smile nervously and say, "I have no idea how to respond" (2005) or "I don't know what the answer is" (2009) or "The answer is that I haven't a clue" (2010). He has denied involvement or knowledge of any cheating on the team. Over the course of seven years, I would walk away time and again thinking Ochowicz was either a practiced liar or the most oblivious man ever to walk in cycling's clink-clink world.

It seems to be a stretch to say that Ochowicz wouldn't have known about the team's doping—rumours of it, or the reality of it. He was a member of Armstrong's inner circle, a man Armstrong professed to be his "surrogate father." Ochowicz stood up for Armstrong at his wedding and is the godfather to his first son.

Hendershot said he would consider Ochowicz the most unethical person on the Postal Team if Ochowicz did know about the doping but turned a blind eye to it. If that were the case it would have effectively meant Ochowicz was relying on the doctors and *soigneurs* to make sure the cyclists didn't overdose and drop dead, Hendershot said.

Armstrong said Motorola's EPO use began in May 1995 at the Tour DuPont, America's best-known multistage race. Armstrong, who had finished runner-up the previous two years, became the second American winner after Greg LeMond. With his victory came a big payday, $40,000. Including bonus money, Armstrong collected $51,000. He shared it with his teammates.

Swart said he received Testa's EPO instructions in the spring of 1995 and that he and Andreu subsequently went to Switzerland to buy the drug. They used it for the Tour of Switzerland, which ran shortly before the Tour de France. Swart said he used EPO for the last time after the prologue of the 1995 Tour. Every morning and every night at that Tour, team employees showed up at the team hotel with bags of ice for riders' thermoses, and were sometimes exhausted after an all-day hunt in countries that mostly serve their drinks at room temperature.

During one rest day of that 1995 Tour de France, Armstrong and many of his Motorola teammates gathered in one of the squad's hotel rooms to give blood samples that they would test in a centrifuge. That centrifuge spun the blood to separate it into three categories: plasma, red blood cells and white blood cells. Once the blood was divided, the riders could test their hematocrit levels. Too high a hematocrit level meant they had used too much EPO and might be placing themselves in danger of a heart attack. (Riders had heard stories of some cyclists setting alarms to wake up in the middle of the night to exercise, so that their EPO-thickened blood wouldn't cause them to suffer cardiac arrest in their sleep.)

With half of the Tour and so many punishing miles behind them, the riders' hematocrit levels should have dropped well below normal. With the EPO they had used, though, their bodies were making new red blood cells at that very moment. Their hematocrits soared, as if they had not pedaled a mile. They were fresh.

Swart saw that most of his teammates had hematocrits of more than 50. His, he recalled, was the lowest of everyone's, at 47 percent.

He remembered the others' numbers: Andreu's was at about 50. Andrea Peron, an Italian, had the highest, at 56. (There have been no findings that Peron ever doped.) Armstrong's was either 52 or 54, at least ten percentage points above his norm. Even with that edge, Armstrong, the strong one-day racer, would go on to finish 36th in that Tour, nearly an hour and a half slower than Miguel Indurain, the winner.

The telephone call came to Kathy LeMond in the middle of the night. The wife of the American cycling star Greg LeMond heard screaming and crying when she picked up the receiver in their home in Belgium. Then she heard a voice say, "He's dead! He's dead! I tried to help him, but he's already dead! I touched him—he's cold! He's dead!"

The voice was that of Annalisa Draaijer, the American wife of the twenty-six-year-old Dutch cyclist Johannes Draaijer. That night at the Draaijers' home in Holland, three days after her husband had returned from a race, Annalisa heard Johannes make a gurgling sound as they lay in bed. She tried to wake him, but his body was limp. He had died beside her. She knew no one else to turn to.

Greg LeMond had raced with Draaijer on the Dutch team, PDM. Their wives bonded because both spoke English. Now their friend was dead. As soon as news of Draaijer's death became public, there was speculation that EPO use had caused the cyclist's blood to thicken into mud and cause a heart attack. No one ever proved Johannes Draaijer died because he was on EPO. But to Greg LeMond, nothing seemed more obvious.

"He died for what?" LeMond asks. "For nothing . . . Everybody knew what was going on, but nobody stopped it. Nobody."

CHAPTER 5

In the fall of 1995, Lance Armstrong went in search of Dr. Michele Ferrari. He wanted to work with the man who had transformed the Gewiss-Ballan bikes at Flèche Wallonne into flying machines.

But Ferrari had become a kingmaker in cycling and had grown increasingly selective about his clientele. So even strong riders like Armstrong needed to undergo a physical before any deal was closed. Because he was afraid of going anywhere alone, Armstrong convinced his girlfriend, Monica Buck, a former Miss Hawaiian Tropic from Texas, and J.T. Neal to accompany him to Ferrari's office in Bologna. They climbed into Armstrong's car for the two-and-a-half-hour drive from Como on autostrada A1, due southeast.

It wasn't the most comfortable ride. Neal didn't want him to go, and was cross that he'd gone ahead and made the appointment. All he said, in his soft Southern drawl, was, "Lance, don't get greedy now."

Only twenty-four years old, Armstrong had nearly $750,000 in the bank. But Neal knew that Armstrong idolized people like Ochowicz, the Motorola team manager who ate at the best restaurants, stayed at five-star hotels and ordered only the priciest wines. Armstrong could see only one route to get there—and that was with Ferrari leading the way. He claims he had asked Eddy Merckx, the five-time Tour champion from Belgium, to introduce him to the doctor, and says that Merckx obliged.

Buck, meanwhile, was a petite, voluptuous aspiring actress who had come from Texas to visit Armstrong. Neal worried about her. Lance had a way with women. He had dumped Buck's predecessor, Danielle Overgaag, a top Dutch cyclist who had lived with him in Austin, because she'd been "too opinionated." Neal had the feeling that Armstrong would never have gone to see Ferrari if Overgaag had still been in the picture. But at summer's end, in 1995, Armstrong had Neal remove Overgaag's belongings from the Como apartment to make room for Miss Hawaiian Tropic, who seemed already to be straining her welcome.

Ferrari's office, in the basement of the doctor's Bologna house, was a chaos of wires, tubes, bicycles and machines. Armstrong had heard about some of Ferrari's clients, including Eddy Merckx's son, Axel. Axel had suddenly ridden faster than ever, and Armstrong had asked him if he had a secret. Yes, Merckx apparently said.

Ferrari, the tall, thin Italian with a receding hairline and avian features, had studied at the University of Ferrara under Francesco Conconi, a scientist considered the grandmaster of Italian sports medicine. Conconi, a former member of the International Olympic Committee's antidoping commission, knew his way around EPO. The IOC had paid him handsomely for his research into developing a test for it. But he was double-dealing. Even as the IOC paid him to develop the test, he delivered EPO to Italian skiers and cyclists.

Ferrari learned from Conconi. Now Armstrong wanted to be the hematocrit-rich Plato to Ferrari's Socrates. After evaluating him, Ferrari praised Armstrong as "amazing, amazing, so amazing." But he told him he could improve only if he followed his advice and his plan, never straying. "I will train you," he said, "and together, we can do great things."

Ferrari charged Armstrong $10,000 for the consultation and commanded 10 percent of his salary. Even Armstrong, who guarded money as if he were as penniless as his poor mother said she once was, thought the deal was worth it for what he could earn later, and agreed to it.

The doctor and rider had to keep their relationship secret because Ferrari was then under investigation by Italian authorities for sporting fraud and for doping his riders. He dealt in cash and wrote little down so that he would leave a minimal paper trail. Over time, though, Ferrari grew lax about his rules.

On Armstrong's happy drive back to Como, he talked nonstop about how his career would skyrocket with Ferrari's training and doping help. (Ferrari, however, denies doping any of his riders.) All Buck wanted to talk about was the two-hour shopping trip she and Neal took while waiting for Ferrari to be done with Armstrong. In a kind of lonely melancholy, Neal saw that Armstrong felt no guilt. Neal felt that Armstrong had forgotten the trip they'd taken to see the family of Fabio Casartelli, Armstrong's teammate on Motorola who had been killed during the 1995 Tour. Armstrong had held Casartelli's infant son in his arms and had embraced his widow.

During one stage of the Tour, Casartelli had crashed and hit his head on a cement block along the road. Testa, who allegedly had been overseeing the doping on the Motorola team, allegedly persuaded the forensic doctor in France not to conduct an autopsy because he said it was obvious how Casartelli had died.

Armstrong would eventually say that the day Casartelli died is the day he learned what it meant to ride the Tour. "It's not about the bike," Armstrong said. "The Tour is not just a bike race, not at all. It is a test. It tests you physically, it tests you mentally, it even tests you morally. I understood that now. There were no shortcuts, I realized."

No shortcuts—unless you consider a secret deal with Europe's most famous and infamous doping doctor a shortcut.

From Austin, Armstrong talked for hours by phone with Ferrari. He took training tips and grilled the doctor relentlessly. Once a week, in the middle of the night, the fax machine in Neal's office would come alive with Ferrari's training and doping calendars: when to take EPO, human growth hormone or testosterone so as to avoid testing positive.

Though much of the public thought Chris Carmichael was the coach solely responsible for preparing Armstrong, that relationship was just a cover. Not that Carmichael would admit it. In 2006, he told me he was Armstrong's main coach, then more recently failed to return several of my phone calls and e-mails asking for comment.

As for getting the drugs, Armstrong had different methods. He could coax teammates into buying them for him from pharmacies in Switzerland, or buy them there himself. The *soigneur* Hendershot could procure drugs from his black market sources. Whatever they had to do, however much they had to risk, the winning would make it all worthwhile.

By 1995, Neal, Armstrong's unofficial business manager, couldn't handle Armstrong's contracts alone. Companies wanted to produce Armstrong trading cards. Others wanted endorsements. Neal needed help. Keeping tabs on Armstrong was near impossible. That's where Bill Stapleton came in.

Stapleton, a former Olympic swimmer who had competed at the University of Texas, had a fledgling sports practice at the Austin law firm Brown McCarroll and he needed clients. He needed Armstrong.

When Armstrong reached out in the spring of 1995, Stapleton promised he would shower him with personal attention. He offered a low commission rate: 15 percent of Armstrong's marketing deals. Other agents, including the high-profile super-agent Leigh Steinberg, had asked for 20 percent.

He took Armstrong out for beers to woo him.

"You'll be a big fish in a small pound," Stapleton told him. "There will never be a time when your calls go unanswered. You will be what my world revolves around."

"You'll be there for anything, whenever I need you?" Armstrong said.

"Yes, for anything, all the time."

"For anything?"

"Yes, absolutely anything."

That was exactly what Armstrong wanted to hear. He loved being the most important person in the room.

Back home, Linda Armstrong's third marriage was crumbling because her husband, John Walling, drank too much and was missing work, and Neal thought Armstrong should help his mother with money—a suggestion Armstrong refused.

For some reason unknown to Neal, Armstrong grew increasingly angry at his mother, long his greatest ally, the creator and perpetuator of the fantastic myth that the cycling world had come to embrace. Now he wanted nothing to do with her.

When Armstrong had bought his land in Austin in 1994 for about $240,000, he could have used his mother, a real estate agent, and spread some of the commission to her. But he didn't. The mother-son relationship was so worrisome that Neal and Linda tried to convince him to see a sports psychologist and channel that anger into his riding. Again, Armstrong passed. This was an Armstrong that Neal didn't know or like. He worried that Lance started every relationship thinking, "What can you do for me?"

The year before, Linda Armstrong and Neal had flown to Minneapolis to seek Greg and Kathy LeMond's advice on negotiating Lance's contracts. At the kitchen table in the LeMonds' lakeside estate, they also asked how to rein in the kid's ego.

"How do I get Lance to be less self-centered and actually care about other people during all this?" Linda asked.

The LeMonds didn't know what to say. For a few awkward seconds, they sat speechless. Did they hear her right? Was Linda Armstrong telling them her son had no empathy? That he was out of control? They believed she was genuinely scared. They stuck to business advice—keep a close watch on him, don't let him stray, carefully choose his partners.

Two years after the Gewiss team swept Flèche Wallonne and suggested to the world that its riders were doping—and doing so under Ferrari's watch as the team doctor—Armstrong took the top spot on that podium, the first American to win the famed spring race. That year, 1996, he also won the Tour duPont for the second year in a row. He was the runner-up at Paris-Nice, a one-week race, and his skills as a sprinter and time-trial rider were improving. All that was left to be considered a Tour contender was to boost his performance as a climber.

But as the summer of 1996 progressed, Armstrong could feel himself slow down. He dropped out of the Tour de France after just five days because of a sore throat and bronchitis. He told reporters, "I couldn't breathe."

Neal also hadn't been feeling like himself. Soon, the reason became clear: Neal had cancer. He was diagnosed with multiple myeloma, a rare cancer of the plasma cells that inhibits the production of healthy blood cells. It hit Armstrong like a sinkhole in his path. Doctors gave Neal only two years to live.

Still, an exhausted Neal went to the 1996 Atlanta Olympics with Armstrong. An electric pump fed chemotherapy drugs into his chest. He slept on the floor of the house Armstrong rented for the Games.

"He needed it for privacy," Neal said of the house. "He needed it for all the damn shots he was getting. You needed the privacy because the other players were not on the drug program. They were not getting shots. It looked like a pharmacy in the bedroom."

Neal watched as Hendershot showed up with a bag filled with vials of liquid, syringes and IV bags and tended to Armstrong as if *he* were the cancer patient. He saw Hendershot give Armstrong an IV before and after the races. Armstrong was already using testosterone, growth hormone and EPO, but Neal wasn't sure what substances Armstrong had received at those Summer Games. Whether he took banned drugs at those Olympics, or to prepare for them, Armstrong won't say. When asked about it, Hendershot can't remember the specific substances he gave Armstrong for those Summer Games, but said, "I would be totally surprised if he wasn't" using banned drugs.

Hendershot told me that it was common to give riders different cocktails of steroids with EPO, and to give them aspirin or pharmaceutical-grade blood thinners to make sure their blood didn't turn to sludge. But whatever Hendershot had given Armstrong at those Olympics, it produced no miracle rides. Armstrong finished 12th in the road race and 6th in the time trial, feeling inexplicably gassed as he struggled in each event.

Armstrong ended the professional season ranked seventh in the world, enough to secure a lucrative contract with the highly regarded French team Cofidis for the following two years. His salary: $2.5 million. He had even negotiated to bring Hendershot onto the team as his personal *soigneur*, a privilege granted to only the most elite riders.

By that time, Armstrong also had a stable of sponsors, including Nike, Giro, Oakley and Milton Bradley. His bank account overflowed. Stapleton said that Armstrong was a very wealthy young man who he estimated would make between $2 million and $3 million that year.

It was time for Armstrong to grow up. He finally moved out of the apartment he had rented from Neal for seven years and headed for a bachelor pad commensurate with his paycheck. Armstrong built a Mediterranean-style, 4,950-square-foot house on Lake Austin, with a pool, hot tub, two boat slips and twenty-nine palm trees. Gone was his beloved $70,000 NSX, replaced by a much cooler stable of toys: a $100,000 Porsche 911, a Harley-Davidson motorcycle, a Jet Ski and a powerboat. He threw himself a lavish twenty-fifth birthday party in his new mansion. But something was wrong.

He'd returned from Europe feeling weak, as if he had the flu. His headaches resisted even a handful of ibuprofen, and sometimes as many as three migraine pills. On his birthday, he blamed it on too many margaritas, but a few days later, he coughed up blood. His personal physician said it was likely that Armstrong's sinuses were bleeding, from allergies.

On October 2, 1996, about 1 p.m., Armstrong and Neal had lunch at their usual haunt, The Tavern in Austin. Afterward, they headed to a mall to find a pair of shoes for Neal. This time Armstrong complained about a pain in his stomach.

"I'm having trouble walking," Armstrong said, doubling over.

Neal told Armstrong that the first doctor's assessment of an allergy attack didn't seem right. He warned Armstrong that it could be serious, that he shouldn't wait to see another doctor. He called one for him. Armstrong was in that doctor's office before 3 p.m., as Neal waited nervously back home.

Doctors checked out Armstrong with an ultrasound, then a chest X ray, then gave him the bad news. "Well, this is a serious situation," the doctor, Jim Reeves, said. "It looks like testicular cancer with a large metastasis to the lungs."

Between 5:30 and 5:45 p.m., Neal's cell phone rang. It was Armstrong.

"I have testicular cancer," he said. "I don't know what to do."

Armstrong was distraught, Neal shocked. Now both of them had cancer.

Within days, doctors discovered that Armstrong's cancer had spread to his abdomen and brain. By month's end, he was admitted to the Indiana University Cancer Center in Indianapolis to have the tumors removed. His chance of surviving the cancer was less than 50 percent, according to his doctors.

The news made everyone in the sport jittery. Ferrari was worried that the drugs he'd encouraged Armstrong to take had given him cancer, or had hastened its spread. Armstrong didn't buy into that theory. If doping caused cancer, then many other riders would be dropping dead. All he would say is that he regretted taking growth hormone. "It's bad. It probably caused the cancer to spread more quickly," he told friends. He claims that he never took it again.

Still, as Ferrari had, everyone wondered if Armstrong had dealt himself a fatal hand—especially Hendershot, who said he immediately thought, "What have I done?"

All of the shots, all of the concoctions, the potions and the cleansers he had injected into Armstrong for three years and more must have had something to do with the cancer. "It doesn't take a leap of faith," the *soigneur* told me. "You have to be monumentally fooling yourself to think that it wasn't a factor. It was certainly putting himself at greater risk."

Now Armstrong could die, and it terrified Hendershot that he might be forced to live with the burden of a young man's death.

"I didn't feel guilty," Hendershot says. "I felt complicit."

But everybody knew about Armstrong's doping, Hendershot said. The riders. The team managers. The *soigneurs*. Those guys washing the bike wheels. They all knew. And no one stopped it, certainly not Hendershot.

He and his wife did the only thing they could think of to make themselves feel better. They dumped his supply of drugs. They packed up their personal things. They left cycling. Hendershot never called Armstrong about the cancer. He never called him again, period.

Hendershot simply disappeared.

CHAPTER 6

Ayear before Armstrong and the Motorola riders discussed plans to use EPO, two years before Armstrong's cancer was diagnosed, Frankie Andreu met a fresh-faced brunette at Buddy's pizzeria in their hometown of Dearborn, Michigan. It was 1994. She was twenty-seven and sold water filters while preparing to open an Italian coffee shop. He was the same age and just back from the spring cycling season in Europe.

A quick survey of Andreu's physique—he was 6 feet 3 inches and 165 pounds, with about 4 percent body fat—made the brunette, Betsy Kramar, pause.

"Um, why are your arms so skinny?" she said, pointing to his spindly biceps.

He blushed. "Oh, I'm a professional cyclist."

"A what? So, that's your job, riding a bike? I didn't know people could do that for a living."

He was handsome, with golden brown hair, green eyes and a sexy smile. She was smitten, even though they seemed to have little in common.

She had graduated from the University of Michigan with a degree in theater. He'd only taken a few courses at a community college while pursuing his cycling career. She was outgoing, with a cutting sense of humor. He was more serious. Both were headstrong and opinionated (Andreu's nickname in cycling was Ajax, for his abrasive mien). Each had a parent who had fled Communism—Andreu's father left Cuba, Kramar's left the former Yugoslavia.

Early on, Kramar realized Andreu fulfilled her three criteria for a husband. Catholic? Check. Conservative? Check. Pro-life? Check. She had grilled him on those subjects the night they met. Her inquisition might have scared off other men, but Andreu was attracted to her confidence and straight-shooting nature.

Soon, Kramar was pulled into cycling. Andreu brought her to races and introduced her to his friends. She learned that Andreu had always been a *domestique*—a rider who works to help the team leader win—and that Andreu's team leader was a kid named Lance Armstrong.

She met Armstrong at a race in Philadelphia, and thought he was just another cyclist. But he was already an American star in the sport, for whatever that was worth in 1994. Greg LeMond was then in the final year of his great career, and cycling's popularity in the United States had waned.

Other than through LeMond's success in the Tour de France, Americans knew about professional cycling mainly through a 1979 movie, *Breaking Away*. In it, a recent high school graduate falls in love with the sport and becomes obsessed with the Italian national cycling team, shaving his legs because he's heard that's what Italian riders do and adopting an Italian accent.

When Kramar and Armstrong had been introduced, she treated him the way she treated everyone else—as an opponent in a debate. She argued with him about his agnosticism, trying to convince him that belief in God is the core to a person's happiness.

"You can't control everything in your life, you know," she said, "because that's what God's for."

"Betsy, that's bullshit, I control my own fate," he told her.

After religion, they argued politics. Though he could be charming for a Democrat, she found him cocky and self-centered. When she visited Andreu in Como, they often would go out to eat pizza. Once, she made risotto at Armstrong's lakeside apartment and he pitched in. He called her a wonderful cook, and he asked for recipes and ingredients. Though she knew he was being nice just so she would cook for him again, she fell for the flattery anyway.

In the summer of 1994, Armstrong loaned his new Volvo—which he was given for winning the 1993 world championship—to Andreu back in the States. "Betsy deserves to ride in a nice car," he said, and Kramar was pleased. Sure, Armstrong was loud and obnoxious, full of himself and full of *it* most of the time. But it wasn't like she was going to marry him.

On September 14, 1996, at the 50-yard line of the University of Michigan's football stadium, Andreu told Kramar that he loved her, and proposed. She cried and said yes.

The wedding was set for New Year's Eve.

Two weeks after their engagement in the fall of 1996, the couple learned that Armstrong had been diagnosed with cancer. Neither of them had ever imagined he would be anything less than a powerhouse. Now the thought of him wasting away sickened them.

Two days after Armstrong had tumors removed from his brain, Kramar and Andreu flew to Indianapolis and walked into a conference room in the downtown Indiana University Cancer Center to visit their friend.

Always nosy, she took inventory of her surroundings. To the

left, a bathroom. To the right, a long, rectangular table. Beyond that, a sofa and a television against the far wall. Armstrong was seated at the table with an IV attached to his arm. To Kramar, Armstrong looked like a ghost of himself, nothing like the indefatigable Texan she had come to know so well.

Cancer had stolen his bravado. He was frail and bald with a long scar that bisected his scalp where doctors had opened his head for the surgery. She smiled and said he looked good. In truth, she was startled to see so much life drained out of him.

Kramar and Andreu gathered with Armstrong and four of his other friends in the conference room because his hospital room had been too small. A Dallas Cowboys football game was on TV. Everyone strained to make small talk.

Armstrong had received a juice machine as a gift, and Kramar started there. "Do you like carrot juice?" she asked him, preparing to extol the virtues of what she called "the power of juicing."

"How about apple? You like apple juice? You know, I have a juicer and I make all kinds of juice with it. You can even put vegetables in it. It's so good for you."

"Thanks, I didn't know that," Armstrong said.

The conversation ended abruptly when two men in white coats walked in. They were there to ask Armstrong about his medical background.

"I think we should leave and give him his privacy," Kramar said, nudging Andreu.

"No, you can stay," Armstrong said.

Kramar motioned again to Andreu, trying to get him to leave. She tapped him with her foot.

"No, Lance said we can stay," he said.

One of the doctors asked Armstrong if he had ever used

performance-enhancing drugs. Betsy's pulse quickened. *What did he say?* She snapped her head to look at Armstrong. She saw him scanning the room, looking at the people there.

There was Coach Carmichael, and Carmichael's future wife, Paige. There was Lisa Shiels, a blond premed student from the University of Texas who'd been Armstrong's latest live-in love. Also in the room was Stephanie McIlvain, Armstrong's personal representative at Oakley, the sunglasses company.

These people were in Armstrong's closest circle. With his glance around the room, he decided he could trust them. One hand on his IV, Armstrong answered the question calmly, as if reading a grocery list.

He said, "Growth hormone, cortisone, EPO, steroids and testosterone."

At that point, sensing Kramar's slack-jawed surprise, Andreu pulled her out of the room and into a hallway. Away from the hospital room's door, near the elevators, Kramar addressed Andreu in a raised voice.

"God, that's how he got cancer, isn't it?" she said. "I'm not marrying you if you're doing all that stuff. The wedding's off!"

"I swear to God. I swear to God. I swear to God," Andreu said. He motioned the sign of the cross. "Please, I promise you, I'm not doing all that stuff."

All Kramar knew about steroids was that Ben Johnson, the Canadian sprinter, had been busted for them at the 1988 Seoul Games after winning the 100-meter dash. But she knew enough to know steroids were unhealthy. And illegal. Worst of all, by her measure, using steroids was an immoral act. It was against the rules of competition. It was cheating.

"Is that what cycling is all about?" she said.

Andreu begged her to keep her voice down. "Betsy, please, I've never taken steroids. I've never taken any of that stuff." He told her not to worry: He was clean. "I'm not involved in any of that doping shit."

She stormed off to the hotel, and he followed. The situation was so tense that they didn't go back to see Armstrong that day. While she wanted to know more, he didn't want to talk about it.

Kramar had no idea that her fiancé had just lied to her face about his drug use. Several of his former teammates said Andreu had taken EPO starting, if not before, the 1995 season. Armstrong and the fellow Motorola rider Stephen Swart said the entire team, including Andreu, had used the drug for the 1995 Tour, though this was disputed by others on the team.

In Andreu's little corner of the world, everyone seemed aware that riders were relying on EPO to race.

It's just that Betsy Kramar was the last to know.

Over the next few weeks, Kramar called four friends and two family members to talk about Armstrong's drug admission. One was Dawn Polay, Kramar's college roommate, who had known Andreu since grade school. "You never know what the truth is," Polay said. "Just listen to what he has to say before you decide anything. Just because one person is doing it, it doesn't mean Frankie is doing it, too."

Polay thought it all was one big, complex mess that Armstrong had created. Why had he trusted Kramar? If he paid any attention to her over the years, he knew she was opposed to smoking and drinking, let alone drug use. Polay thought Armstrong had made a monumental mistake—admitting to something so obviously "against the rules" to Betsy Kramar, an unflinchingly judgmental moralist.

For weeks, Kramar and friends dissected what Armstrong's admission might mean for her impending marriage. *If Andreu had doped, would their children have three arms?* They wondered if Armstrong had caused his own cancer. Kramar even asked her doctor as much.

Most oncological experts say it is impossible to definitively say Armstrong's use of PEDs caused his cancer or exacerbated a preexisting cancer. While testosterone has been shown to cause prostate cancer, there is no proof that PEDs cause testicular cancer, one of the most uncommon types of the disease. Men have a 1-in-270 chance of getting it. At twenty-five, Armstrong was in the age group—twenty to forty—with the highest incidence for testicular cancer.

Though it is still unproven, some experts say that EPO and growth hormone use could hasten the development of tumors and cause cancer cells to replicate at a faster pace. Growth hormone stimulates the liver and other tissues to secrete insulin-like growth factor (IGF-1)—according to Dr. Arjun Vasant Balar, an oncologist at NYU Langone Medical Center in New York—and IGF-1 has been shown to increase the growth of cancer.

Lucio Tentori, a cancer researcher at the University of Rome Tor Vergata, produced a research paper in 2007 that explored whether doping with HGH, IGF-1, anabolic steroids or EPO increases the risk for cancer. He was aware of only one described case of a cyclist's getting cancer after using growth hormone, and that cyclist was diagnosed with Hodgkin's lymphoma, not testicular cancer.

After all his studies and analysis, Tentori would only go as far as to say that "athletes should be made aware that long-term treatment with doping agents might increase the risk of developing cancer."

CHAPTER 7

In the picture they are a team. J.T. Neal and Lance Armstrong: two smiling, bald-headed cancer patients. Neal cherished the photo. It was proof they each had someone to lean on through the uncertainty of a grave illness, someone who every day confronted the frailty of life.

In the fall of 1996, Neal had guided his young charge through cancer treatments at the Southwest Regional Cancer Center in Austin. Neal knew the nurses and doctors from his own stint there, knew the cancer ward layout and arranged a private room for Armstrong.

The seclusion of the private room was perfect for Lisa Shiels, Armstrong's new girlfriend, a college senior who was serious about her schoolwork. She could study and give him the support he needed.

Among the friends and family who rallied to Armstrong's side, only a few thought beyond his survival. Bill Stapleton did. To keep Armstrong looking to the future, Stapleton suggested he establish a cancer charity in his name, so he could remain in the news during his recovery. Armstrong and some of his cycling buddies—Bart Knaggs, John Korioth, and Austin chiropractor Gary Seghi—thought it was a brilliant idea and talked it through during dinner one night. The foundation was a good PR move, but it could also raise awareness for testicular cancer, something that Armstrong felt could keep others from suffering his same fate. If he had known something about the disease, if he had caught it earlier, if his testicle hadn't grown to the size of a lemon before he did anything about it, the cancer likely wouldn't have spread to his abdomen or his brain. He thought the foundation could help save others from their own neglect.

In 1997, Stapleton filed official papers with the Texas secretary of state that established the Lance Armstrong Foundation. Korioth, a bar manager in Austin and one of Armstrong's closest friends, stepped up to run it. Knaggs encouraged some of his rich friends, including Jeff Garvey, a venture capitalist in Austin who was heavily involved in USA Cycling, to join the board of directors.

Armstrong wanted all of his friends to help him in his new, off-the-bike endeavor. In searching for a headquarters for the foundation, he decided one of J.T. Neal's renovated apartments would be perfect. Though the apartment may very well have had a market value of $650 a month, he offered $200—and Neal was offended.

Neal didn't want to give Armstrong another cut-rate deal. Armstrong was rich. Besides, Neal wanted to save money for his family's future. Going through chemotherapy in Austin, he had seen death up close, had known people who didn't make it. His own end was coming, maybe not next week, maybe not next month, but soon.

So Neal said no to the $200 offer, and Armstrong was furious. He claimed Neal wasn't doing everything he could to help build the foundation. Neal expected that reaction, because he had seen everyone in Armstrong's life become yes men: Stapleton, Carmichael, Korioth, Ochowicz. He'd also seen all of them benefit financially and/or professionally from their association with Armstrong.

"He had all the people coming around who liked money and who wanted to impress and he wanted to impress, and he got a lot of values and deals from people like that," Neal said. "It was nothing I could handle."

The Lance Armstrong Foundation's first fund-raiser was a race in Austin called the Race for the Roses, which eventually became the Ride for the Roses. The name suggested that Armstrong had learned the hard way about the need to stop and smell the flowers. Korioth's cold calls seeking sponsorships were met by a surprising ignorance: Rare was the person on the other end who had ever heard of Lance Armstrong. But Michael Ward, a guitarist with the rock band the Wallflowers and an avid cyclist, contacted Korioth to say he wanted to help out with the fund-raiser by having his band play there. Korioth quickly agreed. For the fledgling foundation, it was a huge coup.

Armstrong had not yet won the Tour de France, nor was he in the clear with cancer. The one-year mark with no reappearance of cancer would be a key date in his recovery. But Armstrong didn't think that far ahead. No time for that. Besides continuing treatments and assuring the success of the Race for the Roses, he brought a new woman into his life.

He met Kristin Richard at a news conference announcing his fund-raising event. As a public relations account executive, her job was to promote the race. Armstrong liked her looks, but he particularly loved that she was working so hard for him. She was his official cheerleader, paid to convince people to pay attention to him, his foundation and his big cycling event.

He told Neal he had met this "hot new girl" from a stable,

well-to-do family. Her father was a business executive. The family owned a home near New York City. To Armstrong, the Richard family seemed too perfect to be true. He told Neal that he liked the family's normalcy as much as he liked Kristin.

Shiels was history. Neal's oldest daughter, C. C., bumped into her a few months after the breakup and told her she was sorry that the relationship hadn't worked out. Shiels burst into tears. She had sacrificed basically her entire senior year of college for Armstrong and felt he had discarded her when she was no longer of use. Neal's wife, Frances, said, well, that was Armstrong for you. "He treats people like bananas. He takes what he needs, then just tosses the peel on the side of the road."

Heartbreak notwithstanding, the Race for the Roses event succeeded beyond Korioth's early hopes. To the casual U.S. sports fan, Armstrong's accomplishments—a world championship and a couple stages won at the Tour de France—might not have meant much. But to cyclists, Armstrong was a big-time celebrity. Nearly three thousand riders showed up, including the Olympic speed-skating-legend-turned-cyclist Eric Heiden and Dan Jansen, a speed skater who won a Gold Medal at the 1994 Olympics. In the end, Korioth realized he should have expected a large turnout.

Korioth saw how Armstrong's fans felt as if they knew him intimately. They understood the agony of ascending a steep climb, the monotony of traversing long, endless roads. "It's a very personal connection," Korioth says. "They feel like they could go on a ride with him. And the thing is, they probably could."

Armstrong's cancer deepened those emotional connections, intertwining the circle of cycling fans with cancer survivors. It brought together people who looked to him for inspiration, both as an athlete and a symbol of resilience.

And so began Armstrong's surge into the pantheon of American sports heroes. He had risen from his deathbed to a secular sainthood, and Americans were all but salivating to claim him as their own. He was someone the country could cheer for and be proud of, a man on a classic hero's journey that had all the elements of a boy-done-good story. Not only could American cancer patients beat their disease, but in time they would realize that they also could go on to beat the damned French at their own game, the Tour de France. Armstrong would become a cancer-kicker, a France-kicker and an all around ass-kicker, and Americans are suckers for a sympathetic tough guy.

In one sense, Armstrong satisfied a primal human need to create models for our sanctification. He was an underdog-turned-superhero, first in a cancer ward, later on a bike. Those who believed in him saw only the good side, or convinced themselves that was all there was.

Just after Armstrong had been diagnosed with cancer, Kevin Kuehler, a competitive mountain biker, visited a doctor because he had experienced symptoms similar to Armstrong's.

That doctor said it wasn't cancer, but four months later, Kuehler sought a second opinion. That time, yes, it was cancer. On the way home that day, Kuehler spoke to Armstrong on a call-in radio show.

While nervously trying to explain his experience, Kuehler heard Armstrong cut him off. "Did you call for my advice," Armstrong said, "or did you call just to talk?"

Armstrong advised Kuehler to have the affected testicle removed, a surgery that he said would save Kuehler's life. Two years later, Kuehler reached out to Armstrong again when the cancer reappeared in his lungs. That time, Armstrong arranged a conversation between his main oncologist, Dr. Larry Einhorn of the Indiana University School of Medicine, and Kuehler. Within forty-five minutes, Einhorn was on the phone with Kuehler, discussing a treatment option Kuehler hadn't considered.

That new treatment worked, and Kuehler survived to testify before the nation: "I think it's phenomenal, what he's doing. He could be cured and go on with his life, but he has chosen to go the more difficult route and help other people. Most guys don't feel comfortable talking about what's going on in their pants. But with this kind of cancer, the more you learn, the more you're comforted. That gives Lance a mission."

Other believers would come to include people like a man named Jim from Nashville, Tennessee, whose wife had been diagnosed with leukemia. On his blog, he wrote words that many other Armstrong followers considered the truth: "Clearly, God is working through Lance Armstrong."

As the world's Kevin Kuehlers came to worship Armstrong, J.T. Neal waited for his protégé at the Austin airport, calling his cell phone repeatedly with no answer. It was the spring of 1997, and Armstrong was on his way to a full recovery from the testicular cancer. Fans of his, many of them cancer patients, wanted to meet him, talk to him, even just touch him as he walked by. They sent tons of letters to his Nike representative, saying Armstrong was their hero and begging for Armstrong's autograph. His friends had come to call him "Cancer Jesus." Armstrong hated it.

"I don't like that big frenzy," he says. "I don't like crowds. I don't like people. I don't like strangers in general." Neal thought he was closing himself off.

Still, people liked him. They saw in him what they hoped to see in themselves: a generosity, kindness and, above all, courageousness necessary to survive cancer and return to work—and life.

Neal was on his way to Arkansas for his second bone marrow transplant, which he knew would make him gag and vomit and give him oral thrush, a yeast infection of the mouth common in infants. It would further weaken his body. The transplant might even kill him.

He needed help, someone to feed him and drive him to and from the hospital during the weeklong procedure. Trying to spare his own family the pain of seeing him so ravaged, he asked Armstrong to come with him. Armstrong agreed. He would stay at his side for the whole seven days. Until he wouldn't.

At the airport, Neal's cell phone finally rang.

"Where are you?" Neal said.

"Um, I can't make it, sorry," Armstrong said.

He had backstage passes to the Wallflowers (heck, they'd played at the Race for the Roses and all) and didn't want to give them up. Neal felt betrayed. He had been there when *Armstrong* needed *him*. They had gone through cancer treatments together. He had brought him into his family and had kept his mouth shut about all the drugs he took in cycling, the EPO, the injections of who knows what else. He—not Stapleton, not the Wallflowers— was the one Armstrong called before the 1996 Olympics to help figure out how to get the EPO out of a hotel room refrigerator in Milan because Armstrong had accidentally left it there. He had listened to Armstrong's deepest fears and secrets, including those about his biological and adoptive fathers. He had been his business manager and lawyer, without ever charging a fee. Later, Neal would say, "This is not the treatment I deserved or that anyone deserved."

Some of Neal's friends had called their cancer doctors for him and helped him investigate alternative treatment programs. "But not Lance," he said. "He has not done that."

The more Neal thought about Armstrong standing him up at the airport, the more hurt he felt. He took off the Rolex that Armstrong had given him. It stayed off for good.

One day in late summer 1997, Armstrong sat down with Carmichael, who had flown to Austin to meet him. Carmichael wanted Armstrong to start racing again, and convinced Stapleton to argue the point, too. Both men had a financial stake in a comeback.

Carmichael, who had been replaced by Ferrari in 1995 as Armstrong's main coach, said it would be a shame for Armstrong to quit when he was still so young. Stapleton told Armstrong a comeback could mean big money. Sponsors would flock to him, and not just any sponsors—Fortune 500 companies. Armstrong could very well transcend the provincial roots of the sport.

Though Armstrong knew he'd have to dope again, he told me it didn't scare him because he felt safe in the hands of Ferrari and knew from experience that he would use only a fraction of the EPO that he had—ironically—taken as part of his chemotherapy. He doubted his drug use had caused the cancer. So he agreed to get back on his bike.

Problem was, he had nowhere to go.

Cofidis, the French team, had terminated his $2.5 million, two-year contract. Instead, it offered $180,000, plus incentives that would pay him more for an unexpected return to form. The team wasn't confident that Armstrong would be the same rider.

The offer, insulting in Armstrong's eyes, flipped a switch of anger. Those "Eurobastards" had screwed him. A master at holding grudges, he vowed to get even.

Armstrong had one shot at a better deal: the United States Postal Service team. The U.S.-based squad was owned by Thomas Weisel, a San Francisco investment banker whom several Postal Service riders called "a jock sniffer"—a derogatory term for someone who loves to hobnob with elite athletes. He was a good athlete himself. Competing in his age group, Weisel was a national champion speed skater, a world champion cyclist and a competitive skier. His next athletic goal was to build the country's preeminent cycling team.

Armstrong had ridden for Weisel in 1990 and '91 as an amateur on the Subaru-Montgomery cycling team, which Weisel had bankrolled. Weisel had seen his raw talent. With that in mind, Weisel accepted Stapleton's proposal of a $215,000 base salary for Armstrong, heavy with performance-based bonuses.

That was October 1997, about a year after Armstrong's cancer diagnosis. The cancer would turn out to be a financial boon for Armstrong—and for Stapleton, too. Stapleton wasn't embarrassed to call a postcancer Armstrong a marketer's dream. An autobiography was in the works. People who had paid no attention to cycling now wanted to know about its superhero.

"Lance isn't just a cyclist anymore—because of the cancer, the Lance Armstrong brand has a much broader appeal," Stapleton told the *Austin American-Statesman*. "Our challenge is to leverage that now. He's on the verge of being a crossover-type spokesman. He could be just like an athlete who does a Pepsi or Gatorade commercial. If his comeback has success, we hope to take him to a Kodak or Sony and hope they will turn him into a corporate pitchman."

With Stapleton and Carmichael pushing Armstrong to the brink of international fame, J.T. Neal tried to keep him grounded. Perhaps because he faced imminent death, he wasn't dazzled by the portrayal of Armstrong as the poster boy for cancer awareness. He was dealing with Armstrong, as always, as a father would.

A family friend had taken Armstrong's place as Neal's caregiver in Arkansas for his second bone marrow transplant. That whole week, Neal had wondered where he and Armstrong's mother had gone wrong with Lance. He had long recognized the selfishness inherent in Armstrong's naked ambition, but this time, in dismissing Neal when Neal most needed him, he had gone too far But Neal had kind of seen it coming.

Armstrong had ignored those doctors and nurses who had been at his bedside during his cancer treatments in Austin, and then he used his recovery to make money. It was hypocritical for Armstrong to be a spokesman for cancer awareness, Neal said. "Look how he got it in the first place," Neal would say later. "How he flaunts the rules. It's like, 'I have cancer and I'm a good guy' and 'I will use all means to justify the ends.'"

Neal knew Armstrong was doping again. While Armstrong was raising money for his foundation, he was looking for a way to get EPO in the United States after he'd stopped using the drug to fight his cancer. Armstrong went so far as to ask for the EPO that Neal was using in his cancer treatment. Eventually, when Neal repeatedly refused to share the drug, Armstrong said he had developed a source in the southwestern United States.

As weary of Armstrong's machinations as he was, Neal continued asking him to help his mother, Linda. Neal asked him to give her $10,000 a year. Armstrong refused.

So Neal eventually asked Garvey, the foundation's chairman

of the board, to push Armstrong. When Armstrong again refused, Garvey offered to front the money himself. But he had a public relations problem. If news got out that Armstrong wouldn't help his mother in need, how would it look for the foundation? What if America learned that Lance Armstrong was not a selfless hero?

CHAPTER 8

Two years before Armstrong showed up on the Postal Service team, there was a big shake-up in its organization. After the 1996 season, team director Eddie Borysewicz, the 1984 Olympic coach and Armstrong's former mentor, was not asked to return for another season. Prentice Steffen, the team's doctor, wasn't invited back, either.

Steffen had been in a team hotel room during the 1996 Tour of Switzerland when two Postal riders—Tyler Hamilton and Marty Jemison—approached him to talk. Jemison brought up the team's medical program. He said the team wasn't getting anywhere with the current program—the riders were getting crushed at that race, the team's first big European competition—and asked Steffen's advice.

"Do you think there is something more you could be doing to help us?" he said.

Steffen considered this a euphemism, and felt that Jemison was asking for performance-enhancing drugs. He remembers it as a wink-and-nod conversation that he knew would not go anywhere because, having conquered substance abuse himself, he was against the use of drugs.

"No, I can't really get involved in that sort of thing," Steffen answered.

Hamilton has denied that the conversation ever happened. Jemison said they had spoken with Steffen that day, but that they were asking for legal products, things like vitamins and amino acids. Whatever transpired, Steffen felt that the riders and team management began distancing themselves from him. Mark Gorski, the team's general manager and a 1984 Olympian, stopped returning his calls and e-mails. The next thing he knew, he had been replaced by a Spanish doctor, Pedro Celaya.

Steffen had been with the team for several years and was hurt by his unceremonious departure. There were no formal good-byes; the team just let his contract lapse. Fuming, he wrote a letter to Gorski. "What would a Spanish doctor, completely unknown to the organization, offer that I can't or won't? Doping is the fairly obvious answer."

The team's response came from its law firm. In it, Steffen was threatened with a lawsuit if he made public his accusations.

Borysewicz had also lost his job with the team. Though he had been caught up in the blood doping scandal of the 1984 Summer Games, several of his riders on the Postal Service team said he never offered them anything of the sort. He had told them that he didn't want to be involved in another doping scandal. He was replaced in 1997 by Johnny Weltz, a Dane and a former rider who had spent most of his career with the Spanish ONCE team, which was known as one of the dirtiest teams in the sport. Weltz would join Celaya, a doctor who some riders claimed knew his way around the doping of athletes. (The United States Anti-Doping Agency would eventually slap Celaya with a lifetime ban for doping athletes, but Celaya denied being involved with any drug use. The case was in arbitration in early 2014.)

A new regime was in place that would lay the foundation for

Armstrong's return to the team the next year after he survived cancer. Nothing about the sport's doping culture had changed since he left.

As soon as their teammates left their apartment in Girona, Spain, Darren Baker and Scott Mercier went to work. They looked under beds, in drawers, inside jacket pockets—any and all possible hiding places inside the bedrooms of Tyler Hamilton and George Hincapie, their roommates and fellow Americans on the United States Postal Service team. Finally they stumbled upon a shoebox filled with small pill bottles at the bottom of Hincapie's closet. Tucked among bottles of vitamins was a small tan bottle of testosterone.

"No way!" Mercier said.

"What? That's it? I was sure there would be more," Baker said.

That's all they found, but they'd found an answer to their question: Were their teammates doping? Yes. At least one of them was.

In 1997, Hincapie was only twenty-three, but had long been one of the top cyclists in the United States. The son of Colombian immigrants, he grew up in Queens and began cycling when he was eight. His father, Ricardo, had been a competitive cyclist. George Hincapie would train with his older brother, Rich, in Central Park. On weekends, the Hincapies drove to races in New Jersey, Connecticut and all over New York. Unlike Armstrong, who was a late bloomer as a pure cyclist because he had been concentrating on triathlons, Hincapie was only twelve when he won his first national championship.

In school, he daydreamed about racing in Europe, maybe even in the Tour de France. Ignoring homework, he planned training schedules. He tried one semester of college, at Hofstra University, but decided academics weren't for him.

He took his first vitamin shots with the United States national team, in Italy. In Europe, he said, injecting vitamins was so common that supermarkets sold syringes "next to the apples." At the 1992 Olympics, he received injections from national team trainer Angus Fraser—later accused of doping young riders, though Fraser denies ever doping anyone—but Hincapie assumed his injections were legal supplements, like vitamins B12 and C.

Early on as a pro on the Motorola team, he saw a teammate inject what he assumed was EPO. Another teammate had a drawerful of drugs that he bequeathed to Hincapie when he left the team with an injury. The team's *soigneurs*, including Hendershot, gave Hincapie injections, but he never questioned what was in them. He said his mentor, Frankie Andreu, who'd already been a pro for several years and later raced for the Postal Service team, introduced him to EPO.

"It was just standard," Hincapie says, referring to the doping in Europe's pro *peloton*. "It was shocking, but I didn't have a Plan B. At that time, it wasn't like, 'Well, shit, I've got to cheat.' It was, like, 'I'm not going to let myself get cheated. I have to do this.'"

At his first Grand Tour—the Vuelta a España in 1995, when he was still clean—Hincapie struggled to stay with "the fattest, most out-of-shape guy in the race; that's how hard it was." He realized then that no matter how hard he worked, he would never succeed unless he doped.

For thirty years, his father woke up at 4 a.m. to work in the baggage department for United Airlines at LaGuardia Airport. His mother drove a city school bus for ten years. "That focus and commitment to something was really passed on to me," he said.

"I was going to do what I wanted to do, one hundred percent."

So when faced with the decision of whether or not to take performance-enhancing drugs, Hincapie followed his close friend Armstrong's lead: He went all in. In a year's time, Armstrong would be back on a team with Hincapie and the two would race together and dope together. It was a partnership that would take them places they'd never imagined—places marked with both glory and grief.

Baker and Mercier were two riders on the Postal Service team—perhaps the only two top riders—who said no to doping. Though they had never seen their teammates use performance-enhancing drugs, they were suspicious that their roommates, Hamilton and Hincapie, had gained ground on the EPO-fueled Europeans. How could they do that?

Hincapie, the tall, lanky sprinter whose strength was his speed and power on flat roads, had grown stronger in the mountains. Hamilton, a small guy with freckles, icy blue eyes and wavy auburn hair, had also been climbing better than ever.

Neither had seemed like the type who would dope. Hincapie, nicknamed Big George, was quiet and an all-around nice guy who was as well liked in the *peloton* as he was with fans.

Hamilton might have been plucked from a J. Crew advertisement featuring a boy and his golden retriever. He was a New Englander and former prep school ski racer whose family dressed him in button-down shirts and taught him to be kind and polite. At a glance, Hamilton came across less as a professional athlete and more as a teenager on a bike who tossed your morning newspaper onto the roof instead of the porch.

Armstrong would join the team in 1998. In his year or so away from the sport, the doping culture had not changed. Just because the squad was sponsored by the Postal Service, an independent agency of the United States government, didn't mean the team would follow the rules. Perhaps the opposite held, with the high-profile sponsor putting even more pressure on riders. In charge was Weisel, the financial wizard with a fierce competitive streak, so fierce that he has been said to hire some employees not for their financial acumen but for their ability to help his company win corporate track-and-field competitions.

Baker said one night he and a top Russian rider debated whether there was any justification to dope. The Russian had a good argument. He had been shipped to a sports camp when he was around eleven or twelve, leaving his family and friends behind. He was fine with it, considering the alternative, which would have been a factory job. At camp, three shifts of kids rode ten bikes, and those kids dutifully took "vitamins." It was a life chosen for them. Most American cyclists, for that matter, had nothing to fall back on if they failed. Only a handful attended college.

Baker and Mercier were a couple of rare exceptions. Baker had been a finance major at the University of Maryland, Mercier an economics major at the University of California, Berkeley. So they didn't look at doping as a life-or-death decision. They were in the sport because they loved it.

"It's a bike race," Mercier says. "It's a fun way to make a living, but it's a bike race, c'mon!"

Hincapie hated hearing that, and he hated Mercier because of it. Sure, Mercier had options, but riders like him and Armstrong did not—at least, they felt they didn't. Armstrong feared that he'd have to work at Starbucks if cycling didn't work out for him.

While teammates cursed them under their breath, Mercier and Baker joked about the rampant drug use. Mercier would shake the locked refrigerator on the team truck to hear the glass vials rattling inside. "Hmm, I wonder what's in there? Oh, the special lunch. These are my special B vitamins," he'd say to Baker, laughing as EPO vials made their cheater's music.

To Baker and Mercier, it was obvious the sport had been taken over by doping. Mercier noticed riders in their twenties and thirties with acne, a common side effect of steroids, and some who seemed to have developed big brow bones, a possible side effect of human growth hormone.

At the Tour DuPont in 1994, Mercier had walked into a bathroom and noticed two Spanish riders sharing a stall. He heard one say, "Poco más, poco más," then saw a syringe fall at the riders' feet. "I thought it was gross," Mercier says. "It felt to me like heroin addicts. I felt like, wow, if I have to do that, this is not the sport for me."

At the same race, Mercier had pulled up at the start of one stage along Armstrong, who had such brawny arms that he had to cut his jersey sleeves. His legs rippled with muscles. Mercier said, "Man, Lance, you could be a linebacker, you're so huge. You could play for the Cowboys."

Armstrong's answer: "You think?"

Three years later, Mercier was confronted with doping head-on. At the Postal Service team's training camp in 1997, the Spanish team doctor Pedro Celaya withdrew blood from the riders so he could test their hematocrit levels. Mercier's was 40.5.

"To be professional in Europe, maybe 49, 49.5," Celaya told him.

"*Gracias,* Pedro, how do I do that?"

"Special B vitamins. We can talk later, OK?"

Mercier walked away from it knowing EPO was in store.

In the spring of that year, Mercier had a four-week break during which he was going to his wife's home country, South Africa. He would travel there after competing in the Tour of Romandie, in Switzerland, take two weeks off and train for two weeks. Before the race ended, he met Celaya in a hotel room to discuss the upcoming training schedule.

Celaya handed him a calendar with several little circles and stars marked on certain dates. Next, according to Mercier, came a Ziploc bag filled with pills and vials of liquid. Though Celaya says he was never involved in doping, Mercier claims that Celaya was very much a part of the team's doping scheme. Mercier said he could recall exactly the exchange he had with Celaya when the doctor allegedly handed him the bag of pills and vials.

"What's this, Pedro?" Mercier asked.

"These are steroids," the doctor answered.

"Are these going to make my balls shrink up?"

"No, no," Celaya said, laughing. "You go strong like bull. No racing, for sure you test positive. But it will make you go stronger than ever before."

Mercier alleges that Celaya told him to buy some syringes once he arrived in South Africa, and showed him how to extract liquid from the glass vial. Then he advised Mercier to put the drugs in his front pocket for his flight. If a customs officer stopped him, Celaya said, just say the drugs were vitamins.

Mercier made it to South Africa without incident. Once his training was supposed to begin, he took out the bag of drugs and the calendar that told him what to take and when. On some days, he was supposed to take the green pills first thing in the morning, then later in the evening. Some days at lunch, too. The instructions told him to stop taking the pills on a Sunday before a race in the United States the following Saturday. That's how fast the drugs would exit his system; he wouldn't test positive. Getting away with doping would be easy, if he decided to take that step.

Mercier's wife, Mandie, said she couldn't make that decision for him. She didn't want her feelings about it to taint their relationship. He looked at her and said, "I'm not going to take these."

Mercier lasted only three days on Celaya's training program. The fourth day, he could only get his heart rate to 70 percent of its maximum instead of the 85-95 percent the program required. His legs were shot. For days after that, he was so exhausted and sore that he could do only 80 percent of his workouts.

Then he needed to take a few days off. There was no way he could make it through the two weeks of workouts without drugs. With steroids, he would've recovered from each hard workout and train to his body's full extent the very next day.

Struggling through those workouts, he knew if he raced the next season, he had to be a doper. Hincapie was right. Riders simply couldn't race clean and be competitive anymore. The drugs seemed necessary. Besides, taking them had a huge upside: better results and bigger paychecks.

But Mercier decided to quit the sport. He'd finish the season, but would turn down a contract extension from the Postal Service. His dream was over.

While people have called him courageous and morally strong because of that decision, he is, on one level, embarrassed. He says quitting the sport showed that he was too weak to resist temptation.

"I don't think I'd ever be able to stop doping," he says. "I thought it was a slippery slope."

Mercier finished that season and his career at the Vuelta a España. Even though he had been a strong climber, the sprinters—known for their bursts of speed on straightaways—were outclimbing him. The *peloton* was flying up mountain passes. He had been in third place going into a massive climb early on in one stage. But one by one, riders were overtaking him, as if he were moving in slow motion.

The Vuelta a España also claimed Baker, whose retreat from the sport was thought to be tragic for the fact that he was considered by many to be an amazing natural talent. Jonathan Vaughters, a rider from Denver who would join the Postal Service team the next year, said Baker was good enough to be a top 10 rider at the Tour—"if he would've doped, of course." At that final Vuelta, Baker himself told Sam Abt of the *New York Times* that he once had been as good as Armstrong. "I was strong most of the time, I was just as strong as Lance Armstrong, maybe even stronger on the climbs. But he was always more hungry for the win than I was."

Baker knew, when he was selected for the national team, that riders at the top of the sport were doping. "Everybody knew it," he said, "and everybody talked about it." Riders recited five-time Tour winner Jacques Anquetil's famous line—"Leave me in peace, everybody takes dope"—and repeated what Fausto Coppi, a two-time Tour winner, had told a television reporter. He said he only took dope when he needed to, "which is almost all the time." Baker understood those sayings to be the truth, and he felt pressure to use drugs, but declined.

He had been constantly challenged. At the world championships in 1995, he claims that the doctor working with the U.S.

national team slipped Baker several pills after Baker complained that other riders seemed so much more energized than he was. Baker did not want to reveal the doctor's name, but several team members said that the doctor was Max Testa, who worked on Motorola with Armstrong and other top American riders.

"Here, this will help with the pain in your legs," Baker claims the doctor told him. "It's just cortisone."

"Well, isn't that banned?"

"Yes, but it's not enough to make you test positive."

Baker tossed the pills into a trash can.

At the 1997 Paris-Nice race, a high-pitched buzz had sliced through the air inside Baker's hotel room. He was not amused. He had been fast asleep in his bed when he woke up to see an Italian teammate holding a centrifuge. The guy was testing his own hematocrit. Baker pulled a pillow over his head.

Some French riders had even brought their own doctor to races, and that doctor turned out to be a veterinarian who worked in horse racing. "It was the most ridiculous thing in the world," Baker said. "The guy didn't even work with humans!"

Baker lectured teammates about the dangers of doping. "If you red-line an engine forever," he once said, "it's not going to be good for your car, and doping isn't good for your body, either." Also: "Hormones are what regulate every single thing that happens in your body. When you start messing with those basic building blocks of life, you don't know what's going to happen."

Nobody took him seriously. By then, the management of the team had changed. Systematic doping had already been made part of the Postal team's strategy.

At the conclusion of the 1997 season, Baker and Mercier packed up their things in their Girona apartment. Baker would move to

San Francisco to work in financial services, Mercier to Hawaii to help run one his father's restaurants, where he made $45,000 a year. He and his wife scraped by with their newborn baby.

It's unclear whether Kristin Richard thought about how doping would affect her future family when she married Armstrong in May 1998. She did not respond to requests for an interview for this book.

Their whirlwind romance had begun in early 1997 and he proposed just six months later. Immediately afterward, she took over Armstrong's finances and took control of the household—duties previously handled by Armstrong's mother and J.T. Neal.

In time, she would profess to being a Catholic with a very strong faith, but Armstrong's friends didn't see that side of her early on. Korioth, the former bar manager who became chief of the Lance Armstrong Foundation, had been friends with both Lance and Kristin. "She'd say dirty things to me all the time, crack dirty jokes," he said. "That's her shtick—try to become one of the guys and say things that would shock you."

Korioth saw Kristin Armstrong change from an independent, confident woman into a subservient wife working at her husband's pleasure. Whatever Armstrong wanted, whenever he wanted it, she was there to make his life easier. At the 1998 world championships, there are claims that she even helped him dope. But she didn't stop there. She supposedly helped the entire Postal Service team dope. As the riders exited their hotel to head to the race, several teammates saw her wrap cortisone tablets in tinfoil. One by one, she handed them the tiny packages.

Christian Vande Velde, a rider from suburban Chicago, thought it was funny. "Lance's wife is rolling joints!" he said.

Armstrong was in Bend, Oregon, when the biggest drug bust in Tour de France history unfolded five thousand miles away. The Festina team, one of the Tour's best, had been kicked out of the 1998 race for doping. Willy Voet, one of its *soigneurs*, was caught driving a team car that could have passed for a mobile pharmacy. He carried 234 vials of EPO, 80 doses of human growth hormone and 160 capsules of testosterone.

Armstrong had skipped the Tour that year because he had not been strong enough for a three-week race so soon after his cancer treatments. So, while the top Postal Service team raced in France, Armstrong competed at the Cascade Classic, a multiday stage race in Bend. Officials at the Cascade Classic were excited that a second Postal Service team, starring Armstrong, had come to their event. Without three-time Tour winner Greg LeMond in the sport anymore, cycling's popularity in the U.S. was at a standstill. The officials hoped that Armstrong, the 1993 world champion, could attract a crowd.

He began the race week with one of his oddest victories. In the lead-up to the Cascade Classic, dozens of children, whose average age was about five, competed in the annual kids' race. They arrived on tricycles, skateboards and bicycles (most with training wheels). To give the event a big-time feel, Armstrong had been asked to line up with them and usher the kiddie *peloton* down the road.

The starter's gun kick-started everyone down a short course, a couple of hundred yards long. Some kids swerved diagonally down the road, others meandered toward their parents at the roadside. Some took it so seriously that a group formed at the front, and Armstrong followed.

As that pack moved down the course, Armstrong pedaled alongside the leader, a particularly plucky boy maybe ten years old. Then, with a final quick turn of his pedals, the world champion Lance Armstrong edged the boy at the finish.

Paul Biskup, the Cascade Classic's technical director, saw it and didn't believe what had happened. He said to other officials, "Why did that guy have to cross the finish line first? Why didn't he let that kid beat him?"

They all agreed on one thing: It looked as if Armstrong was such a cutthroat competitor that he simply couldn't help himself.

He won the Cascade Classic.

From his side of the world, Armstrong joked about Voet's arrest. "Maybe the reason that they stopped him was because the exhaust pipe was dragging from the weight of the trunk," he said to teammates at the Oregon race.

In France, no one was laughing. Voet's arrest spurred the police into an all-out war on drugs in the *peloton*. They raided team buses, hotels and equipment warehouses. In Festina's headquarters in Lyon, France, they found drugs labeled with riders' names.

At the start of Stage 8, riders on the Postal Service team had panicked when they saw French police outside a camper used by the team's top riders. Celaya, a mild-mannered doctor, allegedly cursed under his breath. *Mierda. Mierda. Por qué? Por qué? Qué debemos hacer? Qué debemos hacer?* He had a lot to be worried about. The police were raiding team buses and campers, and the Postal Service's bus contained banned substances, including EPO, testosterone and growth hormone. However condoned in cycling, the drugs were a criminal offense in France. Festina's team doctor had already gone to jail, and it was likely that Celaya didn't want to join him.

The camper had been stocked with $25,000 worth of the team's doping products. As riders took off down the starting ramp of the time trial nearby, as thousands of fans cheered, the doctor allegedly gathered everything—all the EPO, all the testosterone, all the growth hormone and all the cortisone. The word was that the police were raiding teams and he worried that they'd be next. So Celaya, according to two team members who would testify under oath to it later, was dead set on flushing the drug stash down the toilet.

Before the doctor pressed down the toilet's lever, though, Hincapie, who was second overall going into Stage 8, took what one rider called "one last huge dose" of EPO. He would need the added boost for the rest of the Tour—a Tour in which some riders would compete clean for the first time because many teams had gotten rid of their drugs one way or another. The prospect of a drug-free ride was so painful that Viatcheslav Ekimov, a Russian rider on Postal who has continually denied ever doping, allegedly joked about diving into the toilet to retrieve the stuff. One teammate looked at the desperate Ekimov and thought, "My God, I thought he'd actually do it."

Armstrong read the newspapers and received dispatches from Hincapie and other friends at the Tour about the Festina case.

He immediately decided Festina had operated so professionally as to make the United States Postal Service team's drug program seem amateurish. While the drug busts moved some teams to run drug-free, or to at least tone down their programs, the Festina scandal inspired Armstrong to build a more complex operation.

When Celaya received a more lucrative offer to work for another team the next season, Armstrong wasn't crushed to see him go. He told a teammate, "He wants to take your temperature just to give you a caffeine pill." For a man who had walked through the valley, in the shadows, Celaya's alleged attitude about drugs was supposedly not aggressive enough.

Jonathan Vaughters was a goofy kid in wool blazers and tight-fitting European pants. He rocked extravagant sideburns—shaved to a sharp point—and plastic-framed nerd glasses, and had raced in Europe since 1994. He and Armstrong had competed against each other since they were teenagers. They also shared the belief that cycling success was built on a foundation of EPO.

He was one of Armstrong's most trusted acolytes. Another, Christian Vande Velde, was a friendly saxophone-playing Midwesterner who would marry his high school sweetheart. Both were *domestiques* whose job it was to usher Armstrong to a victory.

Both Vaughters and Vande Velde feigned laughter when Armstrong joked about the Festina affair. In truth, they said later, the scandal put them on edge. Vaughters, a world-class climber, and Vande Velde, a rookie, were freaked out that riders and team officials were going to jail because of doping. Vaughters knew that drugs were ingrained in the sport's culture at the highest levels. Vande Velde was still figuring that out.

The two shared an apartment in Europe. Vaughters one day

in mid-1998 blurted out, "Hey, do you want to see EPO?" He opened the refrigerator to show Vande Velde a water bottle containing ice and several tiny glass vials. Already feeling guilty about doping, Vaughters didn't want to make it worse by lying to his teammate. So he told Vande Velde everything, a veteran's tutorial about cycling's secrets. He explained the benefits of EPO and how it raised one's red blood cell count. He said all the top riders were using the drug.

Vaughters explained to Vande Velde that Celaya prepared water bottles for each rider and he claimed that each bottle contained EPO on ice. The bottles were labeled with names and dosages: Armstrong. Livingston. Andreu. Hincapie. Vaughters's bottle read, "Jonathan—5x2," meaning the bottle held five vials of EPO with 2,000 units in each.

Vaughters told Vande Velde that riders needed to take other substances to make the EPO more effective. B vitamins. Vitamin C. Testosterone. He showed Vande Velde EPO syringes and testosterone patches. "You're going to need to do all this stuff one day," he told him.

"Really, all of it?"

"Yep, pretty much all of it, if you want to keep up. If you want to stay in the sport."

It was all news to Vande Velde, who'd fallen in love with cycling when he was five years old. His father, a two-time Olympian in track cycling, inflated the tires on their bikes at 6 a.m. so they could ride around their suburban Chicago neighborhood. His elder sister Marisa was a serious cyclist, too.

For the Vande Velde kids, cycling was far more than a hobby. Their father, John, became known in the sport as the P. T. Barnum of track cycling, traveling around the country with what was called "the Vandedrome." It was his own wood-and-steel velodrome, a circular cycling track on which he held competitions. John Vande Velde even had a bit part in the cult cycling film *Breaking Away*, playing one of the bad guys on the Italian pro cycling squad, Team Cinzano. Christian felt he lived with a real celebrity who took him and his sister on long rides through the Chicago suburbs. He was born to be a bike racer.

Over and over, he watched the pivotal scene in *Breaking Away* when Team Cinzano came to race in Indiana and challenged the local riders. Dave, the protagonist, hangs tough with Team Cinzano until one of them thrusts a tire pump into his wheel, causing him to crash. "Everybody cheats," Dave says later. "I just didn't know."

After Vaughters's primer on doping, Vande Velde thought back to training camp earlier in the year when he had noticed Armstrong carrying a mysterious thermos in his duffel bag. Odd: Armstrong had never taken a sip.

During that training camp, he'd asked Armstrong if doping was a problem in the sport, but Armstrong just said he shouldn't worry about it. Looking back, Vande Velde felt stupid for asking. Now he understood why Dylan Casey, a teammate, had scolded him for coming to breakfast one morning at that training camp with a thermos in hand. Casey said, "What the hell are you doing? Are you nuts?" Vande Velde didn't get it. In his thermos, he actually had *coffee*.

Vaughters taught Vande Velde about doping because he wished someone had done it for him when he first raced for the small professional Spanish team Porcelana Santa Clara.

He had never expected to be faced with the decision of whether or not to dope. The team manager, José Luis Nuñes, was a member of Opus Dei, a conservative group within the Catholic church that focuses on simplicity and piety in daily life. He was celibate and went to Mass twice daily. He had told Vaughters and Vaughters's parents, Donna and Jim, that his goal was to develop young cyclists naturally and drug-free because that was what God would want. They put their trust in him.

If that had been Nuñes's goal, he fell short of reaching it. As his team struggled and fell behind on payments to riders, Nuñes allegedly gave in to the sport's reality and allowed the team's doctors to introduce Vaughters and the team's other riders to EPO.

"We're going to use EPO, but we're not going to do it to increase your hematocrit, OK?" Nuñes supposedly told his riders. "We're just going to keep it from dropping below where it would be normally, you know, as if you were just a normal healthy person. This will help you from getting anemia."

Vaughters convinced himself to believe the rationalization. "OK, cool, that sounds fair. I'm not cheating anyone." He agreed to take his first shot of EPO, letting a trainer slip the tiny needle beneath the skin of his arm.

Everyone in the sport knew about the drug and that it was widely used. Vaughters called it "the worst-kept secret ever."

With no test for EPO, he told me, riders were basically "walking around with it taped to their head." He'd once heard Spanish riders chatting about EPO during a race, as casually as they might talk about dinner. "How many units of EPO did you take?" "Oh, really, was it good? Hmm, maybe I'll try that." Vaughters thought, "Wow, I guess all of these guys are doping. *I guess it's not that big of a deal.*"

Even so, the cheating always bothered Vaughters. He was a churchgoing Lutheran and grew up in a conservative family. His father was a Navy lawyer, his mother a teacher. When he did something wrong as a boy, his parents sat him in a yellow tweed chair in the living room until he came up with a resolution for the problem he had caused. His life was entirely rational.

Vaughters felt so conflicted about doping that he took college classes relating to the choices riders made: Ethics I and II. Morality. Endocrinology. If he had to be a doper, he wanted to study up on it. Like Armstrong, Vaughters knew how the drugs worked, how the body processed them and why riders decided to use them.

When it came to doping, Vaughters was pretty sure Armstrong got more out of it than he did. Vaughters had a naturally high hematocrit level, which fluctuated between 48 and 51 percent depending on whether he was at sea level or a high altitude. That meant his EPO doses had to be small or he would fail a new blood test implemented in the spring of 1997 by the International Cycling Union. (The organization goes by the initials UCI for its French acronym.)

At that point, there was still no test for EPO—it would be four years before one was used at the Tour de France—so to try to limit the drug's use in the sport, the UCI began taking blood samples from riders at races and testing their hematocrit levels. Any rider with a level of 50 percent or more would receive a fine and a fifteen-day suspension. Hein Verbruggen, the UCI's president, called it a "health check" because it discouraged riders with dangerously high hematocrits (and thick blood) from competing and possibly risking their health.

Under the new testing, Vaughters could use EPO to improve his hematocrit by only a few points, but Armstrong could gain a much bigger advantage because his normal hematocrit level was 42 or 43. Though each rider's reaction to EPO was different—some were natural responders to the drug, while others didn't respond to it at all, Armstrong could improve his level by at least 7 or 8 points, and likely more. That was much more than Vaughters could.

Vaughters could raise his hematocrit with EPO to about 52—an improvement of 4 points at most—then he would temporarily lower it for UCI's health check by infusing a bag of saline into his blood—a common practice among riders manipulating their blood with EPO. After using the drug, Vaughters saw the numbers tick upward on his power meter, the electronic machine affixed to his bike's handlebars that measured a rider's power output.

Vaughters noticed that many times EPO would give him a 4 to 6 percent increase in power. That translated into a few percentage points of speed. That translated into better finishes.

In time, Vaughters would become one of the best climbers in Europe.

And all of that depressed him.

At the 1998 "Festina" Tour de France, as gendarmes swarmed the race, one team hid its EPO in a vacuum cleaner. One rider had his family members smuggle it into his room at the team hotel. Late in the Tour, in an act of carelessness, a Postal rider left a thermos filled with vials of EPO in the refrigerator of the team bus. So much for a clean race.

The Tour ended with only fourteen of the twenty-one teams that had started. Others had quit or been thrown out. Only 96 of the starting 189 riders finished.

Bobby Julich, an American, finished third, the highlight of his career. He shared the podium with the Italian Marco Pantani, who had recently won the Giro d'Italia, one of cycling's Grand Tours, and the German Jan Ullrich, who had won the Tour the year before. Years later, all three would either be implicated in doping scandals, test positive and/or admit doping. Julich seemed to know it was coming. After the race, he said, "Ten years down the line, you may see an asterisk" next to the 1998 finishes.

Later that year, Armstrong and Vaughters rode in the Vuelta a España, a three-week race and Grand Tour. Armstrong and Vaughters knew each had pushed their hematocrits to the UCI limit by using EPO, but they didn't talk about it.

When Celaya checked each rider's hematocrit to make sure none were going to fail the UCI's blood test, he'd write the rider's initials and hematocrit number on a paper napkin. Vaughters always peeked at those napkins. Armstrong made it his business to know everyone's number.

"Hey, 49, JV? Getting pretty close there, dude," he'd say. If someone's EPO was low, he would chastise him.

Armstrong spoke freely about his doping back then. During that Vuelta he even asked Vaughters and Vande Velde to fetch him a cortisone pill. Near the end of a particularly difficult stage, he asked, "Can you get it from the car for me?"

They looked at him like he'd lost his mind. *He wanted cortisone? Right in the middle of a race? And we have to get it for him?* But he was the boss, so they dropped back to the team car. The team director, Johnny Weltz, didn't have cortisone. To keep the boss happy, he whittled down an aspirin pill, wrapped it in tinfoil and gave it to Vande Velde for Armstrong.

When the race stopped in Andorra, the small principality in the Pyrenees, Vaughters needed to send an e-mail to his mother, so he went to Armstrong's hotel room to borrow his laptop. Armstrong walked out of the bathroom shirtless, brushing his teeth with one hand and holding a tiny syringe in the other. With a deft wave of his hand, Armstrong grabbed a fold of his stomach and—click!—shot himself with EPO.

"Now that you are doing EPO too, you can't go write a book about it," Armstrong said.

PART THREE

LIES OF THE MEDIA

I n the weeks before the 1999 Tour de France, Jean-Marie Leblanc, the Tour's race director, made a pilgrimage to ask for a miracle. He went to Notre-Dame-des-Cyclistes—Our Lady of Cyclists—a tiny stone chapel in southwestern France that is considered the sport's spiritual headquarters. It has ten wooden pews, five on either side of the aisle. Three rows of multicolored cycling jerseys, more than eight hundred in all, line its walls. Tucked in the back are cycling trophies and even bikes.

Leblanc met with the parish priest and they prayed for the 86th running of the great national race. Leblanc needed more than just divine intervention—he needed the race to be clean. The Festina scandal still hung over the Tour. One newspaper in France called it "the Tour de Farce." The French president, Jacques Chirac, had even asked if the race hadn't become too difficult for a normal, nondoping human to endure.

Leblanc promoted the 1999 race as the "Tour of Renewal." Not that every fan, sponsor and journalist bought in. There had been clues that the label was wishful thinking. A month earlier, the 1998 Tour champion, Marco Pantani, had been ejected from the Giro d'Italia. His hematocrit level had reached 52, a number that suggested doping. Suspended for fifteen days, Pantani decided not to defend his Tour title.

Into this drug-induced hellscape rode Lance Armstrong. He appeared on the first day of the Tour, in a theme park called Le Puy du Fou that is like Disneyland for history buffs, and established that his cancer was just a blip on the radar of his career. In an individual time trial held around the park, he won the 4.2-mile prologue, shocking the sport. In his broadcast, Phil Liggett, the longtime television commentator, was giddy: "What a way to make a return to big-time cycling after having had a near-death visit from the dreaded cancer!"

Armstrong said he was surprised at how fast he had ridden—seven seconds ahead of the second-place man. "I gave everything and I felt good," he said. He gave credit to his oncologists for saving his life and said it was amazing that he could even race. Addressing Festina, he said cycling fans shouldn't worry about such a thing ever happening again. It was safe, he said, to fall in love with a man and his bike.

The Postal Service team had a new doctor, a new team manager and a new way of thinking. To win cycling's most prestigious race, it needed to be more aggressive than ever. Some teams might have been scared straight by the Festina scandal. But Armstrong saw an opportunity.

When he won the prologue, he expected doping questions to follow. That was the price of being the team leader, that was the price of winning the yellow jersey in the first Tour post-Festina. While his teammates sat in the shadows, the man in front had to answer reporters' questions every day.

"It's been a long year for cycling," he said, "and as far as I'm concerned, it's history. Perhaps there was a problem, but problems exist in every facet of life: sport, cycling, politics."

He continued, "You come to training camps to assume we are all doped. That's bullshit. We're not."

As Armstrong spoke to reporters after the prologue, his urine samples were en route to the French national antidoping laboratory in Paris to be analyzed for banned substances. For the first time, the drug testers at the Tour would look for corticosteroids—drugs that riders had long abused, primarily because they eased a rider's pain. Cyclists were confident that the Tour didn't test for them.

Corticosteroids, according to Antoine Vayer, the head trainer of the infamous Festina team, were the drug of choice for most riders. He told David Walsh, a reporter for the *Sunday Times* in London, that cyclists had grown to rely on the drug as if they were addicted to it.

"Riders take them when they are stressed, they take them when they are down, they take them if they mess up," Vayer said. "For them, life must be without stress. It is a junkie mentality. Many of the best riders have become psychotic. They want to win money, to screw others because compared to them, everybody else is small. They want to have a nice house, a nice wife, a nice car and they will do whatever to get these things."

For the 1999 Postal Service team, the aggressive new doping program had begun with the team's new doctor, Luís García del Moral. Del Moral, a balding, gruff chain smoker, ran a popular sports clinic in Valencia, Spain, and had replaced the soft-spoken Pedro Celaya as the team's head physician. Celaya is accused of having given riders performance-enhancing drugs, but many felt he was dispensing the bare minimum. Some, like Vaughters, felt he was holding them back. Del Moral had the pedigree of having worked for the ONCE team, which had a reputation for being rife with doping.

On the doctor's suggestion, Armstrong and his teammates experimented with a plasma-expanding drug—none remember the name of it—made to boost their blood volume and, consequently, increase their endurance. The substance, normally used in patients who had lost blood after being burned or going into shock, was supposed to accomplish the same thing as a transfusion or EPO, only on a smaller scale and in a slightly different manner.

"Um, I'm peeing purple," Vaughters once told del Moral. "Are you sure this is OK?"

Despite del Moral's assurances, Vaughters felt an increasing anxiety about the new drugs. He had been using EPO and testosterone. But those were drugs he had researched. Now del Moral was introducing more and more unknowns as he expanded the team's arsenal of pharmaceuticals. In addition to the plasma expander, he gave Vaughters a drug he said would increase circulation. Vaughters lost sleep imagining the imminent arrival of testers who would discover those new drugs, as well as the old standbys, in his system. But that was life on the new Postal Service team.

It was part of the team's preparation for the so-called Tour of Renewal. Armstrong later called the program "conservative." With del Moral and the new team manager, Johan Bruyneel, in charge—Bruyneel had just retired from the ONCE team as a rider—it seemed that the squad's doping regime began to operate like a cold, hard business. While Bruyneel and del Moral say they were never involved in any sort of doping—and would vehemently deny it in later doping cases against them, saying that their accusers were pressured into pointing fingers at them—Vaughters called the new drug program "no-holds-barred." The drugs were supplied by the team and were free. The Italian doctor Ferrari watched over Armstrong and two of his top teammates, Tyler Hamilton and Kevin Livingston. The rest of the team was left to deal with the team's new administration.

"There was no moderating anyone's drug use," Vaughters said. "It was like a freakin' flood of, 'Hey, let's do that. OK, let's do that, too'; the more drugs the better."

While Celaya may have given Vaughters 6,000 international units of EPO for him to use over a two- or three-week period, del Moral gave him 15,000 to 20,000. "Yeah, just be a little careful. You don't want to use it all or your hematocrit will be too high," he would tell Vaughters, who was astonished at the doctor's nonchalance.

Organized and unemotional, del Moral kept everyone's doping plan on a Microsoft Excel spreadsheet. He wasn't interested in coming to riders' homes to discuss how and when to use the drugs he had brought. In Vaughters's case, del Moral usually dropped off drugs in Girona, Spain, when he was on his way to see Armstrong in Nice, France. He wouldn't bother driving into town. He would meet Vaughters next to a tollbooth and make the handoff.

Vaughters would ride his bike there and stuff the package of drug vials and syringes up his jersey for the ride home. Once, on his way back, he put his foot onto the road at a stop sign and the package inside his shirt crashed onto the pavement, vials and syringes flying everywhere, as a group of old ladies looked on. With del Moral in charge now, Vaughters was more stressed out than ever. One thing that bothered him was that the good doctor used preloaded syringes, leaving riders guessing what was inside because there was no label to inspect. When cyclists asked, "Hey, what's that?" he'd say, "It's a professional secret. Do you want it or don't you?"

Already numb to the doping in the sport, Vaughters always said yes. Getting injections, sometimes five in one sitting, had become part of the job—to ensure that Lance Armstrong won the Tour de France.

Johan Bruyneel had worked with del Moral on the ONCE team. While Bruyneel had won two stages of the Tour de France, he was better known for riding off the side of a mountain in the 1996 Tour. (He was not injured and, muddy and shaken, got back on his bike.)

Bruyneel and Armstrong had met at the Vuelta a España in 1998, the year Armstrong finished a surprising fourth after coming back from cancer. Bruyneel was a race commentator then, and there was an instant connection. Bruyneel suggested that Armstrong could be the kind of rider who could win the Tour someday, something no one had ever told him, and that belief in him piqued Armstrong's interest. Bruyneel said he looked at Armstrong and that it "was like looking in a mirror." The two men had the same single-minded will to win.

Armstrong used his power on the team to arrange for Mark Gorski, the head of the Postal Service team's business matters, to call Bruyneel and offer him a job as team manager. Bruyneel took the job and devised a plan.

Armstrong would focus on just one race: the Tour de France. Forget the warm-up races beforehand—those would expose him to unnecessary drug testing. The International Cycling Union had no out-of-competition tests at that time, so he would be safe from testing positive while he used drugs to train harder.

The difference between Bruyneel and the former team manager Johnny Weltz was that riders claimed that Bruyneel was obsessed with the nuances of doping and getting away with it. He allegedly kept tabs of every rider's doping program and knew everyone's hematocrit level. Once, when Vaughters had returned to Europe after spending time at home in the mile-high city of Denver, his hematocrit was 48. He claims that Bruyneel laid into him.

"You are doping on your own, aren't you?" he said, according to Vaughters. When Vaughters said his hematocrit was just naturally that high at that altitude, Bruyneel didn't believe him and stormed away. He wanted control over all the riders who would be escorting Armstrong, the team's star, up and down the roads of France.

On the more stringent doping program—in which the drugs came directly from the team and became necessary, like a bike part—Vaughters was going faster than ever. Before the Critérium du Dauphiné Libéré, one of the warm-up races to the Tour, he had used enough EPO to jack up his hematocrit to 53. A saline drip helped thin his blood for him to pass the UCI's blood test.

He won the Dauphiné's uphill time trial that finished at the summit of Mont Ventoux, a mountain that soars above the Provence region of France and requires an impossible outlay of strength and endurance to reach the top. But Vaughters didn't just win it, he won it in record time—56 minutes, 50 seconds—nearly 43 seconds ahead of the second-place finisher. Armstrong was fifth, about a minute back. It was the first time that Vaughters actually felt he had cheated. All those other times, he was using EPO just to keep up, to survive in a *peloton* that was racing at abnormal speeds. This time, after winning the glory and the prize money, he felt dirty.

"I got to see the strings in the puppet show. OK, I get it now," Vaughters told me nearly fourteen years after that victory. "My question was, am I really good enough to be the best in the world if I doped to the limit? The answer was yes. It was like the mystique was gone."

A few weeks after that, he won the Route du Sud, another big pre-Tour race. But out of fear that he'd be caught doping, he began to dial back on his drug use. He couldn't understand how Armstrong and his wife would live in Nice, when France's anti-doping laws were so strict. He asked Kristin Armstrong how she dealt with the daily possibility of police raiding their house when vials of EPO were chilling in the refrigerator next to the milk.

"The code word is butter, as in, 'Do you have any butter in the refrigerator?'" Vaughters claims she told him.

Vaughters also was starting to annoy Bruyneel because he kept asking him questions about how the doping would work at the Tour. He'd ask, "How is the team going to get drugs into France? Should we be afraid of testing positive? If we get caught there, it's seven years in jail, don't you know?"

According to Vaughters in his testimony to USADA, Bruyneel would answer, "Don't worry, Jonathan. Everything is taken care of."

While Jean-Marie Leblanc prayed the morning of the 1999 Tour de France, the International Cycling Union did its usual dance to rid the race of anyone using EPO. It conducted a blood test on all of the riders to measure their hematocrit levels. Anyone whose level was over 50 percent—unless they, like Vaughters, had a dispensation from a doctor—would receive a two-week suspension right then and there. But, as it often is with drug users and their pursuers, the dopers were one step ahead.

Vaughters remembers that eight of the team's nine Tour riders were dangerously close to the UCI's limit. He claims that they had del Moral and Ferrari to thank for it. Vaughters's hematocrit was 0.001 away from being over. Hincapie, the sprinter, was also that close, with a level of 49.999. Armstrong's was 49.4. "The whole team is ready," Armstrong said.

Just a few weeks before, at the Dauphiné, Armstrong's hematocrit had been 41. He had told his *soigneur*, Emma O'Reilly, about it. When she asked him what he was going to do, he laughed and said, "You know, Emma. What everybody does."

O'Reilly, a feisty Irishwoman trained as an electrician, was in the middle of her fourth season as a *soigneur* with the Postal Service team. It was a thankless job, but she enjoyed seeing the world on the Postal Service team's dime and liked being a part of a team on the rise. She found much less pleasure in playing a part in the team's doping scheme.

For her first year and a half, she was kept out of the drug loop, but in April 1997, she claims she had seen a fellow *soigneur* preparing syringes of a liquid to administer to riders at the Circuit de la Sarthe, an early-season race in the northwest region of France. She was in awe of the dexterity and quickness with which he injected the riders in the buttocks. Then it dawned on her: her colleague had been a mediocre-at-best *soigneur*, giving weak massages and doing a poor job at basic duties like preparing the riders' food and keeping their water bottles clean. But those tasks weren't his main function. Not even close, actually. His real job was to help the riders dope.

The next season, O'Reilly was easing herself into that role. In early summer 1998 she found herself acting as a drug courier for Hincapie. The education of Emma O'Reilly had begun. By the time the Festina scandal rolled around, O'Reilly was tangentially involved in the team's systematic doping plan. She saved the team from being busted by customs agents before the start of that 1998 Tour, which began in Dublin. She had traveled to Ireland early to spend time with family and met the team at the airport as they arrived past midnight one night. When customs agents showed up, she convinced them that "they would have a riot on their hands" if they tried to search the team cars because the riders were tired and cranky. The customs agents finally let the vehicles go without a search.

Armstrong liked working with O'Reilly because she had a sharp sense of humor and took her job very seriously. She was a tough, no-nonsense big sister who wouldn't take his crap and would get the job done. "Someone had to put him in his place, and on the team, that was me," she said in 2012.

Still, O'Reilly would bring Armstrong ice for his EPO thermos, and claimed she once drove to Spain to pick up a bottle of pills from Bruyneel before delivering them to Armstrong in a McDonald's parking lot in France. With his wife sitting in the passenger seat of Armstrong's car, O'Reilly said she remembered slipping the bottle into his hand, as if they were making a drug deal.

Armstrong trusted her enough that he asked for her help to hide evidence of his doping before the 1999 Tour. Just before the team's pre-race medical checkup and press conference, Andreu noticed a bruise on Armstrong's arm, a black-and-blue mark that came from an injection he had received. Afraid that journalists would notice and pummel him with questions, Armstrong asked

O'Reilly for some concealer, and she went out of her way to help him.

As Armstrong churned his way to the Alpine mountaintop finish in Sestriere, Italy, he looked like he was on a Sunday afternoon training ride in Austin. It was Stage 9 of the twenty-stage Tour, the first mountain stage, and the Postal Service team was crushing everyone in its path. Andreu and Hincapie laid down a grueling pace for Armstrong through the early climbs, forcing other teams to struggle to keep up. When Andreu and Hincapie could go on no more, the climbing specialists Hamilton and Livingston took over. Both crashed on one tricky descent, though, leaving Armstrong to fend for himself.

With no teammates around to shield him, Armstrong attacked with about six miles left to go in the final climb. It was a remarkable show of strength, and the television commentators made sure their viewers realized it. One said it was astonishing to see Armstrong's composure during the ascent. His face never once showed a grimace and his pace didn't slow for even a millisecond. He looked like a machine.

Armstrong had won the prologue of the Tour, then didn't wear the yellow jersey again until Stage 8, when he won the individual time trial. But it wasn't until Stage 9 that he showed everyone he was a completely new Lance Armstrong. Never before had he been so strong in the mountains.

Now, near the end of the stage, as the crowds along the route cheered him on, Armstrong the cancer survivor yelled into his microphone, so the people in his team car could hear him loud and clear, "How do you like them fuckin' apples!" He crossed the finish line 31 seconds ahead of the second-place Alex Zülle of Switzerland, and more than a minute ahead of the rider in third.

The next day, French newspapers launched an attack on his credibility, hinting that he couldn't have produced that performance in the mountains without pharmaceutical help.

The French newspaper *Le Monde* raised questions about the ride, pointing out that Armstrong's best in the mountains, before the cancer, had left him no closer to the stage winner than eighteen minutes behind and as far back as half an hour. Headlines read, "Armstrong, the Extraterrestrial of the Tour," "Stupefying Armstrong," "On Another Planet" and "Hallucinating Armstrong."

And then came the first doping charge of his career.

Le Monde reported that Armstrong had tested positive for cortisone after the Tour's prologue. One journalist at a press conference asked if he had been taking it for medical reasons. Over two days, Armstrong denied using the drug. "They want me to crack on the bike and I'm not going to. It's vulture journalism. I have been persecuted," he said.

O'Reilly already knew that Armstrong's comments about the cortisone test were lies. While giving him a massage one day, she claims that she heard him, team owner Thomas Weisel and team business manager Mark Gorski brainstorming to devise an excuse for Armstrong's failed drug test. Weisel and Gorski deny having the conversation or knowing anything about the doping on the team, but O'Reilly alleged that she heard the three of them come up with the idea to produce a backdated prescription for saddle sores, an injury for which cortisone cream is used. She claims they had said that they would just have del Moral create a prescription for Armstrong to hand to the UCI, and that would explain why Armstrong had tested positive for cortisone. Gorski supposedly left the room to get it. "Now, Emma, you know enough to bring me down," Armstrong said.

Armstrong alleges that the UCI was also trying to help him out of the tough spot. According to Armstrong, UCI president Hein Verbruggen contacted him and said, "This is a real problem for me; this is the knockout punch for our sport." Armstrong alleges that Verbruggen—who strongly denies that he was involved in any cover-up—told him that he wanted nothing to ruin Armstrong's magical comeback story, particularly post-Festina. So according to Armstrong, Verbruggen endorsed his plan for a backdated prescription. But it was up to Armstrong to find a saddle sore cream or eye ointment that contained Cemalyt, the drug for which he had tested positive. Verbruggen vehemently disputes those facts. "It's a bullshit story and nothing else. Never, ever would I have had a conversation saying, 'We have to take care of this,'" he said.

None of Armstrong's teammates believed his saddle sore story. They knew the positive test had come from Armstrong's injection of cortisone several weeks before at the Route du Sud.

Several days after news of his positive test was published, the cycling union released a statement saying that Armstrong had been using a cortisone cream to treat allergic dermatitis. He had tested positive for "minimal traces" of the drug, it said, but Armstrong's use of the cream "was authorized by the rules and cannot be considered a doping practice."

The statement came with a request: "We would like to ask all press representatives to consider the complexity of these matters and the regulations and legal aspects before publishing their articles. This will ensure that superficial and unfounded claims are avoided."

Defending his sport and its biggest race, Verbruggen would eventually declare that the Tour was "mostly clean." He said the proof was that the UCI's blood tests on the riders during the Tour had shown that all of the competitors were way under the cycling union's limit of a 50 percent hematocrit, unlike in past Tours when riders' hematocrits were mainly 48 or 49. Verbruggen said the 1999 Tour tests didn't not reveal any "such a level."

But had he misspoken? At the start of the Tour, according to Vaughters, nearly all of the nine riders on Postal Service had hematocrits that were dangerously close to 50. And it was just one of twenty teams in the race.

The improbably fast speed of the Sestriere stage had not been ignored by some of the riders trying to keep up. Former Postal rider Jean-Cyril Robin told fellow Frenchman Christophe Bassons, "This has got to stop! We can't go on racing like this!" (The speed at the Tour was 25.2 miles per hour. Never before had it exceeded 24.9.)

Robin and Bassons had finished in the back of the pack that day, and both knew why: doping. Bassons was said to have been the only clean rider on the Festina team the year before. He has said he turned down a salary that would have been ten times his normal paycheck if he'd agreed to a program of EPO. This earned Bassons the nickname Monsieur Propre, or Mister Proper, and other riders gave him a hard time about speaking out against doping in the *peloton* and breaking cycling's code of silence. Armstrong had berated him so much at the Dauphiné the month before the Tour that Vaughters once patted Bassons on the back and said, "Sorry what you've had to go through." Armstrong saw the gesture, and excoriated Vaughters: "What are you, another fucking Bassons?"

During the 1999 Tour, Bassons wrote a daily journal for the newspaper *Le Parisien* in which he said the Festina scandal had changed nothing. Riders were still doping, and doing it without remorse. After the Sestriere stage, he told the newspaper *Aujourd'hui* that Armstrong's ride had "disgusted him" because it was so suspicious that he had ridden so fast, so easily. He thought it was the perfect moment to speak loudly about the "*cyclisme à deux vitesses*" or "two speeds of cycling."

During another mountain stage the next day, with the world watching, Armstrong tapped Bassons on the shoulder and told him to shut up. If Bassons thought that negatively about the sport then he had no right to be a professional cyclist and should quit.

"What you are saying is no good for cycling," Armstrong said. "Go home! Fuck you!"

After that, the power of Lance Armstrong, the sport's new *patron*, ripped through the *peloton*. Many riders stopped talking to Bassons. Nobody wanted to be seen with him.

Leblanc, the race director, told *Aujourd'hui* that Bassons spoke as if "he is the only rider who is beyond reproach." Leblanc said EPO use "has practically disappeared." Bassons's own team called him a coward and said he spoke about doping for his self-glorification, and that he should get out of the sport. He was a marked man, and in a day's time, he would indeed quit the Tour.

"If I made a mistake, it was believing that others would support me," Bassons said, adding that riders not using EPO were likely taking cortisone or lesser drugs, so they weren't in a position to join him in his antidoping crusade.

The French newspaper *L'Equipe* said Bassons "died at the stake" and had been "burned by his passion," like Joan of Arc.

Every day for six months, Bassons woke up crying for no reason. The next year, he raced with several former Festina teammates, who refused to speak to him. In 2001, he was racing at the Four Days of Dunkirk and several competitors tried to ride him into a ditch. He finally quit the sport entirely.

Armstrong—the sport's newly christened leader—had said the words: *No more Bassons*. And his will was done.

After the Festina scandal, the top climbers on the Postal Service team didn't want to travel with their EPO, lest the French police decide to raid their team bus or hotel rooms. So they hired someone to do it for them: Tyler Hamilton claims that a Frenchman named Philippe Maire, who was Armstrong's handyman and gardener in Nice, would be their drug courier during the Tour.

Maire supposedly would follow the Tour on a motorcycle, earning him the nickname "Motoman." When Armstrong, Hamilton or Livingston needed EPO, the team trainer Jose "Pepe" Martí allegedly would call Motoman on a prepaid cell phone and Maire would weave through traffic to meet him at a handoff point. Maire and Martí deny any involvement. If the Motoman story were true, the scheme would have been as simple as ordering takeout.

Hamilton and Livingston supposedly would room together so that Bruyneel and Armstrong could come to their room to talk about doping. That exclusive group, nicknamed the "A" team, used the team's nicest RV, while the other riders squeezed into a shoddy secondary camper.

Del Moral or Martí allegedly would bring the preloaded syringes into the camper or hotel room, so that the A team could inject EPO every third or fourth day until the third week of the race. When the deed was done, one of them would shove the syringes into a bag or a Coke can and slip out of the room to dispose of the evidence.

The "B" team received their syringes wrapped in aluminum foil and del Moral gave everyone injections without telling them what the substance was. Though some riders didn't know it, one of the substances the whole team was taking was Actovegin, the calf's blood extract that was used for stroke patients and supposedly helped with blood circulation. It was just one of the many drugs in the Postal Service squad's medicine cabinet.

Vande Velde, in his first Tour, was so exhausted that he agreed to have del Moral give him testosterone. In my interview with him in early 2013, he said he had been getting a massage from a *soigneur* who was "a big Dutch dude named Ronnie," when del Moral came into the hotel room. The doctor said, "I have testosterone. Do you want it or not? Yes or no? I can come back."

Vande Velde was lying there, thinking, "Holy shit, he's giving me my first talk about doping in front of somebody else. Man, oh, man, I'm losing my mind." He considered the consequences of saying yes. (It would be cheating and he could test positive.) Then he thought of the consequences of no. (He might not be able to ride out front and help Armstrong; he might be so tired that he couldn't finish the Tour.) Finally, he said, "Yeah, screw it, I'll take it." Del Moral asked him to open his mouth, then dropped a few drops of testosterone mixed with olive oil onto his tongue. He told him, "It will be out of your system by tomorrow morning."

Vande Velde told me, "It could have been a placebo, for all I know. It was a minute amount . . . Maybe I slept better because my hormones were actually decent."

Vande Velde said having an organized doping program wasn't the only reason the Postal Service team excelled. "To put it concisely, the biggest thing was that we were going to train harder than everybody else, we were going to have a better diet than everyone else and we were going to dope better than everybody else."

Vaughters would've been on the same doping plan as the B team if he hadn't crashed in the race's second stage. The *peloton* was riding in western France along the slippery Passage du Gois, which is covered by water during high tide. The rider in front of Vaughters tumbled to the ground after skidding on a mossy section. Vaughters hit him, and went flying.

He hit the rocks along the road so hard that he was knocked out. He opened his eyes to see a woman, screaming. Blood poured from his face. Yet he climbed back onto his bike and rode gingerly down the course, alone and pensive.

He had taken a shot of EPO in Spain just before the plane's door closed on his way to the Tour. Because of that he had nearly gone over the hematocrit limit during the UCI's testing. Now he worried that he would break the limit if he was tested again because his body was so sensitive to EPO. The more he thought about it, the more nervous he became and the slower he rode.

Vaughters took his crash as a sign to stop doping. Nothing good could come of it. He stopped pedaling, and waited for the ambulance behind him.

"I'm never, ever going to dope again," he said, to no one in particular.

* * *

Riders like Vaughters and Hincapie watched Armstrong from afar, thankful that it was Armstrong—not them—who had to lie for the entire sport.

"What can I do, I've been on my deathbed and I'm not stupid," Armstrong told reporters at that 1999 Tour. "I've never tested positive."

In one poststage television interview, he said, "I can emphatically say I'm not on drugs. I'm sure that there's been some looking and prying and digging . . . You're not going to find anything. If it's *L'Equipe*, if it's Channel 4 or if it's a Spanish paper, Belgian paper, Dutch paper, there's nothing to find. And I think once everybody gets done doing their due diligence, everybody realizes that they've got to be professional and can't print a bunch of crap, then they'll realize that they're dealing with a clean guy."

In an interview with Australia's SBS television, he was blunt, saying, "There's no secret here. We have the oldest secret in the book—hard work."

He denied doping in dozens of ways, insisting that he wasn't suddenly the "new rider" some journalists had suggested. Those reporters pointed out that the best he had done in the Tour before his cancer was 36th. Armstrong explained that if there was something he needed to hide, he wouldn't be living, training and racing in France, which has such strict antidoping laws.

When a *Le Monde* reporter asked why Armstrong initially denied presenting the UCI with a prescription for the cortisone to justify its use, Armstrong shot back, "Monsieur Le Monde, are you calling me a doper or a liar?" The question went unanswered. None of the other journalists in the room chimed in.

Armstrong used his survivor's story to gain sympathy, something his critics would eventually dub his "cancer shield." He said, "They say stress causes cancer so if you want to avoid cancer, don't come to the Tour de France and wear the yellow jersey."

While European writers remained critical of Armstrong, most of the American press defended him. Reporters from the United States were streaming into the Tour to write about the new American hero who had rescued cycling from drug use. Almost a thousand journalists were accredited for the race, two hundred more than usual. Lost amid the hoopla was the Tour's long history of doping.

USA Today said Armstrong couldn't enjoy his success and blamed the French media. "He's understandably upset about their brand of shoddy, jealous and jingoistic journalism."

The *Philadelphia Inquirer* said that the Tour de France had found "its healer after last year's drug scandal." "The French press, in which objectivity is scant, has hinted cynically, through ambiguous headlines and quotes from unnamed doctors, that no mortal could rise so phoenix-like without artificial help."

The *Detroit News* wrote that Armstrong was "doing his best to ignore the silly whispers among the French press corps," and that many journalists who'd never covered cycling were continuing to "search for another doping scandal such as the one that rocked the Tour last summer."

The *Washington Post* dubbed him "a cancer survivor and a man who almost single-handedly has revived a sport tarnished by widespread doping." It also called the French media "prickly."

The *New York Times* wrote that Armstrong was "an outspoken opponent of the use of performance-enhancing drugs in the sport" who has given the Tour "a resoundingly positive image" and has "provided an inspirational, feel-good story."

Americans were inundated with pro-Armstrong propaganda.

Phil Liggett, the Tour commentator for ABC television, pointed out that the French were having their worst showing at the Tour since 1926 and were just envious of Armstrong's success. "No way he's taking drugs," he said. "They're just knifing him over there."

Even Armstrong's cancer doctors piped up. "This guy is so clean-living you wouldn't believe it," Dr. Lawrence Einhorn of Indiana University Cancer Center told the Associated Press.

People who pay attention to sports—journalists included—want to believe in the miracles of athletic competition. Reporters wrote what they were told by the Postal Service team, by Armstrong and his agent, Stapleton. Gorski, the business manager, said that because of the Festina scandal, clean riders like Armstrong finally had the chance to make it to the top. "It's like a miracle!" he said.

They explained how Armstrong became a three-week stage-race rider after years of being a cyclist whose strength was one-day events. It was the cancer. It caused him to shed fifteen pounds from his 5-foot-9 frame—though some news outlets reported it to be ten pounds, and yet another, ten kilos (22.2 pounds). His weight loss became his defense: With fewer pounds on his body, it was so much easier for him to propel himself up steep mountains.

The American press also gave credit to Armstrong's "coach," Chris Carmichael. Even if Carmichael did not know it at the time, he was in essence a prop to cover Armstrong's involvement with Ferrari's drug program. According to *USA Today*, Carmichael helped Armstrong by using "cutting-edge techniques to develop tremendous aerobic capacity and pedaling efficiencies." The *Washington Post* said Carmichael's techniques used "more revolutions at a lower gear speed instead of power riding at a higher gear." Carmichael once boasted that Armstrong's training results were "even better than if he had used EPO."

Betsy Andreu was at home in Dearborn, Michigan, with her two-month-old son, Frankie, watching Armstrong's phenomenal stage to the mountaintop of Sestriere. She was aware that doping existed in the *peloton*, but thought her husband was clean, considering he had told her so that day in 1996 when the two of them had overheard Armstrong's drug confession to his doctors in Indianapolis. But as the Sestriere stage unfolded on her television, the truth dawned on her.

Not only was Armstrong chugging up the mountain like a train, her husband was out in front, too, pulling Armstrong up some of the toughest climbs in the Alps. She called her friend Becky Rast, the wife of cycling journalist and photographer James Startt.

Becky Rast thought Betsy was calling to preen over her husband's accomplishments. She said, "Oh my God, Betsy, Frankie's doing it! He's going so great!"

"Great, my ass," Andreu said. "What the hell is he doing pulling? He's not a climber! He should be just trying to make the time cut."

Betsy Andreu knew that her tall, lanky husband was a born sprinter, made to go fast and use his power over short distances. She was seeing something that was not physically possible. She had left Europe at the end of March to settle in back home to have her first baby, and had seen Frankie only briefly for the birth. In their entire time together, she had seen him inject himself with something only once, and he said that had been a vitamin B12 shot. Now it seemed obvious he had been doing some type of drug in her absence.

When she called him later that day, she skipped the pleasantries.

"What the hell was that?" she said.

By the 1999 Tour, Betsy suspected that their good friend Lance was cheating in more ways than one. When Betsy talked to Armstrong one morning before she left Europe that spring, it only complicated her image of him. They had seen each other the night before at a party at Armstrong's house in Nice, France. He called Betsy upon waking up and told her he had found a woman's clothes and jewelry strewn next to his pool.

"Who'd I end up with?" Armstrong asked.

Betsy jumped to conclusions. "You have to be kidding me. You have a pregnant wife at home [in the United States]! How could you?"

In a lather, she called Kevin Livingston's wife, Becky, who said she was the one who had left her clothes and jewelry at Armstrong's pool after changing into her bathing suit. She said nothing had happened between them. Still, Andreu decided Armstrong had "no moral compass."

For years, she told only family and friends about Armstrong's doping confession in the hospital room, but never went public with it because the cycling family protected its own. Frankie didn't have a college degree and needed to work in cycling because he felt, like Hincapie and many others, that it was his only way to make a living. So Betsy kept her counsel, believing Armstrong's confession "exposes cycling to a certain extent. It was a secret we all had to keep quiet about."

Armstrong was confident that she would keep his secret. On one training ride the year after the Andreus overheard his doping confession in the Indianapolis hospital, he asked Frankie about Betsy's reaction to it.

"Did she say anything about it?"

"She freaked out a little bit, and, you know, we got into a couple of arguments. But then it kind of went away."

"Good, good, we don't want anyone asking too many questions."

Armstrong rode on, unconcerned and comfortable with his buddy's assurance that it kind of went away.

On the final ride in the 1999 Tour de France, Armstrong and his Postal Service team led the *peloton* into Paris, a red, white and blue blur as they whooshed to the finish line in the fastest time ever recorded—better than 25 miles an hour. En route to completing the 2,404-mile odyssey, they posed for photos and drank champagne. After three weeks of eating right, Armstrong ravenously licked an ice cream cone.

The streets were lined with nearly 500,000 fans, including a bigger-than-ever contingent from the United States. Armstrong rode imperiously beneath American and Texas flags as he became only the second American—Greg LeMond was the first—to win cycling's crown jewel.

Standing atop the podium, with the Arc de Triomphe as a backdrop, Armstrong listened to the "Star-Spangled Banner" play as he held his right hand over his heart. His pregnant wife stood to the side, and he stepped over to her for a moment to wipe tears from her eyes. He said, "I'm in shock, I'm in shock, I'm in shock."

He said he hoped his victory inspired those fighting cancer: "We can return to what we were before—and even better." Then he gave credit to those who helped him achieve a previously unthinkable goal.

"Fifty percent of this is for the cancer community—the doctors, the nurses, patients, their families, the survivors and those unfortunate ones who haven't made it," he said. "Twenty-five percent was for myself, my team. And the other twenty-five percent was for the people who did not believe in me."

George W. Bush, then Texas governor, called Armstrong's cell phone and said, "We're so proud of you. It's unbelievable."

Kirk Watson, the mayor of Austin and a testicular cancer survivor, was in the process of arranging a parade and a festival back home in Armstrong's honor.

Armstrong's oncologists boasted. Dr. Einhorn, one of his doctors in Indianapolis, said, "If Hollywood makes a movie of this, most people will leave the theater shaking their head with incredulity. Even the name, 'Lance Armstrong,' it just sounds too good to be true."

Armstrong's march to victory immediately ignited the sport's popularity in the United States—TV ratings for the Tour's final day had jumped by 80 percent over the prior year. Viewers got their first glimpse of Armstrong as a Nike spokesman as he starred in one of the company's "Just Do It" commercials. The company cast him as the first dead man to ride the Tour: "According to the latest cancer survival rates, Lance Armstrong is neither alive nor is he racing in the Tour de France."

One Chicago sports columnist, Bernie Lincicome, said fans should not feel guilty about cheering for Armstrong in the wake of the drug insinuations, which he called "petty slander" created by jealous journalists. Followers should believe that Armstrong is an inspiration and an honest athlete, he said in his column.

"I mean, a guy beats cancer and the Alps," he said. "Did they give Hannibal a drug test?" He continued, "We have every right to feel good about it, about him and his place at the top of the American summer."

An army of people rallied to Armstrong's side because of his victory. Fans who had considered bike racing an exotic, niche sport and who never even knew there was a big race in France every summer—much less nearly every summer for the past ninety-six years—bought bikes and looked to Armstrong for motivation. Trek promised its dealers a signature Armstrong bike by Christmas. One shop owner in suburban Dallas said she couldn't keep Postal Service jerseys on the shelves because they were selling so fast, at $70 each.

Armstrong would soon be on the cover of not one, but two Wheaties boxes, and General Mills said those boxes outsold others by about 10 percent, meaning millions of dollars in extra sales. The Postal Service said it won "millions and millions" of dollars of business from its rivals because of its relationship with Armstrong.

Some marketing experts, like David Carter and Rick Burton, told *USA Today* that Armstrong could be as big an American sports star as Michael Jordan and Tiger Woods.

Carter called Armstrong an "all-American, Norman Rockwell-like embodiment of what people want their heroes to be." Burton said, "He's the kind of guy you want your son to become—or your daughter to marry."

Armstrong, in turn, was about to become very rich as the new American sports hero. His agent, Bill Stapleton, had already negotiated a book deal with $400,000 in guaranteed money for Armstrong, and two movie deals were in the works. Stapleton said Armstrong had signed close to $1 million worth of new sponsorship deals before the Tour was even over. "And we haven't even started hearing from the soft drink and fast-food companies," he said.

Bristol-Myers Squibb, the company that manufactured Armstrong's chemotherapy drugs, had signed him to a $250,000 endorsement contract. The Postal Service boosted his salary to $2 million. His public speaking fee increased from $30,000 to $70,000, plus first-class expenses for two.

He would go on to write a best-selling autobiography, *It's Not About the Bike*, in which he told his story of surviving cancer and winning the Tour against all odds. Of performance-enhancing drug use, he said in the book, "Doping is an unfortunate fact of life in cycling, or any other endurance sport for that matter. Inevitably, some teams and riders feel it's like nuclear weapons—that they have to do it to stay competitive within the *peloton*. I never felt that way, and certainly after chemo the idea of putting anything foreign in my body was especially repulsive."

The book launched him into another stratosphere altogether when it came to marketing. For the year 2000, he would make $5 million in endorsements, plus a $2 million salary, which put him on the level of top NFL football players—those athletes once revered by his classmates back in Texas.

In the days after the 1999 Tour, Armstrong flew on Nike's jet to New York City, where he hit all the morning and talk shows, including *The Late Show with David Letterman*, during which Letterman called the European press "idiots" and said their doping accusations were "just crap." Armstrong's next stops included the White House, where he presented President Bill Clinton with a bike.

Armstrong and Stapleton were right: Armstrong's cancer was

the best thing to ever happen to him, marketing-wise. He was turning down offers of endorsement deals that were for less than $1 million. Armstrong said he was now "a business entity, instead of a person."

But on that final day of the Tour, Armstrong had a moment to savor his triumph, and all that it would mean to him. After stepping off the podium, he grabbed a giant American flag and rested its pole against his shoulder as he and his teammates climbed onto their bikes. A team Armstrong had dubbed "The Bad News Bears" rode up the Champs-Élysées for the honorary lap around the Arc de Triomphe. Seven of the nine riders were American, and the team had done what it needed to do to succeed in an unscrupulous sport.

During the ride, a French journalist pulled beside Armstrong on a motorcycle and asked him what he thought of his achievement.

"If you ever get a second chance in life," Armstrong said, "go all the way!"

I n preparation for the 2000 tour, Armstrong, Hamilton and Livingston flew by private jet from Nice to Valencia, Spain. Three weeks later, Armstrong would try to win his second straight Tour. But one important task had to be completed first, according to Hamilton.

There in Valencia, in a deserted luxury beach hotel, Bruyneel and Martí allegedly watched as del Moral slid wide-gauge needles into the veins of these three Postal Service stars. In just fifteen or twenty minutes, 500 ccs of blood from each rider had flowed through tiny tubes into plastic IV bags atop a white towel on the floor. The blood bags were then stored in a blue cooler.

The next month, two days before the Tour's hellish Mont Ventoux climb, those blood bags reemerged just when many of the riders needed them most. As those riders lay on beds in a spacious suite at the Postal Service team's hotel, the blood bags were affixed to the wall above them with athletic tape. Out came the wide-gauge needles and IV tubing. The teammates shivered as the chilled blood dripped into their veins.

Riders had heard that the Tour might be using a newly developed test for EPO, so the Postal Service team fell back on the old-school technique of blood transfusions. No test could determine whether riders had transfused their own blood. The UCI still measured each rider's hematocrit level to ensure it was below 50 percent, but now the riders were raising their hematocrit with transfusions instead of with a drug.

The process was "Frankenstein-ish," Hamilton said later, "something for Iron Curtain Olympic androids in the '80s." He also thought it smacked of "a junior-high science experiment."

By the time the riders put the blood from those bags back into themselves at the 2000 Tour, Armstrong was already wearing the leader's yellow jersey. He had made his move on Stage 10, going from 16th place to first, gaining an improbable ten minutes on his competition. Hamilton, Livingston and Russian teammate Viatcheslav Ekimov had ushered Armstrong to the final climb of the stage. With about eight miles to go, Armstrong took off on his own, ascending with such speed that rivals called his efforts "otherworldly," as if his bike had a hidden motor.

Armstrong extended his overall lead with a swift climb up Mont Ventoux. He bolted up the mountain to finish inches behind the stage winner, Marco Pantani, a skinny, compact Italian, one of the era's best climbers. In the media room, reporters gasped.

Aside from some French fans yelling, "Doper! Doper!" as he pedaled past them, Armstrong won the 2000 Tour without being thwarted by controversy.

Only later that year did he learn he was in trouble again.

Hugues Huet, a journalist from the state-sponsored television station France 3, had followed an unmarked Postal Service team car for more than a hundred miles. At one stop, two team staff members had tossed trash bags into a Dumpster. Huet filmed them doing it, then later looked inside the bags and found used syringes, bloody gauze and empty boxes of medical products, including

Actovegin. The drug wasn't a banned doping product, but anti-doping experts said the calf's blood derivative could improve the performance-enhancing effects of blood transfusions or EPO.

The footage of the team staffers throwing out that trash would make it into a France 3 documentary. But even before that film appeared, the Paris prosecutor's office opened an inquiry into whether Armstrong's Postal Service team had broken antidoping laws in France.

Armstrong and his team acted surprised by the investigation. Dan Osipow, a Postal Service spokesman, said the squad had a zero-tolerance policy regarding doping. Armstrong was so upset that he threatened to boycott the 2001 Tour and not defend his back-to-back titles.

"The substances on people's minds—Activ-o-something is new to me," Armstrong said. "Before this ordeal, I had never heard of it, nor had my teammates."

He said he was innocent, his team was clean, no one on his team had tested positive. Later, he said the doping charge could have been devastating for his reputation and his family if it had stuck.

"Everything I had worked so hard for, my reputation, what I'd done as an athlete, everything I had could go away, all the things you lose when people don't think you're a good guy," he wrote in one of his books.

Eventually, Armstrong accepted that the team had kept Actovegin so the team doctor could treat road rash. Then he claimed the drug was for a staff member who was diabetic. Gorski insisted that none of the team's nine riders had taken it.

Vaughters was at home in Denver during the off-season when he heard about the French criminal investigation. Out of curiosity, he researched the drug on the Internet and surmised that it was the same one del Moral had injected him with at the 1999 Tour. *Extract of calf's blood?* He felt like vomiting.

His first wife, Alisa, came home to find her husband balled up on the floor in the foyer, clutching his knees and crying.

"I didn't know what it was," he said. "They wouldn't tell me." He spat out the words as he sobbed. "And now, what if I have mad cow disease? What have I done? What have I done?"

Alisa Vaughters had heard her husband cry only once before, and that was after he had cheated with EPO to set the course record on Mont Ventoux in the Dauphiné. But mad cow disease? People had died of it in France. She worried about her husband, the father of their infant boy, Charlie.

Unlike Betsy Andreu, who was duped by her husband during that 1999 Tour when he had used EPO to help Armstrong win, Alisa Vaughters knew her husband had been doping. She was shocked by the suggestion that any of the wives or girlfriends didn't—they had to know if their men were using EPO. Her husband kept EPO in the refrigerator, same as Armstrong. "You'd have to be pretty dumb not to know," Alisa said.

When Alisa had met Jonathan, he had been open about his drug use and seemed educated about the possible side effects. Later, he told her that some wives helped their husbands dope, but—to her relief—he said he didn't want her to do that.

She wasn't like Kristin Armstrong, who allegedly casually referred to EPO as "butter" and supposedly handed out cortisone to riders at the 1998 worlds like bottles of Gatorade. And she wasn't like Haven Hamilton, who many on the Postal team noticed seemed ultra-involved with her husband's career and just as invested as he was in his success. As Tyler Hamilton trained for hours every day on the roads of Spain, his wife often drove a pace car. (Tyler would later allege that Haven was "a team player," at times ensuring that his blood stayed cool in their refrigerator, where they stored it in a soy milk container.) No, Alisa Vaughters was a flight attendant, rarely available for such training support and not interested in it anyway.

The first time she spoke about doping with another wife was in 2002, at a bachelorette party for Christian Vande Velde's soon-to-be-wife, Leah, who fought constantly with Christian about the presence of needles in their house. (Vande Velde had become a client of Ferrari's in late 2000.) He hid the injections from her by taking them in the bathroom with the door closed, but she'd find stray evidence anyway and blow up. She worried about drug use affecting his ability to have children. Finally, at her bachelorette party in Boulder, Colorado, Leah turned to Alisa with tears in her eyes.

Above the heavy beat of the dance-floor music, and after several drinks had lowered inhibitions, Leah shouted, "It's just so hard! All the needles! It's just so hard!"

Alisa yelled back, "I know!" They hugged. Both cried. They felt relieved that they could finally commiserate with another wife about the doping. Both felt helplessly entangled in the sport's lies.

Like Mafia wives who enjoy the spoils of the business but never discuss their husbands' dirty work, the two women had never before even broached the subject of doping. Like other riders' wives, they would gather for lunches in Girona or meet for coffee. They would spend hours together, weeks together, turning to each other for support in a foreign country when their husbands were on five-hour training rides or at weeklong races. While their husbands spoke freely among themselves about their doping regimens, wives like Leah and Alisa remained awkwardly silent.

Once the bachelorette party was over, the two friends went

back to their old ways. They never mentioned the subject of doping again.

It seemed implausible to Betsy Andreu that Armstrong could use drugs after nearly dying of cancer. She couldn't understand how Armstrong's wife, Kristin, and other wives apparently accepted their husbands' doping regimes. She would confide in Angela Julich, the wife of Bobby Julich, an American rider who had competed with Armstrong on the junior national team and had finished third in the 1998 Tour. When she told Angela about Armstrong's confession in the hospital room, Julich replied, "I'm not surprised."

The two hated the doping, but could prove nothing. They did know, however, that Armstrong, Hamilton, Livingston and Axel Merckx were clients of Ferrari, then under investigation in Italy. Betsy Andreu considered that connection to be evidence enough for what was going on with the Postal Service team.

"If your husband comes out of a hotel room wearing only his underwear and there's another woman inside the room in bed, do you need more proof to know that he's cheating on you?" she said. "I'm not stupid, you know."

She asked Haven Hamilton about doping and heard Tyler's wife say, "I don't want to hear about it." Andreu dreaded bringing it up with Livingston's wife, Becky, because Becky seemed too naive. The way she talked about Ferrari made it seem as if she really thought her husband would drive all the way to the doctor's office in Bologna, Italy, to get stretched out or massaged. When Andreu told her that she once overheard Armstrong admit his drug use, Becky Livingston grew sheepish. "Wow," she said in almost a whisper. "Wow."

But Andreu was most annoyed by Kristin Armstrong, partly

for her Gucci-wearing, Louis Vuitton–toting, condescending snobbery, but mostly because she appeared to so casually accept the doping. "It was kind of like a necessary evil," Kristin Armstrong apparently told her when Andreu asked her about EPO.

Just the thought of EPO made Andreu upset. In early 1999, she recalled, she was at dinner in Nice with the Armstrongs and Livingstons when Pepe Martí, the supposed trainer/drug courier, arrived late. She claimed that Martí supposedly had driven from Spain, crossing the border at night, to deliver EPO to Armstrong. As Armstrong allegedly took the drug from Martí, he apparently said, "Liquid gold!"

Weeks later, Betsy and Frankie Andreu drove to the Milan–San Remo race with the Armstrongs. They made an unusual pit stop in a parking lot of an Agip gas station just off the highway, on the outskirts of Milan, so Armstrong could meet Ferrari in a camper van parked in the lot.

Betsy asked Armstrong, "Why are we stopping here? Isn't it weird that you're seeing a doctor in a parking lot?"

"It's so the fucking press doesn't hound him," Lance said, referring to reporters who wanted to ask Ferrari about his involvement in doping riders.

Waiting for Armstrong that day, Betsy Andreu said, felt like she had fallen into a spy movie. An hour or so later, Armstrong bounded out of the doctor's camper, saying, "My numbers are great!" Back on the highway, Armstrong told Frankie Andreu he would get better results himself if he weren't too cheap to use Ferrari.

Frankie had told Betsy, "Sure I don't want to spend the money, but I don't want that shit in my body." He told her about Ferrari's fee, 10 to 20 percent of a rider's salary, way too much for him.

Armstrong had also been pressuring him to "get serious" about his training, which he took to mean he should use EPO regularly.

With all that in mind, Betsy Andreu had shown up at the very end of the 1999 Tour de France on a mission to find out what drugs her husband had taken to climb so fast during the mountain stages. Their first time alone was the night of the Postal team's lavish post-Tour celebration party, held on the banks of Paris's Seine River, inside the Musée d'Orsay. She wanted to talk about the doping. He didn't. He begged her to shake Armstrong's hand and congratulate him on the victory. She wouldn't.

"I want to know what in the hell you did," she said. "Why did you climb the way you did? There's no way that Lance won this thing clean."

"Please go shake his hand, Betsy, please."

"No."

"Please, for me?"

"No. Get it through your head—I'm not doing it."

It took a trip back to their home in Nice to finally get Frankie talking about his drug use. Betsy found a thermos and a thermometer in their refrigerator, telltale signs her husband had been using EPO.

"You don't understand—I can't even keep up if I don't use EPO," he said. "The speeds are so fast that I wouldn't even make the time cut."

"You can't tell me that everybody is doing something, Frankie. You know that's not true. But I don't care what other people are doing. If you need to use EPO to stay on Postal, then I want you off of Lance's team. Get off the team, Frankie; we don't need to deal with this shit."

Frankie Andreu remained on the team for the 2000 season,

but told me he didn't participate in the team's new blood doping scheme. He said he rode the Tour clean. His contract was not renewed. He would never again compete in the sport.

For Postal Service's top riders—Armstrong, Hamilton and Livingston—duplicity and secrecy were part of the game they played with the public. What began as an innocent love of riding bicycles became a life of code words, clandestine meetings and furtive conversations. They received their drug cocktails in white paper bags, like packed lunches, and each had a secret, presumably untraceable cell phone, which they used to discuss their doping and plans to avoid drug testers. To avoid being heard talking about doping, they often referred to EPO as "Edgar Allan Poe," or just "Poe." They flew to races on Armstrong's private plane, to avoid nosy airport security agents.

Once, on a training ride in Girona, Vaughters heard Armstrong say into his cell phone, "I had an ice cream with sprinkles."

"Who was that?" Vaughters asked.

"None of your business," came the reply.

To Vaughters, exchanges like that made it evident that Armstrong enjoyed "the cloak and dagger" part of doping. It was just another way of competing.

Blood transfusions put the Postal team far ahead of the other cheaters in the *peloton*. Those teams didn't have Postal Service's money. Armstrong's team also had Motoman—Armstrong's motorcycle-riding personal assistant—transporting their chilled blood into France and to the riders' hotels when they needed their transfusions. Bruyneel was allegedly in charge of the whole plan, Hamilton claims, with del Moral watching over the medical process and Ferrari in charge of the top riders.

"The systemization of it gave them the edge," according to Vaughters. "While other teams maybe had one or two guys doping like that, nobody but Postal had every top guy on a sophisticated plan."

The riders paying for Ferrari's private services often used testosterone patches. He told them the drug would be detectable for only a very short time after the patch was removed from the skin. Ferrari also had advised them that using EPO was OK, even in 2001, when the UCI first started testing for it. They could inject a smaller amount of the drug into their veins instead of subcutaneously, so it would clear their systems faster. They could use that small amount more often, too, a process called microdosing. Even when they used blood transfusions to cheat, they still needed to use EPO to mask the effects of the transfusions.

Blood transfusions would flood the body with red blood cells, blocking its need to produce immature cells called reticulocytes. EPO then would stimulate the production of those reticulocytes, a value that drug testers examined closely for signs of doping. So by using transfusions coupled with EPO, riders could fool drug testers with blood test results that looked normal.

Not that it was very difficult to beat the drug testers, anyway. At that time there was little if any out-of-competition testing for professional cyclists, so they didn't have to worry much about surprise drug tests.

The United States Anti-Doping Agency, a quasi-governmental agency formed to handle antidoping in Olympic sports in the United States, was in its infancy, created as an independent agency only in October 2000. Until then, USA Cycling and the UCI were in charge of the drug testing, but it seems those entities couldn't be trusted. They had an interest in making it look like their sport was clean.

In 2001, Armstrong was tested by USADA twice. Hincapie was tested three times, Hamilton once, Livingston not at all. For the next two years, USADA tested Armstrong once a year, though he was tested by other entities during the Tour.

The UCI didn't perform many out-of-competition drug tests until the mid-2000s. That lag in testing made it easier for riders to dope in previous years because most drug use was done in preparation for a race. Doping before the competition would allow them to train harder and recover faster.

Back then, it wasn't hard to avoid testing positive even when riders were tested in competition. They weren't properly chaperoned before the drug test and were given way too much time to possibly manipulate their urine so it wouldn't produce a positive sample (by drinking tons of water, or even using a hidden catheter filled with clean urine at the moment of collection).

When drug testers showed up at the team hotel during a race, or at someone's house, Armstrong and his teammates seemed to know they were coming. In 2000, at a race in Spain, Hincapie—the loyal sidekick—saved Armstrong from testing positive by warning him that the drug testers were in the hotel's lobby. Armstrong had just taken testosterone oil, and so he dropped out of the race to avoid testing. Other times, it was as if Bruyneel knew the testers' schedules, as if someone had tipped him off.

At the Hamilton household, when testers came knocking, Haven Hamilton allegedly knew enough to ask her husband, "You're good?" If he had taken drugs recently—if he was still "glowing," as he called it—they supposedly huddled on the floor until the testers left.

During races, the winner is usually tested along with three random riders. Postal Service never had anyone test positive—at least officially. According to Hamilton, Armstrong allegedly tested positive at the 2001 Tour de Suisse.

"You won't fucking believe this," Armstrong supposedly had told him. "I got popped for EPO."

Hamilton claims that Armstrong wasn't worried about the positive test because "his people had been in touch with the UCI, they were going to have a meeting and everything was going to be OK." Armstrong allegedly also told Floyd Landis, a rider who would join the team in late 2001, that "he and Mr. Bruyneel flew to the UCI headquarters and made a financial agreement to keep the positive test hidden." Verbruggen, the UCI president at the time, later said that neither he nor the UCI was ever complicit in a cover-up. "You will never, ever find any cover-up in the UCI while I was president, and I'm sure afterwards neither," he told Ben Rumsby of the *Telegraph* in London.

Armstrong bragged to those teammates that he had so much power in the sport that even a positive test couldn't stop him. The funny thing is that his EPO test result was never an official positive, according to several people who worked on the case.

The EPO test was so new that Martial Saugy, the director of the antidoping laboratory that analyzed the 2001 Tour de Suisse urine samples for the drug, did not deem Armstrong's urine positive because the threshold to flag a sample as positive was so high. Instead, he labeled Armstrong's samples as suspicious for EPO. About a year later, another antidoping lab director, Jacques de Ceurriz, also tagged Armstrong's urine sample as suspicious. That time, the sample came from the Dauphiné, and UCI was notified about it.

The lab directors Saugy and de Ceurriz did not realize they were dealing with Armstrong's urine sample until much later because they had been working with anonymous samples. But the

UCI officials were able to match the sample number with Armstrong's name. They quickly called Armstrong to notify him that he had come perilously close to testing positive. It was a slap on the wrist that said Armstrong should be careful about being so sloppy.

Armstrong was in disbelief. He also didn't understand how his test result could be considered questionable, and considered the test unreliable. So he set out to learn how the new EPO test worked, and asked the UCI for help. It arranged a tutorial.

The UCI set up a meeting that was held at the start of the 2002 Tour, with Armstrong, Bruyneel, and Saugy, so that Saugy could explain the science behind the EPO test. Though the meeting was unconventional—USADA later bristled that Saugy had given Armstrong "the keys" to beating the EPO test—Saugy thought he was proving to the *patron* of the *peloton* that the method of screening for EPO was valid. His hope was that Armstrong, in turn, could warn other riders to stop using the drug. After all, the literature concerning the test was already publicly available. Saugy also was told by the UCI that Bruyneel had a scientific background and had a lot of questions for him. So Saugy explained to Armstrong and Bruyneel that the EPO test entailed scientists putting the urine sample on a thin layer of gel, running electricity through it and waiting for different forms of proteins in the urine to spread out. When those proteins finally did, they left a ladder-shaped pattern that the scientist had to interpret as positive or negative for the synthetic version of EPO. Because the test required interpretation, that left a big gray area that riders could possibly use to their advantage.

Armstrong and Bruyneel listened to Saugy like schoolkids in a classroom, but said nothing. At the end of the presentation, only Armstrong spoke. He crossed his arms and gave Saugy a menacing look. His eyes narrowed.

"Do you realize that you are putting so many careers under pressure?" he said.

Then he stomped out of the room.

According to two antidoping scientists who are not officially authorized to talk about the case because they didn't work on it, if Armstrong's urine sample from that 2001 Tour de Suisse had been examined under 2013 standards, Armstrong would have failed the test.

Heading into the 2001 Tour, the *Sunday Times* of London published a story by David Walsh that claimed Armstrong had spearheaded the use of EPO on his Motorola team in 1995. Walsh was an award-winning writer who had long doubted Armstrong's claims of innocence and was one of the few English-speaking reporters who put those doubts in print. Now he had gathered circumstantial evidence suggesting he had been right to doubt.

Walsh's story said Armstrong was a Ferrari client. It also quoted an unnamed Armstrong teammate saying that several Motorola riders discussed the use of EPO and that "Lance was the key spokesperson when EPO was the topic." (Years later it was revealed that the New Zealander Stephen Swart had been Walsh's source.)

Armstrong was livid. As usual, he fought back. His agent, Bill Stapleton—who would later earn a reputation for threatening reporters with lawsuits after they wrote critical stories about Armstrong—had heard about Walsh's story even before it was published and executed a preemptive strike by arranging for a reporter from the Italian newspaper *La Gazzetta dello Sport* to interview Armstrong. In the interview, Armstrong said he had worked with Ferrari for six years in preparation for a special feat he had wanted to accomplish: a world's record for the most miles a rider could log in an hour while riding on a velodrome.

His teammates thought that was hilarious and ridiculous. They had never heard anything about Armstrong's project, and joked that he probably never even rode on a velodrome.

At the 2001 Tour, after Walsh's story was published, Armstrong considered refuting Walsh's accusations to a small group of trusted journalists. He asked for a meeting with those reporters, but canceled twenty minutes later and sent a statement instead.

In it, he admitted seeing Ferrari and wrote that the doctor "has had a questionable public reputation, due to the irresponsible comments he made in 1994 regarding EPO" (when Ferrari said the drug was only as dangerous as drinking too much orange juice). "I have never denied my relationship with Michele Ferrari. On the other hand, I've never gone out of my way to publicize it." He also said, "He has never discussed EPO with me and I have never used it."

Armstrong said Ferrari only gave him tips "on dieting, altitude preparation" and only used natural methods of improvement, like tweaking his form on the bike.

Despite Armstrong's denials, Walsh's story spread through the sports pages, mostly in Europe, and jump-started the Armstrong PR machine. Stapleton was a big part of the effort. To defend his client, Stapleton also defended Ferrari. He told the *New York Times* that Ferrari "knows physiology, and when he discusses gearing, Lance listens."

"Dr. Ferrari is not a witch doctor," Stapleton said.

Nearly every day at the 2001 Tour, Armstrong was forced to defend his relationship with Ferrari. He told journalists he was "proud" to work with him "on a limited basis" and would rethink using the doctor if a criminal investigation in Italy that focused on Ferrari uncovered any wrongdoing.

"People are not stupid," he said about a week before the Tour finish. "They will look at the facts. They will say: Here's Lance Armstrong. Here's a relationship. Is it questionable? Perhaps. But people are smart. They will say: Has Lance Armstrong ever tested positive? No. Has Lance Armstrong ever been tested? A lot."

He and Stapleton were not alone in their fight. While Armstrong parried with journalists in France, Nike, one of his primary sponsors, took his case to the American people—to those who believed what they saw in television commercials, anyway. The company aired a new TV spot featuring Armstrong.

Armstrong looked into the camera and said, "This is my body. And I can do whatever I want to it. I can push it, study it, tweak it, listen to it. Everybody wants to know what I'm on. What am I on? I'm on my bike, busting my ass six hours a day. What are you on?"

Walsh had a hunch what he was on. And it certainly wasn't only his bike. It was drugs. He just needed solid proof.

For a subsequent story Walsh wrote about the Armstrong-Ferrari connection to kick off the 2001 Tour, Walsh spoke to Greg LeMond. After reading that Armstrong was working with Ferrari, LeMond said, he was devastated because he considered Armstrong to be both a great rider and an inspirational hero to cancer patients.

"If Lance is clean, it is the greatest comeback in the history of sport," he said. "If he isn't, it would be the greatest fraud."

In the last two years of his life, from spring 2000 to the fall of 2002, in hopes of writing a book, J.T. Neal recorded twenty-six hours of audiotape. The tapes re-create and comment on the most exciting times of his life, primarily the years the young Texan Lance Edward Armstrong rose from obscurity to superstardom.

Neal never finished the book. Long after his death, the tapes remained hidden in the bedroom closet of his son, Scott. Nobody in the family had listened to them, but I was given the tapes, along with permission to use Neal's words in this book. While in Austin, to transcribe the recordings, I met with Armstrong and asked him about his former best friend.

"J.T. Neal? Forget about that. Don't go chasing that shit," he told me.

He dismissed Neal's importance, saying Neal hadn't known anything about his doping because the drugs came after the two of them had grown apart. Little did he know that in a matter of just a few hours, I'd be sitting in the Neal household, headphones on, laptop at the ready, listening to the first tape that Neal had recorded. It brought his voice to life: "Today is the twelfth of April, and this is the beginning of my recollections on Lance Armstrong . . ."

In an attic above the carport at J.T. Neal's house—the former church on a hill over Austin—three large boxes and two suitcases sit covered with the dust of more than a decade. The boxes are filled with documents, press clippings and posters featuring Armstrong as a young rider under Neal's care. One of the suitcases, both marked with fading Motorola Cycling Team logos, belonged to Neal and the other to Armstrong, and contain not only old jerseys from the Tour de France, but ones with iron-on felt letters, from tiny local races that marked the beginning of Armstrong's career.

More and more, as Neal realized his death was imminent, Armstrong's behavior upset him. Neal had seen the "What Am I On?" Nike ad. He also had heard Armstrong's denials that he had hooked up with Ferrari and was doping. It was one thing for Armstrong to be a liar, but Neal thought he had gone beyond simply lying to living a life of deceit.

"When he said, 'I've never taken EPO,' he sits up there and denies that he's ever done it, I know he's lying," Neal said. "And I know that kids look up to him; they've always looked up to him."

He didn't like the way Armstrong treated the former Postal Service rider Kevin Livingston, either. Armstrong had basically dumped him from the Postal team in exchange for some Spanish climbers. Livingston was the friend who had been by Armstrong's side on the national team, then Motorola, and especially when Armstrong fought cancer. He was even there in the awkward moment when Armstrong had needed a ride to deposit his sperm in a sperm bank before his cancer treatments. He was there to slowly pedal beside Armstrong on rides when chemotherapy sapped him of his energy. Of all the good soldiers in Armstrong's army, Livingston was as good as they came.

He also had been there to dope with him. Both were Ferrari clients. Livingston, who in 2010 told me he had never doped, had followed Armstrong to the doctor's door. Unfortunately for Livingston, Ferrari wasn't meticulous about hiding the fact that Livingston had been his client. An Italian criminal investigation looking into Ferrari's alleged doping uncovered documents that suggested Livingston had used EPO and a powerful steroid. Those documents were made public.

About the same time Armstrong and Livingston parted ways, Armstrong also refused to help Frankie Andreu get a new deal with Postal Service. He told Hamilton that both Livingston and Andreu wanted too much money and were "not gonna get shit."

Betsy Andreu was convinced that Armstrong got rid of her husband because he refused to join Ferrari's doping program. The way Neal saw it, Armstrong had made conscious decisions to turn his back on two of his most loyal teammates.

Neal thought Armstrong was isolating himself from people who cared about him personally and was associating only with those who could help him win a bike race, become richer, or both. He said the only friends Armstrong had left were "two-fold friends," like Carmichael the coach, Ochowicz the former team manager and Stapleton the agent—friends only because he made them money. "I feel like in the long run, it's going to be a disadvantage to Lance because he doesn't have any other friends. He's cast aside every friend he's ever had," Neal said. "Now all the people Armstrong has around him are yes-men and groupies, and if they don't agree with him, he gets rid of them . . . It's a sad state for him, because once all those go by, he's not going to have anybody. He will be alone with his millions."

In the months after Armstrong's first Tour win, in 1999, Carmichael founded Carmichael Training Systems—a Web-based coaching business with the promotional tag: "Lance Armstrong calls him coach. Now you can, too"—and wrote books based on his affiliation with the Tour de France champion. The first, *The Lance Armstrong Performance Program: 7 Weeks to the Perfect Ride*, was published in the fall of 2000 and became an immediate best seller.

The business started out of Carmichael's home in Colorado Springs. In less than two years, by mid-2001, it had forty coaches, five hundred paying clients and revenues that had jumped 100 percent per year. By July 2002, the company had fifty employees, seventy-five coaches and a thousand subscribers. Like Armstrong, Carmichael had become a sought-after commodity. In newspaper and magazine reports, he described the miracle training program that had turned Armstrong into a Tour winner.

He said he woke up one night and it hit him: Armstrong had been burning out his anaerobic energy system. The same physiological system that helped Armstrong win big one-day races was preventing him from winning three-week races. Carmichael said he had devised an idea that would mold Armstrong into a possible Tour contender. Armstrong would no longer ride in a big gear, but would pedal faster, at 85 to 95 revolutions per minute, to train his body to utilize more of his aerobic capacity and spare his anaerobic energy. His training would entail intervals of brief spurts of power. It was what Carmichael said was one of the keys to Armstrong's success: He pedaled faster than everyone else!

Neal considered it amazing that it took until 2001 for the public to divine that Carmichael might not be the force behind Armstrong. After all, Armstrong's first trip to see Ferrari was way back in 1995, when Neal had accompanied him. Maybe the cash payments had hidden their association, or maybe it was the fact that both Ferrari and Armstrong had taken such care in keeping their relationship a secret.

In November or December 1999, Ferrari visited Austin. He stayed at a home Armstrong owned outside of town. Neal assumed that many people in Armstrong's entourage knew what was going on. Even Armstrong's mother was tangentially involved. One wire transfer, dated July 24, 1996—back when she was in charge of paying her son's bills—came from a bank account that appeared to have both her and her son's name on it. The transfer showed that $42,082.33 had moved from their account to Ferrari's.

It is unclear whether Linda Armstrong—who went by Linda Walling then—knew that Ferrari was doping her son. On his audiotapes, Neal said he and Linda had "a laugh" about Chris Carmichael's pretending that he contributed to Armstrong's 1999 victory, suggesting that Armstrong's mother knew that Carmichael was just a cover for Ferrari. What is clear about that time in Armstrong's life, though, is that his relationship with his mother was on a downhill trajectory. Once he married Kristin in 1998, it took a sharp dive.

"You know how that goes," Armstrong told me, suggesting that his relationship with his mother had soured because of the tension brought on by the stereotypically tumultuous mother/daughter-in-law relationship. He said his mother felt that Kristin and her family looked at her as white trash, and that Kristin didn't like his mother constantly doting on him. Making the situation even worse was that his mother's third marriage was failing: She filed for divorce from John Walling in November 1998.

Neal, one of Linda Armstrong's closest friends, grew increasingly angry. She had told him that she had been supporting herself and Walling for two or three years by working at what she called "a corner office" global accounts manager job at the communications company Ericsson, and by selling real estate.

After her marriage broke up, she told Neal that she had to sell the house she and Walling had lived in. She moved into a rented duplex in Plano. Most of her furniture was in storage because the new place was too small to hold it. A month after her divorce was final, Armstrong won his first Tour.

In 1999, her company paid her airfare to the Tour de France, and Ochowicz put her up in a hotel so she could cheer on her son. She hardly spent any time with Lance after his victory. And even when she and Neal asked Armstrong for signed yellow jerseys, he wouldn't immediately comply. The rift between Armstrong's mother and Armstrong's wife had torn mother and son apart. Kristin Armstrong allegedly urged her husband to cut his mother off so that she wouldn't keep undermining their marriage. Armstrong felt obliged to do it to keep her happy.

In 1993, when Armstrong won the world championships, the son had demanded that his mother come along when he met the king of Norway, saying, "No one checks my mother at the door." In 1996, when he moved into his first house, he named it Casa Linda after her. Now he wouldn't even return her phone calls.

Neal finally asked Armstrong—pleaded with him—to give his mother some money, and tried to explain to him how important it was to take care of his own. Armstrong first told him that his accountant had advised against giving his mother any tax-free money, but Neal took that as a lie. He told Armstrong he should be ashamed that he wasn't helping his mother. "I stood up to him because his mother had nothing and he had millions," he said.

To his wife's dismay, Armstrong eventually listened to Neal and helped his mother to pay her divorce lawyer. But Neal was sure that Armstrong held his intervention against him and that he used it as an excuse to pull away from him.

Neal sensed that Armstrong didn't want to be told what to do anymore. He wanted the people around him to do what he wanted them to do. Some people in Austin who were close with both Armstrong and Neal said, however, that their relationship broke apart because Neal was not corporate enough for the rich venture capitalist guys Armstrong hung out with at Livestrong. Neal was the opposite of materialistic: Though he was wealthy, he often wore baggy, torn sweaters and khaki pants with holes in them.

Neal knew he was dying and might not have much time left. He was on and off steroids for his illness, and they made him irritable and loquacious, eager to let his real feelings be known. He had come to the point that he was tired of giving everything he had to Armstrong without Armstrong ever giving back. It was too late to cry about it now, but Neal regretted that he had spent so much time with him and, at times, neglected his own children in doing so.

Part of Neal was proud of what Armstrong had accomplished and was happy for him. It had felt so sweet for him and his wife, Frances, to hold Armstrong's son, Luke, shortly after he was born. The Neals felt like they had raised Armstrong and considered Luke to be family.

"If we had listened to the warning signs a little sooner, or if he hadn't had drugs, he probably wouldn't even have had the problems he has now," Neal said. "But he gave his soul to Dr. Ferrari for the money. It's a shame, because he could have gone on and not used drugs, not got everybody else on the program, and still would have been an excellent cyclist."

On September 24, 2001, Neal received an invitation in the mail to attend a party celebrating the fifth anniversary of Armstrong's cancer diagnosis, which he called his "Carpe Diem" day. That Latin phrase means "Seize the day," and Armstrong chose it because the diagnosis spurred him to overcome adversity and take charge of his life. A frail, ailing Neal subsequently had written Armstrong a note about the time in 1996 that they both learned they had cancer—Neal in the summer, Armstrong in the fall—a time in which he and Armstrong were inseparable. "It was only like yesterday when we had the first day of Carpe Diem." He never received a response.

Neal had bumped into Armstrong at a restaurant weeks before, when Neal was still recovering from a broken hip and a tumor that had forced him to endure more than a dozen radiation treatments. They hadn't seen each other in a while and Armstrong had seemed excited about reconnecting. He said they needed to get together, and they exchanged cell phone numbers. But it was hard for Neal to tell if the gesture was genuine. "He said he was going to call me, but I haven't heard back," Neal said at the time. "I'm sure he's really busy."

In his final days, Neal called Linda Armstrong. "Always have loved you and that boy of yours," he said. She told him that he had done a fine job at being her son's "surrogate mother" as he stood in for her when she lived three hours away. She wanted to know how he felt. Neal wouldn't say. He hated being asked that.

So, on October 1, 2002, even some people who had been close to him were surprised to hear that he likely would not make it to the next morning. Armstrong's mother had tried to call her son to tell him about Neal, whom she described as "one of the few people who really cared about him [Armstrong] without having anything to gain from it." The story from there differs, depending on who tells it.

Linda Armstrong said in her book that she called Armstrong at home once, but that the answering machine picked up. The next time she called, someone she didn't know answered the phone. She could hear a party in the background.

Her son had been celebrating the anniversary of his cancer diagnosis: It would be six years the next day, October 2. When she asked to talk to Lance, the person on the other line said, "He's out swinging on the rope with Ethel," his mother-in-law. Armstrong's mother told the person it was urgent and that Lance needed to call her immediately.

"Sure, no problem," the person said.

While Armstrong partied, Neal's family and close friends gathered at Neal's house to say good-bye. One of the athletes he had watched over drove straight from Dallas, more than two hundred miles away, doughnuts in hand. Another was out scouring stores for egg-crate foam to put on Neal's bed, so he would feel more comfortable. Another was trying to control her emotions, but was sobbing.

Two people who had been at Neal's bedside said Armstrong had reached out to Neal that night by calling his cell phone. The person who answered the call said he turned to Neal and said, "It's Lance." But Neal, still deeply hurt, waved it off. "I'm not taking it," he said.

Armstrong and Doug Ulman, chief executive of Armstrong's foundation, said they were together in a car en route to a

Livestrong function the next day when Armstrong got the call to say Neal had died that morning. Ulman said that was one of the two times he had ever seen Armstrong cry.

The *Austin American-Statesman* wrote a glowing obituary of Neal, with the headline, "Austin man was athletes' best friend." Neal, who was sixty, helped athletes "achieve health and greatness" without ever taking a penny for it, the story said. Josh Davis, a two-time Olympic swimmer, was quoted as saying, "J.T. was a great example of a true human being who was put on this earth not to take but to give."

Neal's funeral was held in a church on the grounds of the University of Texas. Kevin Livingston and other athletes Neal had helped were among the pallbearers. According to Armstrong's mother, Armstrong stood in the churchyard after the service and "looked shell-shocked and sorrowful."

Neal's family and others at the funeral had different recollections.

Armstrong and his wife had gone to the funeral straight from a photo shoot. He wore a T-shirt, a black leather blazer, jeans and flip-flops. She wore a white flowing shirt with eyelets.

He didn't look shell-shocked or sorrowful, they said. He seemed more dispassionate or irritated. When the service was over, he walked up to Neal's daughter Caroline. Her heart fell when she saw him dressed so casually, but she was too distraught to criticize him.

He told her, "I don't do funerals."

She stood there for a second, amazed at his attitude and holding back tears.

"Lance, what do you want me to say? This is not about you."

PART FOUR

LIES OF THE BROTHERHOOD

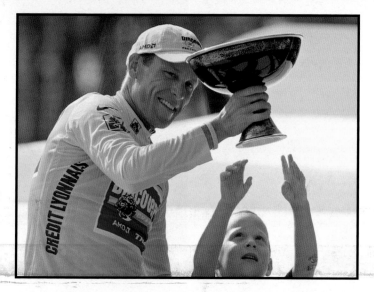

Lance Armstrong said he would never dope because it would reflect so poorly on his children, including his oldest son, Luke *(right)*, seen here reaching for his father's Tour de France trophy after Armstrong's record seventh victory.
(Peter Dejong/AP/Corbis)

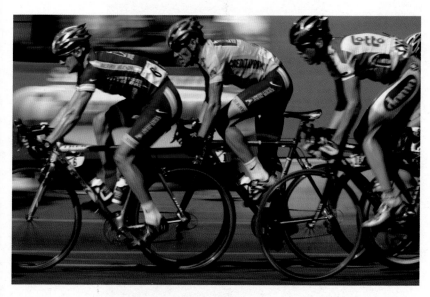

Floyd Landis *(left)* leads Lance Armstrong *(center)* down the Champs-Élysées in July 2004, as Armstrong won his sixth consecutive Tour de France.
(Andrew P. Scott)

His grandmother Willine Gunderson *(left)* and his father, Eddie *(right)*, lost touch with Armstrong when Lance's mother took him and moved away, breaking all contact.
(Courtesy of Micki Rawlings)

Terry Armstrong adopted Lance when he was a toddler and remained a forceful presence in his life until Lance was sixteen. *(Olan Mills)*

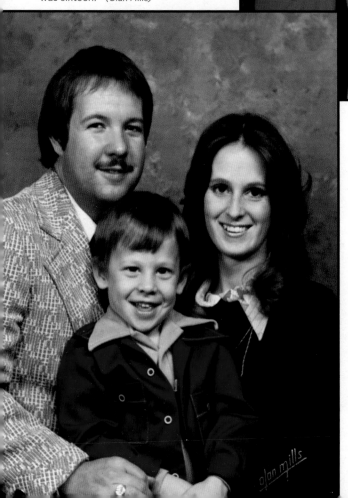

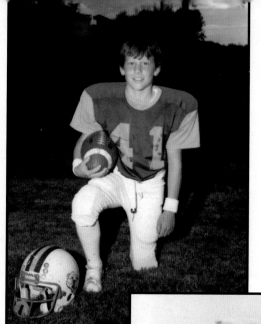

Terry Armstrong coached Lance's youth football teams and read fire-and-brimstone Vince Lombardi speeches to him at bedtime. *(Courtesy of Terry Armstrong)*

When it came to winning, both Terry and Lance could be ruthless. Terry would call Lance a loser if he didn't try hard enough in competitions. *(Courtesy of Terry Armstrong)*

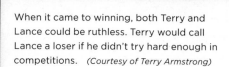

Linda Armstrong was a teen mom who practiced permissive parenting, at times acting more like a friend than a mother. *(Courtesy of J.T. Neal family)*

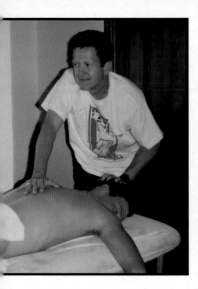

For more than a decade, J.T. Neal *(above)* was Lance's *soigneur*, lawyer, business manager, and father figure. *(Courtesy of J.T. Neal family)*

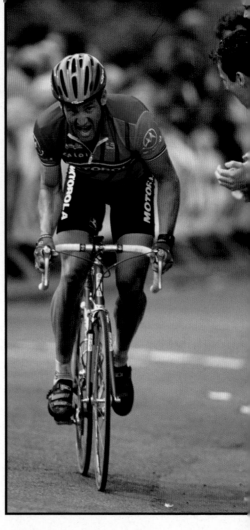

In 1996, one year after becoming a client of the Italian doctor Michele Ferrari, Armstrong became the first American to win the prestigious one-day Flèche Wallonne race. *(Joe Patronite)*

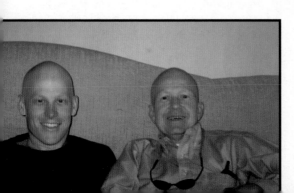

J.T. Neal and Lance Armstrong were diagnosed with cancer only months apart. Armstrong was the lucky one. Neal died in 2002. *(Courtesy of J.T. Neal family)*

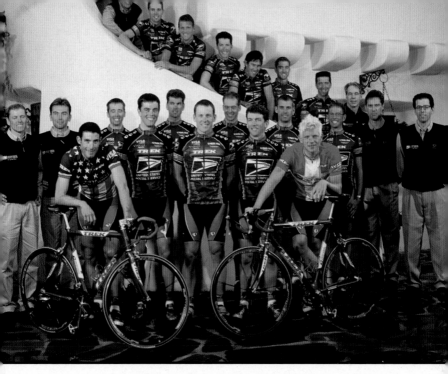

A year after Armstrong returned to cycling, the 1999 United States Postal Service team was built around him, and featured the top American riders of that era: Tyler Hamilton *(to Lance's right)*, Frankie Andreu *(second row, fourth from left)*, and George Hincapie *(front row, left, leaning on his bike)*. Owner Thomas Weisel is on the stairs, third from right. For years, the team would dominate the Tour, with an unsurpassed doping program. *(Joe Patronite)*

Betsy and Frankie Andreu, seen here cooking with Armstrong in Como, Italy, in 1995, were part of his inner circle Betsy would become one of Armstrong's fiercest enemies when she spoke out against his doping and bullying. *(Courtesy of Betsy Andreu)*

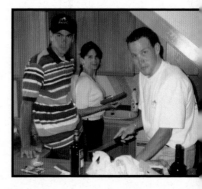

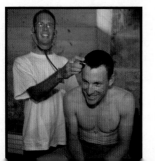

Jonathan Vaughters, an enigmatic Postal Service teammate, quit because he was sick of doping and convinced other riders to testify against Armstrong. *(Michel Spingler/Associated Press)*

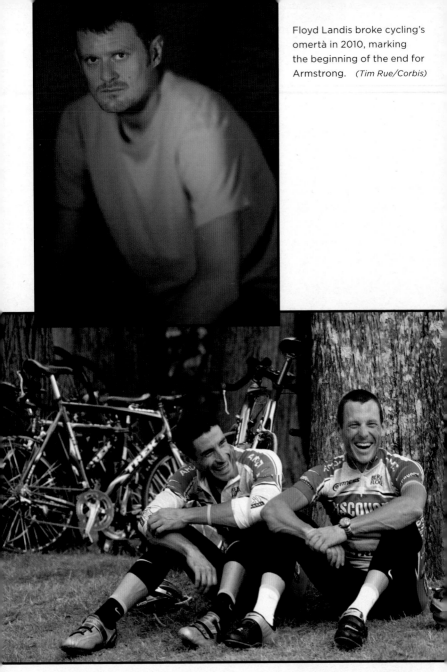

Floyd Landis broke cycling's omertà in 2010, marking the beginning of the end for Armstrong. *(Tim Rue/Corbis)*

George Hincapie was the only rider by Armstrong's side through seven of his Tour victories. His testimony sealed Armstrong's fate. *(Eric Gaillard/Reuters/Corbis)*

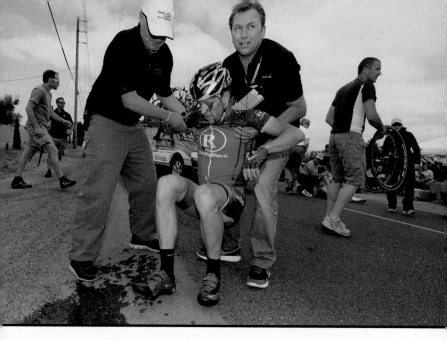

On the day Landis's allegations of Armstrong's doping were made public, Armstrong crashed out of the Tour of California. Team manager Johan Bruyneel *(right)* helped him to his feet. *(Tim De Waele/ TDWsport.com/Corbis)*

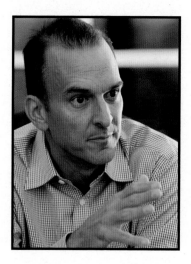

Travis Tygart, the chief executive of the United States Anti-Doping Agency, received several death threats when he brought a doping case against Armstrong. *(Ed Andrieski /AP/Corbis)*

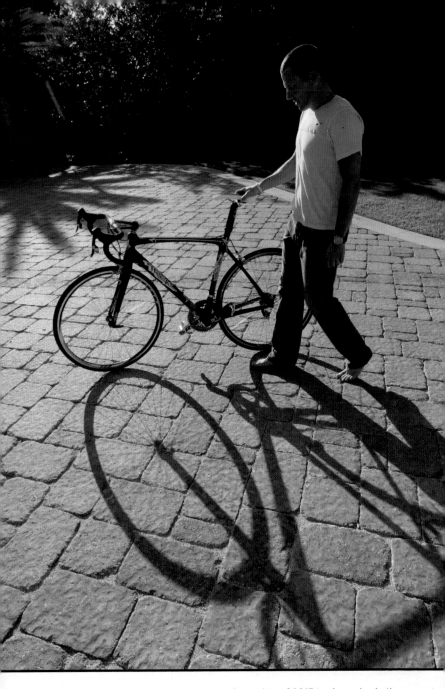

Armstrong sold his Texas dream house in the spring of 2013 to downsize in the shadow of several multimillion-dollar lawsuits. (*Erich Schlegel*)

CHAPTER 13

David Zabriskie wanted to get up from the table at the coffee shop in Girona, Spain. He wanted to push back his chair, stand tall and say, "No, thanks, drugs aren't for me," and walk away from Johan Bruyneel and Dr. Luís García del Moral. It was May 2003. Zabriskie was in his third year as a pro, and was the youngest member of the Postal Service team, a team he almost didn't make in the first place because Armstrong thought he was, like Vaughters, too weird. He imagined striding away from that café with the swagger of a Western-movie gunslinger. But he didn't move. He couldn't.

Instead, Zabriskie felt as if his hand were welded to the tiny espresso cup in front of him. He'd gone to the café with Postal Service teammate Michael Barry to pick up injectable vitamins—which the team called "recovery"—when, he claims, Bruyneel had handed him much more than that.

"We brought the recovery products for you, and some EPO," Bruyneel allegedly said, as casually as one might ask a fellow diner to pass the salt.

"Uh, what?" Zabriskie said. To buy time, he put questions to Bruyneel and the team doctor, del Moral.

"If I take this, will I be able to have kids?"

"Yes, you will, you can still have kids," Bruyneel said.

"Will they be retarded?" Zabriskie said.

"No, they will not."

"Um, will my ears grow bigger?"

"No, no they won't," Bruyneel said. "You know, you don't have to take it."

Zabriskie was a skeletal figure atop his bike, all elbows and kneecaps. Six-foot and maybe 150 pounds. His haircuts alternated between rock-star shaggy and jarhead buzz cut. He'd once nurtured a brawny mustache that would have been too much even for Wild Bill. Many of his teammates found him odd, and not just because he had one green eye and one blue. He believed in, or at least talked about, certain conspiracy theories, such as the one that had the U.S. government creating processed foods to kill off its own people. He worried that his cell phone was giving him brain cancer. A shy man among strangers, Zabriskie was comfortable enough on the team bus to sing aloud, crack jokes and talk about the world-saving lineup of superhero statues that decorated his house.

In 1998 Zabriskie, then an amateur, had been invited to Austin to ride with Armstrong and Livingston. He pedaled in their shadows while listening to Armstrong talk about his sexual exploits. Zabriskie was so intimidated that he didn't say a word, at first. He finally accelerated to ride alongside them and show that he was a Casanova, too. Listen to this: He once met a girl in a 7-Eleven, "and, oh yeah, I banged her." The story was a fabrication, Zabriskie's sophomoric way of trying to be one of the guys.

But it didn't sit well with Armstrong. Years later, when Bruyneel considered bringing Zabriskie onto the Postal Service team, Armstrong recalled Zabriskie's strange behavior that day. He told Bruyneel not to hire him. Zabriskie got the job only after several people connected to USA Cycling convinced Armstrong that Zabriskie wouldn't be a distraction.

Still, on that day in May 2003 at the Girona café, Zabriskie's innate awkwardness presented itself when, he claims, Bruyneel set down the package of EPO. Every top Postal Service rider had likely come to such a moment. With Zabriskie, though, it was different. He had never ridden for any other team and had no real knowledge of the drug culture. Of all the riders who went through Postal Service, none was more naive, none as trusting.

So he was rattled by what he claims was Bruyneel's offer of EPO. Even the mention of drugs disturbed Zabriskie. He had grown up around drugs and learned to hate them. He had seen what drugs could do. He'd seen what they had done to his father.

Michael H. Zabriskie's obituary in the *Salt Lake Tribune* said he passed away peacefully on September 7, 2000, had "enjoyed music, fishing, sports, and he loved the Utah Jazz." It was a kind remembrance of a man who had lived in darkness.

He spent days in his basement, stoned and drunk, selling marijuana and cocaine from his La-Z-Boy recliner. He fought so much with his family that they often sought refuge in a bedroom, cowering as he tried to force his way in. He terrified his wife, Sheree, with threats of physical abuse. She believed her husband might try to kill her or her children someday. She had seen such horror before. Her father had killed her mother with a shotgun before turning the gun on himself.

In defense, Sheree Zabriskie created a world for her children away from their father. She checked them into a hotel or took them camping. On better days, she took them to movies while her husband cooled off. It was the family's version of normal.

For Zabriskie, the symbol of the family's dysfunction was his father's old brown recliner. *That chair.* That worn-out, thread-bare, dingy, godforsaken chair that sat in front of the television in the basement. Zabriskie's father went through at least three of them. Zabriskie was sure that his father would die there, legs kicked out in front of him, the air thick with stale marijuana smoke, a glass of Lord Calvert whiskey swirling in one hand, TV remote control in the other.

Zabriskie was in elementary school when his father told him he worked in construction. For a long time, Zabriskie didn't know any better. He knew his dad stashed envelopes filled with $500 each into the tubing of a brass hat rack, and he knew that the basement smelled funny but didn't know what the smell was. He started to suspect something wasn't right while doing his seventh-grade homework one night on the bar in the basement, as his father watched a Larry King segment on medical marijuana.

"Look, some guy's lighting a joint on Larry King!" his father said to a friend on the phone. When Zabriskie heard his father speak about drug use so casually and use the word "joint," like it was a staple of his vocabulary, it finally hit him: *Oh my God, Dad is a drug dealer!* After years of building up his courage, Zabriskie finally confronted his father. Michael Zabriskie explained that he had started to sell drugs as a young father who dropped out of school to support his family.

That didn't make Zabriskie feel any better, especially when his life was so tumultuous. Where his dad had punched holes in walls and threatened his family with violence, Zabriskie had become withdrawn and timid. He retreated to a basement room where he kept superhero statues of Batman, Spider-Man and He-Man. They were symbols of his yearning to protect his mother and sisters and save himself from torment. He was a non-Mormon in Salt Lake City, a city of Mormons, and more than once his schoolmates and neighbor kids told him he was bound for hell.

He was a good student who received mostly As and Bs. Yet he ate his lunches alone in a nearby field and never went to school dances. He was an outcast. After school, he Rollerbladed on the parking lot of a Mormon church. There he tuned out the world, dancing on his wheels while the mix-tape in his Walkman played *West Side Story*, *Camelot* and The Who's *Tommy*. He would stay for hours, singing the shows' lyrics and dreaming about doing something—anything—that would make him famous. He didn't want to be known forever as some ne'er-do-well devil kid from a bad family. Then he would skate home and be snapped back to the reality of his father, drunk and sprawled out on that miserable La-Z-Boy. He had begged his father to stop drinking, written him letters about how much he meant to him, but he had gone unheard.

In eighth grade, a woman rang the doorbell at the Zabriskie house. She told David she had knocked the side-view mirror off the Zabriskies' camper, parked on the street. She wanted to talk to his father about it, but Zabriskie couldn't coax his father upstairs. Suddenly, the woman stepped aside and in stormed a SWAT team. A stream of officers rushed by in helmets and riot masks with their black automatic weapons at the ready. They shouted, *Police! Police!* They pushed the fourteen-year-old Zabriskie aside and raced toward the basement.

His father was ushered out in handcuffs, quipping, *What took you so long?* David screamed at him through his tears, "This is all your fault!" The police had seized marijuana, cocaine and thousands of dollars in cash. Michael Zabriskie was off to the county jail for drug trafficking.

When David Zabriskie returned home after the raid, he found the house torn apart. His mattress had been slashed and thrown askew on the floor. Earlier, when the police had asked him if there was any money stashed in the house, he was so nervous that he told them the truth. Yes, yes, he told them. It was Christmas money, and it was hidden inside his mattress. Under duress, whenever the pressure seemed unbearable, Zabriskie was unable to keep a secret.

Cycling saved him. Zabriskie's therapy was to race a mountain bike on the city streets. The faster he pedaled, the farther it took him from home. He used his rage to propel his bike up steep canyons. The more his legs and lungs hurt, the more he pushed himself. *I'll never be like my father. I'll never be like my father.*

Eventually, when he felt he had become a pretty good rider, he attended a meeting at the Rocky Mountain Cycling Club. A local sports physiologist, Steve Johnson, spoke about race tactics and how cycling was far from an individual sport. Johnson moved paper clips around a projector to show how a team worked. One rider could lead the *peloton*, move and open the door for a rider behind. Another could shield a teammate from an attack. You need teammates, and they need you, he said, and that's the only way to win. Zabriskie liked the sound of that.

He showed up an hour early for his first group ride with the cycling club. His new clip-in shoes couldn't help him on the sixty-mile ride. His seat was too low, and he hadn't brought any water, only a pack of gum. Though he barely made it home, needing much encouragement from other riders, he'd relished every minute of the experience. On those roads, battling his own physical and psychological pain, he had finally found peace.

After the ride, he fell into his bed and felt his heartbeat pulsating through his body. All he knew about cycling competition was the name of its biggest event, the Tour de France. He didn't know it was a three-week ride, two thousand miles, climbing mountains, flying in sprints, all of it asking more of a body than most bodies can give. He didn't know anything about it, really. But after that ride with the Rocky Mountain Cycling Club, he knew one thing for sure.

There on his bed, the boy who wished he was a superhero told himself, "I just took the first step to the Tour."

Zabriskie was lanky and lean, perfect for cycling. At sixteen, he won his first national event, the Iron Horse Classic in Colorado, and later that year won the state championship for his age group. At seventeen, he won a junior race in Colorado named after Lance Armstrong, already a world champion. That victory qualified Zabriskie to train at the United States Olympic Training Center. The next year, he finished fourth in the individual time trial at the 1997 junior world championships and decided, with the guidance of Johnson, who had become his mentor, to forgo college for a shot at riding professionally.

When the Festina scandal hit in 1998, it prompted Zabriskie and teammates on the junior national team to gossip about PED use. They thought they might have to use drugs to succeed. Zabriskie once asked Johnson about doping. "Don't worry, you won't have to dope," his mentor said. "The sport is cleaner than ever."

"So, you think I should keep going?"

"Yes. You will be fine, I promise."

Levi Leipheimer, who had attended the University of Utah and had known Zabriskie for years, told him it was a perfect time to turn pro because doping was on the way out.

But then Zabriskie met Matt DeCanio, a professional rider, and took a long ride with him in Colorado Springs, Colorado, home of the Olympic Training Center. Zabriskie asked him what it was like to race in Europe, and if drugs were a problem there.

"Oh man, it's bad, really bad," DeCanio said.

"Like, how bad?"

"Those guys are taking veterinary grade pills, horse pills, all kinds of pills."

For an hour and a half, DeCanio told so many wild tales of drug use in Europe that Zabriskie thought the veteran was playing with him, trying to scare him. In fact, DeCanio's talk was Zabriskie's first warning: Pro riders use drugs, and if you want to ride in the top levels, you will use them, too.

It wasn't as if Zabriskie could seek his father's advice. When he left training camps and went home, he saw his father drinking more than ever. The week after he turned twenty-one, he decided he'd had enough.

The breaking point came when he and his mother were on the phone to make a plane reservation for a trip to the national team's training base in Europe. His father kept picking up the line in the basement, trying to disrupt the phone call; he had propped a bar stool against the basement door so no one could enter. David snapped. Screaming and cursing, he kicked the basement door off its hinges, charged his dad and ripped the phone from his hands and straight out of the wall. Never before had he challenged his father, and his aggression frightened both of them.

Seven months later, Michael Zabriskie died. The barrels of Lord Calvert whiskey had ruined his liver and turned his skin yellow. David's many pleas had been well founded—his father would not live to see his son become one of the world's best cyclists. The drugs and the drinking had done it, David told himself. *Those damn drugs*.

There had been no good-bye or reconciliation between David and his father. David had been indignant when he'd visited him in the hospital where he was being treated. He'd never dreamed it would be his last chance to make peace with him.

He skipped the funeral to race in Europe, at the Grand Prix des Nations in France. At that race, his anger, resentment, regret and sadness coalesced with his talent to propel him past the physical pain. He won that race for riders under twenty-three, his first big European victory, while Armstrong won the professional race. The day would be remembered for something else, too. At the finish line, Zabriskie met a man who would, for the next several years, guide and mold him: Johan Bruyneel.

Bruyneel was big-time, savvy and slick after leading Armstrong and the Postal Service team to two Tour victories. Zabriskie was impressed that such an important person could be so nice. Bruyneel told him how good he was, how good he could be and how he could be rich if he signed with the right team. Zabriskie needed no sales pitch. He wanted money and the independence it brought, and he wanted all of it now. So weeks later, in Izegem, Belgium, in a back room of a jewelry shop owned by Bruyneel's brother, he signed with Postal Service for $40,000 a year. He was joining a team led by Lance Armstrong, already one of the most well known and popular athletes on earth.

Right away, he learned that his world was not Armstrong's. No private jets, no multimillion-dollar contracts, no screaming fans. Riders like Zabriskie were drones around the hive. Zabriskie started at a training camp in Tucson, Arizona, during which the team celebrated his twenty-second birthday by buying him shots of vodka. He ended up room-spinning drunk, throwing up behind the bar. Hincapie snapped photos of him, while Bruyneel urged him to have one more shot, just one more.

"Take it or I'll fire you!" he said, according to Zabriskie.

Zabriskie wanted to say no, he couldn't possibly have more alcohol. But it was Bruyneel, the top boss, the man who held his future in his hands and wielded his power within the team. So Zabriskie, as he had with his father, caved. At night's end, after vomiting for hours and enduring violent diarrhea, he passed out in his hotel room bathtub.

With that initiation, he had become part of a new family— one just as dysfunctional as his family back in Utah. Bruyneel, the father figure, was always off with Armstrong and ignoring the young riders. Zabriskie again felt lost. He also was homeless. Marty Jemison, a fellow Utahan, had asked Zabriskie if he wanted to take over the lease of his $400-a-month apartment in Girona, but Bruyneel said, "Don't take that apartment, nobody is going to live in Girona anymore, I'll help you find a place."

Zabriskie was temporarily dumped at the apartment of two older riders, including the Australian cyclist Matt White. The place was a mess, with food and clothes everywhere. On a training ride that day, White told him he had taken "tons of human growth hormone" while riding for an Italian team and it made his feet several sizes bigger. It was sensory overload for Zabriskie, the new guy who was still exceedingly shy. He asked himself, "How did I end up with these delinquents?"

Zabriskie searched for an apartment, but saw only one dingy, huge building after another. Finally, he chose a one-bedroom apartment above a coffee shop in a town thirty miles away.

Even the sweet smell of coffee from the shop below provided no comfort to Zabriskie. His loneliness hit an all-time low. He lived on pizza. He didn't race much because his training was going so badly. He spent hundreds of dollars on phone calls to Randi Reich, a beautiful, brainy blonde enrolled at the University of California, Berkeley, whom he had met before leaving Utah. She had been a high school classmate of one of Zabriskie's sisters. He told her the pressure to dope was rising slowly but steadily. She said if he ever took drugs, she'd leave him. He assured her he never would.

He tested Armstrong on a training ride, trying to see if the two-time Tour winner would admit that doping was part of the sport. "I think I'm a pretty strong bike rider," he told Armstrong. "I just don't understand how if I'm at my maximum, guys are just flying by me."

Armstrong said only, "You got to train harder."

Zabriskie was skeptical. He had heard foreign riders talk about doping, casually chatting about what they were taking and what other riders were on, as though the stuff weren't banned. He had seen what went on inside the team hotels on a daily basis. Sometimes the injections came from syringes with a green liquid inside, sometimes the liquid was yellow, other times it was clear or red. Del Moral told him it was a mix of vitamins and that he shouldn't be afraid to take them. That first season, every time he was offered a shot of that different colored "recovery," he politely declined.

By fall 2001, Zabriskie believed some top riders could be clean, and that included Leipheimer, who had finished third in the Vuelta. His finish sparked rumors that he was a doper, but Zabriskie didn't believe it, even going as far as to defend Leipheimer to naysayers.

"I know Levi, and he trains his ass off," he said, only to see the doubters laugh in his face. He told Leipheimer, "Dude, I know a lot of guys are saying that you're dirty and taking drugs and stuff, but I know how hard you train, and I think you deserve it."

The next year, Zabriskie made only $15,000 because of his performance the season before. His training had gone so terribly—he was eating poorly and was unfocused because he was so lonely—that Bruyneel didn't even trust him enough to enter him in races. Zabriskie returned to the team only after begging Bruyneel to give him another chance. In his desperation to remain in the sport, he started to feel that some performance-enhancing substances were OK. At the Redlands race in April 2002, he felt so beat down and exhausted that he asked a teammate, Dylan Casey, for a shot of those "recovery" vitamins. Casey took out the vial and Zabriskie inspected it. Yep, the label said vitamins, so he let Casey inject the liquid into his arm. Zabriskie couldn't tell whether it had worked or not, but it didn't feel that nefarious—he was always taking loads of vitamins orally anyway.

He eventually learned to inject himself and search for a proper vein in which to deliver the "recovery." Nobody had offered him any doping products yet.

Later in the 2002 season, Bruyneel told him he would have to inject all the vitamins the team offered to him. Zabriskie agreed. He thought it was strange that his teammates didn't comment on the fact that he injected himself regularly, like a junkie. Once, when he missed the vein with the "recovery," prompting a huge bubble to form beneath his skin, Zabriskie ran to get Frankie Andreu's help. Andreu laughed and said, "Don't worry, it'll go away," as if he'd seen it many times before.

Zabriskie remained reluctant to blindly take what other riders got from the doctors. At the Spanish Vuelta in 2002, del Moral had a group of riders line up on the team bus before the time trial for an intramuscular shot that no rider could identify. Zabriskie wasn't sure if it was legal or not, but no one complained.

"OK, stand on one leg and relax your butt," del Moral said before jamming a needle into each rider's buttocks. Zabriskie wanted to lie down for the shot because it would be less painful. The doctor refused the request and demanded that he remain standing, so he declined the injection altogether. "No, thanks."

Afterward, del Moral was annoyed that Zabriskie had not gone along with the plan.

"You are a pussy, you are a fucking pussy," the doctor said.

In his second year on the team, Zabriskie became more comic relief than just an awkward young kid. Occasionally, he broke into song on the team bus to elicit laughs. Once, Zabriskie serenaded Bruyneel with a song he'd learned from another pro cyclist, belting it out to the tune of Jimi Hendrix's "Purple Haze."

> *EPO all in my veins*
> *Lately things just don't seem the same*
> *Actin' funny, but I don't know why*
> *'Scuse me, while I pass this guy.*

At the café in Girona that day in May 2003, after finishing fifth in the Four Days of Dunkirk, and feeling good about his clean success, Zabriskie allegedly listened to Bruyneel and del Moral talk about the need for doping in elite cycling. To succeed in the sport, he claims they said, Zabriskie needed to start shooting up EPO and taping testosterone patches to his body.

"Look, Dave, those guys that just beat you at this race in Dunkirk? They were all on it," Bruyneel supposedly said. "Even the guys behind you were all on it."

Zabriskie wasn't sure if he was telling the truth. He said, "I know the team is in trouble right now with points, and you guys just want me to score you some easy points."

"No, it's not like that," Bruyneel said, laughing.

Zabriskie looked to Barry, with whom he had talked about EPO while rooming together earlier in the season. He needed some backup. Just weeks before, Barry had told him that he wanted to find a way to quit the sport because of the doping.

"Are you not going to ask any questions?" Zabriskie asked Barry. "Are you going to do this?"

"It's just how it is," Barry said.

Barry, who had joined the team the year before, was once one of the riders asking doctors about their injections. Del Moral would respond, "Don't you trust me?" or "You guys ask too many fucking questions." Yet by the time he and Zabriskie were offered EPO that day, Barry had already decided that he would join in. He had seen too much doping to believe he could succeed without it.

When Barry moved into Jonathan Vaughters's room in Girona the year before, in an apartment now shared by Vande Velde and another rider, he had found empty ampules and used syringes under the bed. Later, he had discovered EPO and human growth hormone hidden inside a bag of coffee in the fridge, and saw chemical burns that testosterone patches had left on Vande Velde's body. The more time Barry spent on the team, the more brazen his teammates became with letting their doping be known. Hincapie, who became close with Barry, encouraged him to use EPO and testosterone to "make him feel better," and said that he wouldn't have to use much of either drug to see results. Barry trusted Hincapie's advice.

So supposedly the four of them—Zabriskie, Barry, Bruyneel and del Moral—rose from the café table and made the short walk to Barry's apartment. The way Zabriskie saw it, two new riders were about to graduate from the clean class of Postal riders and be inducted into the team's doping program.

Once inside, the riders claim that Bruyneel and del Moral rushed through the ceremony, with del Moral walking them through what they needed to do to use EPO.

> Be careful when you inject it. Needs to be directly into the vein. If accidentally injected into fat, the EPO can be detected for more than a week and you could easily test positive. You will receive a coded text from me with instructions on how much to use.

As the administrator of this ever-growing club based on secrecy, cheating and lies, Bruyneel allegedly emphasized the importance of paranoia. Wash your syringe out, so if anyone finds it, the substance will be undetectable. Throw away the ampule far from your apartment and make sure you are not being followed when you do it. If a drug tester shows up, don't answer the door. And never, ever tell anyone.

Both riders held out their arms so del Moral could prick them with the needle.

"It went in just like the other stuff, the 'recovery,'" Zabriskie said. "It just didn't feel any different." It was one more step in a series of tests toward making the Tour team. Just another step toward helping Armstrong win and become richer, more powerful, more beloved by millions.

To Zabriskie, it all happened so fast—the café meeting, the walk to Barry's apartment (a relatively safe place to dope because he was Canadian and USADA wouldn't show up there), the instructions, the needle prick. It felt like he was a passenger in a plane crash and he had no time to save himself. He wondered: "Is this how it felt for everyone their first time? For Armstrong? For Vande Velde? For Hincapie? Is there anyone strong enough to resist the suffocating pressure, to stop time and walk away?"

Zabriskie felt betrayed by Bruyneel, a man he claims was the gatekeeper to his drug use and someone he trusted, someone who had swooped into his life and helped him rebound from the loss of his father. In his apartment, alone, he threw down the EPO, testosterone patches and "recovery" he alleges Bruyneel had given him, collapsed onto the floor and melted into a fetal position. After several hours, he finally rose to call his mother and tell her what had happened.

"I just, I just, used drugs, I just became Dad," Zabriskie said.

Her son repeated that sentence several times before the mother understood the words through his tears. He had just cheated. He had just broken his promise to the woman he considered the love of his life.

"I think you need to leave right now and be done with this," his mother said. "Come home. Come home. Just come home. These are not good people."

Zabriskie went home the next week to train for the rest of the season. On Memorial Day, he rode alone down Millcreek Canyon, a popular hiking and biking area. Speeding down the main road, he saw a white Nissan SUV stop to turn into a parking lot. He thought the driver had seen him coming. She had not. Zabriskie crashed head-on into the SUV. He flew more than twenty-five feet through the air and landed on sharp rocks along the road.

His entire left side was torn up. Several fingernails had been ripped off by the SUV's headlights. His left lower leg was positioned at an unnatural angle, badly broken and afire with pain. His left wrist was broken and began to swell.

Covered with blood, Zabriskie pulled himself to a seated position and considered what had just happened. It was more than an accident, he thought. This was a sign from God.

CHAPTER 14

At the end of the 2001 season, Lance Armstrong wanted another strong climber on his team. He got one all right: a slight, redheaded, fair-skinned Kid Rock look-alike from a community of religious fundamentalists in Pennsylvania. His name was Floyd Landis, and he was smart, witty, and more than a touch paranoid. Given to extremes, he might drink a case of beer every night for a week before switching to nothing but a bowl of cereal for days. But Landis could really ride.

When Zabriskie was healthy enough to return to Postal Service, in 2004, he shared an apartment with Landis and another rider, Tony Cruz. Both Zabriskie and Landis were enigmatic, and both had distinctive senses of humor. They became fast friends. But Landis battled depression. In 2002, his first season, he had popped antidepressants to get by. He didn't like living in Girona, apart from his wife, Amber, and his stepdaughter, Ryan, and he didn't like the hierarchy on the team. He thought it was unfair that he made only $60,000 a year.

In their Girona apartment, he grumbled to Zabriskie about Armstrong's wealth: "His fucking money, his fucking jet." Frustrated and angry that he had not achieved Armstrong-level success, Landis once walked onto the balcony and threatened to jump. He said he wanted to "end it all."

"Floyd, have you ever had a good day?" Zabriskie asked.

"Yes."

"Well, you will never have another good day if you end it all right now."

Chances are, he wouldn't have ended it right there. The balcony was on the second floor.

The two men became inseparable, almost literally. They squeezed together on a little scooter, because they didn't want to buy a car. Zabriskie would sing Lynyrd Skynyrd's "Simple Man": "Forget your lust for the rich man's gold/All that you need is in your soul." Armstrong called them "Dumb and Dumber."

One rainy day, Landis convinced Zabriskie to skip their daily training ride. They sat at a café and ingested enough caffeine to kill a small mammal. The story became part of the team's folklore: Landis drank thirteen cappuccinos in a row, Zabriskie stopped at five.

The pair's version of life as a cycling pro was nothing like Armstrong's. They were out to have fun, which included throwing darts at a team poster they had taped to their apartment wall. Armstrong treated cycling like a serious business of which he was the CEO. A lot of money was at stake. Armstrong's top *domestiques*, like Hamilton and Vande Velde, would come to earn salaries approaching a million a year. Armstrong was pulling in millions annually.

Armstrong looked at Landis like he was a bad employee who could keep the company from reaching its potential. He didn't like Landis's lack of discipline. Worse was Landis's lingering conflict with the UCI, which held the bank guarantees for the teams in competition, and as such was responsible for paying out if one of them ever went belly up. Landis, who was owed his salary from his previous team, was telling reporters that the UCI wasn't protecting its riders.

Verbruggen, president of the UCI, replied with a letter rebuking Landis. "Such an aggressive approach might perhaps work in the U.S.A.," Verbruggen wrote, "but it does not in Europe and most definitely not with me."

Armstrong told Landis that he needed to apologize to the UCI chief. He said, "Look, Floyd, you have got to do what this guy says because we're going to need a favor from him at some point." Armstrong claimed that he'd needed the UCI's help when he had apparently tested positive at the 2001 Tour de Suisse. Landis needed to apologize to Verbruggen so the Postal team could remain on the UCI's good side.

Landis apologized rather than further antagonize Armstrong and Verbruggen. It was a rare moment that reached back to his childhood when, as a good Mennonite boy, he bowed to authority. But those days had come and gone.

Floyd Landis had grown up in Ephrata, in the heart of Pennsylvania Dutch country, where many of the residents are either Amish or Mennonite. His parents, Arlene and Paul, raised him and his five siblings as Mennonites, following a branch of the Anabaptist Protestant religion that believes in a literal interpretation of the Bible and preaches pacifism. For his first nineteen years, Landis shared a double bed with his brother, Bob, in a two-story white house with a white picket fence, a radio tuned to a local gospel station and a television used only to watch home movies.

Paul Landis made his living from a self-service laundry, a car wash and odd jobs. Money was tight, but they didn't need much. Clothes were simple—the women wore plain cotton dresses and head coverings; the men wore white shirts and cotton slacks held up by suspenders. Life on Farmersville Road included no rock music, no cursing and no alcohol.

Landis grew up with strict definitions of how a person should act and what he should do with his life: Give all glory to God. Live simply. But Landis was an independent thinker, and full of questions like, "Why is it that half of the world has never heard of this religion and they are going to go to hell?" He could recite passages from the Bible, but, like Armstrong, he struggled to keep the faith.

He left home for California at the age of twenty, on his bike. Six years later, he joined Postal Service and headed for Europe. As a professional, he continued to question convention. He didn't understand why some people thought it was OK to snack on pastries during a race but it was taboo to eat a doughnut. He found it hard to believe the accepted wisdom that a rider who didn't wear socks could catch a virus through his feet. And why were riders allowed to eat cheese but not ice cream? Landis gained a reputation as a man stirring the pot just to stir it—or drinking thirteen cups of cappuccino just to drink thirteen cups of cappuccino.

He tried to fit in when it became clear that he risked being ostracized. He agreed to undergo blood transfusions to gain an edge, and accepted testosterone patches from Armstrong, which he claims happened in full view of Armstrong's wife. He was rewarded for following rules. Landis made Postal Service's Tour team for 2002. A week into the race he lay on the opposite side of a bed with Armstrong as they received blood transfusions the day before an individual time trial, in which Armstrong finished second, and Landis fifteenth.

As one of the feared members of the Postal Service's Blue Train—the team's nickname because it often rode together, creating a blur of blue—Landis helped Armstrong to strong finishes in the mountains, including back-to-back stage wins in the Pyrenees. Those daily victories helped set Armstrong up for his fourth Tour title.

By 2002, Armstrong had replaced Livingston and Hamilton with Landis and Spanish climbing specialists who did what they were told.

All but two of Armstrong's band of brothers on that first Tour-winning team had left. Hincapie and Vande Velde had remained. By then, they had hired Ferrari to help them dope, often meeting in Hincapie's apartment—because he lived alone—to inject themselves with EPO. They wore long sleeves to hide bruises and track marks.

From Armstrong's perspective, his team had changed but the doping program ran as smoothly as ever. Upon winning the 2002 Tour, he said his body "was remade" after his cancer, but it was his team that deserved the credit for his success. "It's the organization, the team, the program," he said, adding that it was a "sick mentality" to think he'd dope.

Yet the French newspaper *L'Equipe* published a story with the headline, "Must We Believe in Armstrong?" The story reported, "There are too many rumors, too many suspicions. He inspires both admiration and rejection."

The *Washington Times*, meanwhile, reported that the French were just jealous: "France's motto: If you can't beat them, investigate them."

In addressing reporters, Bruyneel praised the U.S. Postal Service for its laissez-faire attitude with the team. "We have a sponsor that doesn't tell us, 'You have go to this race or that race because we have commercial interests there.' What Postal wants is that we arrive at the start of the Tour 100 percent. How we get there is our problem."

The Postal Service enjoyed the PR boost Armstrong had given it, but was also wary of the doping allegations in the air since Armstrong's return. When it renewed its sponsorship in 2000, it included in the four-year deal a "morals turpitude and drug clause" that said the Postal Service could suspend or fire any rider for failing drug tests or for inappropriate drug conduct prejudicial to the team or the government agency.

Stapleton stayed in front of any suggestions that Armstrong cheated to win. He told one of the team's sponsors, Coca-Cola, "Look, he doesn't take drugs, OK? I will stake my entire career on it."

Armstrong began working on a sequel to his autobiography. The book, *Every Second Counts*, denounced all doping allegations. He wrote about the French government's investigation into the medical waste Postal Service team members had tossed into a Dumpster at the 2000 Tour. The investigation had made his sponsors nervous, but Armstrong said he was bothered most by its effect on his reputation.

He worried for his son, Luke. "Luke's name is Armstrong and people know that name, and when he goes back to school I don't want them to say, 'Oh yeah, your dad's the big fake, the doper.' That would just kill me."

Armstrong and Kristin had put forth an image of having the perfect marriage: two beautiful people with money, fame and celebrity friends—kind of like the Kennedys' Camelot, one pal said. But Armstrong wanted out. The two were on a beach in Santa Barbara, California, on Valentine's Day when he told her he was leaving. He wanted a divorce.

Kristin had signed a nondisclosure agreement that kept her from answering questions about her husband's doping, a rule she followed even during legal proceedings. Later, she said she had become "a yes woman" who was just trying to keep herself happy at her own expense.

Mike Anderson, who had taken a job as Armstrong's bike mechanic/personal assistant in 2002, said Armstrong wanted out of the marriage because he wanted to enjoy all the spoils of being a celebrity—and that included the "countless girls who had knocked on the windows of the team bus."

Eventually, Armstrong would kick out Anderson, too. In 2004, Anderson found steroids in Armstrong's medicine cabinet in Girona, and sensed that Armstrong was pulling away from him because he had stumbled upon Armstrong's secret. Unexpectedly, he was fired.

The two then butted heads in court. Anderson claimed that Armstrong backed out of a promise to finance a bike shop Anderson had wanted to open; Armstrong claimed Anderson was extorting him. They settled out of court.

Anderson, an American who was married to a fellow American, couldn't get away from Armstrong fast enough. Feeling harassed by Armstrong, he felt that he couldn't flee far enough. So he moved his family to New Zealand.

The French dropped their investigation of Armstrong in late 2002. But a certain Irish journalist wasn't as easy to shirk. Jonathan Vaughters first heard from David Walsh in the fall of 2003, more than a year after he had left the sport, presumably for good.

Walsh—"that fucking little troll," to quote Armstrong— wanted to meet with Vaughters in the United States for a book about cycling. Nothing on the record. Just for background.

Vaughters, working as a real estate agent in Denver, agreed.

Over burritos at a local Mexican restaurant, Walsh said he thought it curious that Vaughters had retired so suddenly, in his prime at the age of twenty-nine and with another year left on his contract with the French team Crédit Agricole. Walsh said the former Postal Service *soigneur*, Emma O'Reilly, told him Vaughters could be trusted and might have a story to tell.

"I just want you to be honest with me," Walsh told Vaughters. "I know you doped, but at the end of the day, I feel like you are one of the good guys. You left the sport at the peak of your career. I want to know why. And I want to know about the doping that happened on Postal. Tell me about Lance Armstrong."

Vaughters didn't say a word. Walsh pressed him. It was time, he said, to end the lying and cheating that had begun in cycling a hundred years before. He said Armstrong needed to be stopped.

"Jonathan, you've got a chance to stand up for your sport and make things right," Walsh said.

Vaughters was torn. After he'd left cycling, he wanted nothing more to do with it. He was sick of the lying and the cheating. He wanted to start a new life.

After winning the time trial and setting the course record on Mont Ventoux in the 1999 Dauphiné, he promised himself that he'd never again use EPO. He didn't keep the promise. He left Postal Service after that season, then doped occasionally, though without the success virtually guaranteed by his old team's well-organized, centralized program.

About a month before the 2002 Tour, Livingston—in his final year with Jan Ullrich's Telekom team—suggested that Vaughters try a new drug called Albumin. It was a concentrate of plasma proteins from human blood and would increase a person's hematocrit.

Vaughters wasn't sure if Livingston had ever used the drug, but he thought he'd give it a try after reading a pamphlet about it that he found on the Internet. He bought the Albumin from a pharmacy in Spain.

Vaughters—and many other top riders in the *peloton*, for that matter—had to resort to using drugs like Albumin because they had no system in place to reinfuse their own blood at the Tour. There, Armstrong and Postal Service had a huge advantage. They had the funding to do what they wanted, and a plan in place that had been fine-tuned over years. If something went awry, they gambled on having the protection of the UCI officials.

Teams that wanted to race clean, like Crédit Agricole, had no chance. Vaughters learned that firsthand. When he raced for that team in the 2001 Tour, he was stung in the face by a wasp or a bee during a training ride. His right eye swelled shut, yet he couldn't take cortisone because he hadn't declared it to the UCI before the race and couldn't get an exemption to use it because it hadn't been approved for an allergic reaction.

He begged the team doctor to give him a cortisone shot and say it was for a knee injury, which would have been a lie but would have allowed him to continue racing. But the team manager, Roger Legeay, said no, because the team would be breaking the rules. Vaughters walked off in a huff, saying, "Screw this, this is hypocrisy from all angles."

He showed up at the stage start the next day, thinking that probably half the riders were taking cortisone against the rules, and Armstrong said, "What the fuck is wrong with your face?"

"Bee sting."

"Why wouldn't you take cortisone for that?"

"Because it's actually not allowed for an allergic reaction."

"You're on the wrong team, dude."

In 2002, Vaughters regrouped for the Tour. While Armstrong had Bruyneel, del Moral and Motoman allegedly working out the logistics of his doping, Vaughters was the mastermind of his own little plan. He would continue using testosterone patches and microdoses of EPO. But he would also use Albumin to dilute his blood before the UCI's hematocrit screening. That way, it would look like his hematocrit was low, when it was actually well over the 50 percent limit.

It seemed like a brilliant idea, until he looked again at the label a few days before the Tour. It said the drug carried a 1 percent risk of causing hepatitis C. He thought of his son, who was about two, and said enough is enough. He threw all his drugs into a garbage bag and tossed it in a Dumpster.

Vaughters dropped out of the Tour about halfway through and told Legeay that night that he was quitting the sport to be with his family. He said the team didn't have to pay him his salary—$350,000—for the remaining year of his contract. He just wanted out.

Back in Girona, he left his apartment to head back to Colorado in such a rush that he forgot to discard the testosterone patches under the bed and the centrifuge in the living room.

And now, Walsh was with him, looking him in the eyes, telling him he could see genuine goodness in him. No one does anything to clean up cycling, Walsh said, but Vaughters could be different. He could expose its secrets. Maybe young riders of the future wouldn't have to face the decision that Vaughters once had to: dope or quit the sport.

"Do we really have to do this?" Vaughters asked. "In all honesty, if you take down Lance, someone else will just take his place."

"Yes, Jonathan, but if you cut off the head, maybe the body will fall."

Vaughters paused, let out a huge sigh and said, "OK, OK, I'll do it."

Betsy Andreu had put a dent in the shield around Armstrong's secrets. She had contacted Walsh in 2001, after he had written about Armstrong's involvement with Ferrari, and became one of Walsh's best sources for information about doping in the sport.

Now Vaughters shattered that shield by answering every question Walsh asked.

After the interview, Vaughters realized what he had done. "Either I'm going to be pushed out of the sport," he said, "or Lance is going to be."

The ninth stage of the 2003 Tour de France was run on a day so hot in southeastern France that the road's asphalt bubbled. The Spaniard Joseba Beloki led Armstrong by three bike lengths down a steep descent toward a sharp right turn. Beloki's rear wheel skidded from beneath him. He grabbed the brakes. His rear tire exploded and the bike collapsed. Beloki was thrown against the road. Medics found him in pieces, his right femur, elbow and wrist broken.

And what did Armstrong do in the milliseconds between Beloki's spill and his own certain disaster? If he flinched, no one saw it. He veered left of Beloki's screams and headed off the road. Off the road? In the Tour de France? Only Lance Armstrong would fly past a startled gendarme at roadside and head into a farmer's fallow field.

Down the French farmland made hard by drought, Armstrong's bike shook and rattled as if crossing the ties of a railroad track. He careened a hundred yards, perhaps, and at the bottom of the hill saw a ditch. So he hopped off his bike, picked it up, leaped with it in his hands across the ditch, then set it down.

He remounted to cross the road ahead of the *peloton* bearing down on him. Former teammate Tyler Hamilton reached out to pat Armstrong's shoulder, as if to say, "Cool, dude." On television, one commentator shouted, "This is unbelievable! I've never seen this before. Armstrong went across the field. There, he's back on the road. At four kilometers to go, what great reflexes from the man from Texas! That man was in complete control there. Oh, this is incredible!"

Those seventeen seconds—from Beloki's crash to Armstrong's remount—tell you Lance Armstrong was born to be on a bike.

He could have ridden straight into a wall of corn or sunflowers, or come to a full stop as the rider behind him did. He didn't. His tires could have sunk into soft earth. They didn't. If he considered all that, no one ever knew it. He simply rode into the unknown, and anyone who'd ever seen him at work could imagine those steel blue eyes narrowed into slits above cheekbones so sharp they could cut you. Watch the move often enough on YouTube and you might even see the bright cape of a superhero billowing from his shoulders.

At the stage's end, Armstrong told reporters, "I was very afraid, I was very lucky . . . I was lucky that the field could've been full of crops, it could've been a drop-off."

With an official's ruling that his shortcut maneuver through the field was unavoidable and thus legal, Armstrong finished the stage strong on his way to a fifth straight Tour victory.

Before the cancer, he said, winning was nice but not essential. After the cancer, "I was pretty fucking laser-focused," he told me.

He expressed that focus in eight words:

"I win, I live.

"I lose, I die."

As the 2004 Tour approached, Armstrong staged a preemptive strike against *L.A. Confidentiel: Les Secrets de Lance Armstrong*, the book Walsh wrote with Pierre Ballester, a Frenchman who had worked at *L'Equipe*. A month before it was scheduled to be published, Nike and the Lance Armstrong Foundation began selling yellow rubber wristbands bearing the word "Livestrong" for a dollar apiece. Proceeds funded the foundation's programs for young people with cancer.

The specific timing was contrived, but the idea for the wristband had been a work in progress for months. Nike wanted to do something to commemorate Armstrong's fifth Tour victory and Scott MacEachern, his personal representative at the company, thought it should be something that people could wear to show their support for the cancer cause. Nike and a team of advertising and marketing gurus then designed the rubber bracelet, after getting the idea from some NBA stars who wore something like it.

Within weeks demand outran supply. Armstrong had created a pop culture phenomenon just when he most needed positive press. Together with his foundation and Nike, he had planned it that way.

They hoped that the wristband's "Wear Yellow" campaign would overshadow Walsh's exposé, which was to be published June 14, about two weeks before the start of the 2004 Tour. (On that date, a Lance Armstrong Foundation press release asked all Americans to wear yellow on June 16 to show support for people living with cancer.)

Armstrong had read a ten-page excerpt from the book in the French weekly magazine *L'Express*. He knew it included the most damaging doping accusations against him yet—that he had doped with various substances, including EPO. The book also described Armstrong telling his cancer doctors in an Indiana hospital room that he had used several performance-enhancing drugs.

Emma O'Reilly, the former *soigneur*, had been a primary source for Walsh. She told Walsh how she had used her makeup to cover Armstrong's bruises from an injection and how she had delivered a vial of pills to Armstrong. She said Armstrong's excuse for the cortisone positive at the 1999 Tour was a lie. He took the drug as a performance enhancer, not for saddle sores as he and the UCI had insisted.

After years of silence, O'Reilly had been paid for the information—"an insignificant amount of money," about $7,500—but she said she talked mostly to cleanse herself of some guilt.

Armstrong immediately came after Walsh. He told a Dutch newspaper that Walsh was the "worst journalist I know," a man willing to "lie, to threaten people and to steal" for a sensational story that had no basis in fact. "Ethics, standards, values, accuracy—these are of no interest to people like" Walsh.

Then he filed suit in Britain against Walsh and Walsh's deputy sports editor, Alan English, at the *Sunday Times* of London, which had published a news story based on revelations in the book. He was asking for 1 million pounds, or about $1.5 million. In France, he had sued Walsh, Ballester and the publishers of *L'Express*, plus the book's publishers, La Martinière. Armstrong also sued O'Reilly for libel—asking the court to grant him "more money than I was worth," she said. Perhaps he thought the threat of other libel suits would silence stories that hadn't yet gone to press.

A day after news of those lawsuits broke, Armstrong announced that his team had secured a new sponsor for 2005, the Discovery Channel. Judith McHale, president of Discovery Communications, praised him as a role model: "There is no better ambassador for quality and trusted information."

At the news conference for that announcement, Armstrong said that he had filed the lawsuits because "enough is enough." He also chipped away at O'Reilly's credibility, saying he hadn't worked with her much and she had been fired when "inappropriate" issues arose.

Armstrong and Stapleton wanted the media on their side. Stapleton told the author Daniel Coyle, who was writing his own book, *Lance Armstrong's War*, that Walsh's effort to expose Armstrong would be futile. Armstrong would never dope and take a chance on losing sponsorships with Coke, Nike and Subaru, companies that had put their trust in him, he said.

"If we're fucking lying, we can kiss it all good-bye," Stapleton said. "Does anybody think for a second that a secret that big wouldn't come out?"

A few weeks later, at the start of the 2004 Tour, Stapleton stood in a parking lot with Bart Knaggs, his business partner, and Frankie Andreu, who had retired as a rider and was working as a commentator for the Outdoor Life Network. In a scene straight out of *Goodfellas*, Frankie claims Stapleton put a hard squeeze on him to get his wife, Betsy, to say she hadn't been a source for Walsh's book. What Stapleton didn't know was that Andreu was taping the conversation.

Stapleton, Knaggs and Andreu ended up in that parking lot because of a story that began in 2001. That's when Walsh reported that Armstrong had seen Ferrari. Betsy Andreu had seen Walsh's work, and was impressed. She asked her friend James Startt if he could tell Walsh to call her. He did, and that was the beginning of a long-distance relationship between Andreu and Walsh that lasted years. Both were obsessed with revealing the truth about Armstrong.

Andreu trusted Walsh enough to confirm for him that Armstrong's hospital room confession had occurred. She told him that he was right to question Armstrong's story about riding clean. "Don't stop digging, David," she said. "You have to expose him. Keep digging."

She couldn't go on the record with him because her husband still worked in the sport and she knew how much power Armstrong wielded over their family and cycling. The Andreus had three children to support. Betsy Andreu was a housewife. Frankie Andreu didn't have a college degree—all he knew was cycling. Armstrong had the Andreus and their livelihood in a chokehold.

But from behind the scenes, Betsy could damage him. For Walsh, she became a clearinghouse for information on Armstrong. She tried to help Walsh track down Lisa Shiels, Armstrong's former girlfriend who was in the hospital room during Armstrong's confession. Her mistake was calling Becky Livingston for Shiels's number, specifically asking her to keep the request from Livingston's husband, Kevin.

A second after Betsy hung up with Becky, Kevin Livingston supposedly called, yelling about Betsy's effort to help Walsh. "He'll bring everybody down. You can't do that. This is Frankie's livelihood; this is my livelihood. Are you crazy?"

The request got back to Armstrong, who then sent Frankie Andreu a scathing e-mail.

"To go around and say to becky 'please don't tell kevin' is as snaky and conniving as it gets," Armstrong wrote on December 15, 2003. "i know betsy is not a fan, and that's fine, but by helping to bring me down is not going to help y'alls situation at all. there is a direct link to all of our success here and I suggest you remind her of that."

So, on that day shortly before the 2004 Tour, Stapleton called Andreu to set up the parking lot meeting. Frankie took along a tape recorder, hidden in his shirt pocket.

Stapleton said, "You know your wife is a source for Walsh."

Andreu refuted it, saying that his wife only spoke to Walsh about some "nitpicky stuff" and that Walsh had asked her help in tracking down Armstrong's old girlfriend. He said he realized that he, the team and everybody in the sport benefited from Armstrong's accomplishments.

"I have fucking protected Lance for a long time," Andreu said. "Every interview I give, I frickin' talk to this stuff, I say everything good and I like him, you know?"

Stapleton was skeptical. He told Andreu that Walsh boasted about speaking to Betsy, calling her courageous, saying she was willing to testify against Armstrong and that "she knows these things about Lance."

He then asked if Betsy would be a witness against Walsh in the libel case in France. Would she be willing to take a strong position and say that Walsh was a liar? Or maybe, for now, could she just make a supportive statement about Armstrong?

"I know Betsy doesn't like Lance, but it's all in our interest not to blow this whole thing up," Stapleton said. He said it was part of the grand plan to get enough witnesses to discredit Walsh so that the *Sunday Times* and La Martinière, the book publisher, would be forced to admit that Walsh's entire premise was flimsy. They would publish an apology and/or pull the book off shelves and Armstrong would drop the lawsuit. End of story.

"The other option is full-out war in French court and everybody's gonna testify. It could blow the whole sport," Stapleton said.

When they parted, Stapleton said they would send something to Andreu for his wife to sign. But Andreu knew that wouldn't work. She wouldn't shake Armstrong's hand after the 1999 Tour victory, and now Stapleton wanted her to support him publicly?

Here's Betsy Andreu's response to Stapleton's idea: "Tell him to fuck off. I'm not signing anything. I'm not fucking protecting him."

Walsh was treated like an outcast at the 2004 Tour. Armstrong made sure of it.

Most journalists covering the Tour form carpools during the three-week race because the days are long and the route covers more than two thousand miles. Walsh had planned to ride, as he had before, with John Wilcockson and Andy Hood, two journalists from the U.S.-based cycling magazine *VeloNews*, and Rupert Guinness, an Australian who wrote for the *Sydney Morning Herald*.

At the race start in Liège, Belgium, though, Wilcockson told Walsh he could not ride with them. If he did, Armstrong would no longer talk to *VeloNews*. For an American publication, that would be suicide. So Walsh squeezed in with several reporters from the French newspaper *Le Monde*. He felt like he couldn't ask any

English-speaking journalist for the favor because Armstrong likely had power over them, too.

While Walsh was being vilified, Armstrong and Postal Service were on a high. Early in the Tour, Armstrong and his teammates won the team time trial to put Armstrong in yellow, with Hincapie second overall and Landis third. It was the first time in the 101-year history of the Tour that American riders were first, second and third in the standings.

Emboldened by their success, the Postal Service team did what was necessary to keep doping. They usually had been so paranoid about their doping that they'd lock down their hotel rooms before performing blood transfusions in them. With plastic and tape, they'd cover the vents, the smoke detectors, the air conditioners and even the toilets in an effort to thwart any attempts at someone taping them with a hidden camera.

But now, on one ride from a stage finish to the team hotel, the team bus came to a halt on the side of a mountain road. It wasn't engine trouble that stopped it. It supposedly was several riders' need for blood. While the bus driver pretended to tend to the bus's nonexistent mechanical problem, some riders on the Postal Service team apparently received blood transfusions, some lying on seats, Armstrong on the floor. Their blood bags were allegedly hooked to the luggage racks above them, letting the blood flow through the tubes and into their veins more easily. Fans and reporters driving by might have seen it for themselves but for the vehicle's darkened windows.

Armstrong also dropped any pretense of benevolence. During the 18th stage of the twenty-stage race, he chased down Italian rider Filippo Simeoni, who was ahead of the pack in a breakaway and 144th overall. Back in the main group, Hincapie thought, "Why is he doing that? He's leading the race by seven minutes!"

Revenge, that's why. Simeoni had testified against Ferrari in the criminal doping case in Italy, saying Ferrari had given him drugs like testosterone and EPO. Armstrong had rushed to Ferrari's defense, calling Simeoni "a compulsive liar" who had doped long before he met Ferrari. Simeoni sued him for defamation of character.

So when Armstrong finally caught Simeoni on that Stage 18, he was trying to teach him a lesson. He simply couldn't help himself.

While the television cameras rolled, he pedaled next to Simeoni and told him in Italian, "You made a mistake when you testified against Ferrari and you made a mistake when you sued me. I have a lot of time and money and I can destroy you."

Simeoni tried to remain with the breakaway, but the other riders asked him not to, because their chances to win the race were diminished with Armstrong there. He gave in. He and Armstrong slowed down to allow the main pack of riders to catch up. French rider Laurent Jalabert said Armstrong's move was "like a child crushing ants."

Once Armstrong was in the *peloton* again, he appeared to joke with other riders and made the universal signal for keeping quiet—he zipped his lips. The television feed caught him doing it, and played it again and again. He even looked into the camera and smiled as he pulled his finger and thumb across the front of his mouth.

Later, Armstrong said he had overtaken Simeoni because he "was protecting the interests of the *peloton*. All he wants to do is destroy cycling and destroy the sport that pays him, and that's wrong."

Simeoni said, "I was surprised by what Armstrong did to me, but he showed today in front of the whole world what kind of person he is. I was the victim of a big injustice today. It wasn't possible for Armstrong to let a little rider like me have a chance for a little glory in the Tour de France. That's a sin."

Armstrong won that Tour by more than six minutes after winning six stages, and dominated more than ever to set the record for most Tour titles. Robin Williams, the comedian and actor, was in the stands at the finish line, wearing a T-shirt that said, "Yellow, front of the race" in French. The singer Sheryl Crow was there, too, to give Armstrong a hug and a kiss. The superhero and the rock star were an item now. She was just one of Armstrong's many female partners who allegedly knew about his doping but kept quiet about it. How could any of them miss it? Armstrong said to me. *For God's sake, the EPO was right there next to the butter.*

On that final day of the 2004 Tour, Armstrong's foundation said it sold 25,000 yellow wristbands in Paris. About 1.37 million viewers watched the Tour's final stage on the Outdoor Life Network, a massive American audience for the French race.

Despite Walsh's evidence, things looked as peachy as ever for Armstrong.

For Simeoni, though, life was about to get worse. Like Bassons, the Frenchman who had been forced to quit the 1999 Tour, Simeoni was first bullied by Armstrong, then the rest of the *peloton* followed. No team wanted him. He was sure that Armstrong had something to do with his team's not being invited to the 2009 Giro d'Italia, even though Simeoni was the Italian national champion. Once again, Armstrong's will was done. Simeoni quit the sport a year later.

Things weren't any easier for O'Reilly. She had become so entangled with lawsuits relating to Armstrong that her relationship with her boyfriend, Mike Carlisle, suffered. Carlisle had been battling multiple sclerosis, and the stress of the situation worsened his symptoms. She felt like Armstrong was trying to bankrupt her, or drive her crazy, or both. "I thought he was going to take everything from me."

For the Andreus, the threats continued. One arrived via Armstrong's former Postal Service teammate, Hincapie, who had always been the do-as-he-was-told type.

"I cannot understand how you can just sit around and let besty [sic] try and take down the whole team," he wrote to Frankie in August 2004. "Yes, she is just saying things about lance, but it effects [sic] us all. You were a part of the team just like us. If he is guilty then so are you. The whole thing is so hypocritical. She is attacking our livelihood. A sport that we love and work fucking hard to be good at. You have not been gone that long. How can you forget?"

Hincapie says he sent the e-mail because Andreu had been part of the doping culture, too—and had even introduced him to EPO. Hincapie said he and Andreu were on Motorola in 1996 when he found a thermos filled with glass vials in their refrigerator. Andreu first said the vials were substances that would help recovery. Hincapie got him to admit that it was EPO.

Andreu said he needed the drug because he was getting older. All Hincapie knew, though, was that his competition was taking a drug to get an edge, so he needed to get it, too.

"He was my role model, and I started doing EPO because of him," Hincapie said. "It was crazy that he was letting Betsy point a finger at Lance, because her own husband had done the same thing. She was threatening everyone's ability to make a living in the sport. I was trying to get him to stop her."

But the momentum was slowly shifting and Armstrong's hold on the sport was slipping. His former teammates and employees were becoming increasingly disgruntled with the way he treated them. Instead of being especially nice to those people who knew his secrets, Armstrong was tossing them aside as if they had been strangers. It would be his fatal flaw.

By the end of 2004, Zabriskie would be gone. Landis would be off the team, too, headed to be the leader of the Phonak team, which had offered him $500,000—more than double his $230,000 salary with the Postal Service squad.

Zabriskie had problems negotiating a new contract with the Postal Service squad. He said he asked for $70,000 a year, but Bruyneel wouldn't go past the $65,000 Zabriskie was making. Bruyneel's argument was that the team had stood by him when he got hit by the SUV back in Utah, so that was payment enough. Zabriskie thought he should be paid more, considering he had just won a stage of the Vuelta a España, one of cycling's Grand Tours. They had reached an impasse.

After finishing fifth in the time trial at the 2004 world road cycling championships at the end of the season, Zabriskie sat on the lawn of the race hotel in Verona, Italy, with Steve Johnson, his longtime mentor and the man who had convinced him to forgo college for cycling. In 1999, Johnson had taken a job at USA Cycling and had moved up quickly—he was now chief operating officer and director of athletics. He also was close friends with Postal Service team owner Thomas Weisel.

Zabriskie says that he complained to Johnson about his contract problems, but in his anger and disappointment over how the Postal Service team treated him, he apparently told Johnson about the team's doping program as well. He claims that he told Johnson, "They were giving me injections, drugs."

Zabriskie explained that he had taken a chance in telling Johnson about the doping. Part of him was anxious that it would leak out that he had broken the sport's code of silence and that he'd be ostracized, because he knew that Armstrong "would just steamroll people in the industry." Still, Zabriskie had hoped that Johnson would notify USADA, and that someone would look into Postal Service's cheating.

But, according to Zabriskie, Johnson didn't even respond. Johnson later said to me that he never heard any "credible, specific claims" about doping on the Postal Service team before 2010, when accusations about Armstrong's doping were made public.

After speaking with Johnson, Zabriskie says that he returned to his hotel room and retrieved the team-issued Livestrong bracelet he kept in his luggage. He placed it in an ashtray and set it on fire. As the acrid smell of burning rubber began to permeate the room, he looked at his roommate, a rider set to join the Postal Service squad the next season, and said, "Have fun on your new team."

By then, Tyler Hamilton had been gone from the Postal Service team for three years. In the summer of 2004, he became the perfect example of what happens to Postal riders who weren't under the protection of Armstrong's team and who weren't a part of an efficient doping program. He tested positive.

After he won the gold medal in the individual time trial at the 2004 Olympics, scientists working at the Games for the International Olympic Committee found evidence of someone else's blood in his system. The World Anti-Doping Agency had just begun to test for blood transfusions in which athletes use someone else's blood, a practice banned in cycling since the late 1980s. Hamilton was the first to fail the test.

The positive test was dropped because of a lab error. Yet even that wasn't enough to scare him into competing clean.

One month later, Hamilton, riding for the Swiss-based Phonak team at the Vuelta a España, again tested positive for a blood transfusion.

He immediately denied wrongdoing. "I have always been an honest person," he said. As Armstrong had done for so many years, Hamilton was stone-cold lying.

In preparation for that cycling season, he had deposited his blood for safekeeping with sports doctor Eufemiano Fuentes in Valencia, Spain. When some of the blood was reinfused into him late that summer, he was likely given someone else's by mistake, accounting for why he tested positive for transfusing someone else's blood. It wasn't the first time Hamilton had problems with blood he had stored with Fuentes, either.

Earlier that year, at the Tour in July, Hamilton reinfused another blood bag that had come from Fuentes's freezer. Minutes later, he came down with a fever and knew something had gone wrong. As his urine filled the toilet, it was such a deep red it looked black, making it seem like something out of "a horror movie."

He was nauseous and shivering. "It felt like my skull was being cracked and peeled off my brain, piece by piece." He placed his cell phone near his bed, in case he needed an ambulance, and told his teammates that he might die. He was convinced that his blood hadn't been stored properly and that he had infused dead cells into his body.

"Either that, or my blood bag was tampered with, or the test didn't work," he said much later, during his testimony in Fuentes's criminal trial in Spain in 2012. Whatever the reason, the error could have killed him.

Armstrong heard about Hamilton's mishaps and shook his head. He considered Hamilton to be too much of a risk taker when it came to doping. In Armstrong's eyes, Hamilton always wanted more, always wanted to push the limits of safety. While Armstrong said he only doped to prepare for races, Hamilton doped all year round.

Hamilton's first public appearance after the positive test in 2004 was in Las Vegas, at Interbike, North America's largest cycling trade show. There he began his effort to salvage his reputation. People had given him the benefit of the doubt. After all, he was known as the most polite person in cycling.

His sponsors and team publicly supported him, with Bell Helmets giving away "I Believe Tyler" buttons. Fans waited hours to get his autograph and offer their condolences for his golden retriever, Tugboat, who had passed away just before the Olympics. Hamilton had ridden to Olympic victory with Tugboat's identification tag tucked inside his helmet.

But other cyclists were losing patience. Bobby Julich, the former Motorola rider, said, "I'm sick of people who cheat, sick of cleaning up their mess and trying to explain it."

Back in Boulder, Hamilton's adopted hometown, Hamilton was introduced to a crowd at the University of Colorado, and his father, Bill, leaped from his seat and shouted, "We believe in you, Tyler!"

The Hamiltons came out fighting, attacking the validity of the test and calling into question the fairness of the system run by the World Anti-Doping Agency and USADA. One theme central to his case was that Tyler had had a "vanishing twin" who shared his mother's womb when he was a fetus and created a mixed population of blood cells in his body, a condition that apparently explained everything.

Vaughters was upset. He knew that Hamilton had lied and that the lies perpetuated the sport's long-standing culture of cheating. He was sick of Armstrong's bullying, especially the zip-the-lips gesture regarding Simeoni. After leaving the real estate business behind, Vaughters had started a cycling team for riders under twenty-three years old and cringed just thinking that they could be headed for drug use and a life of lies in the pros.

So in the fall of 2004, he packed his bags and drove south to Colorado Springs. There, he left his wife and son at the Broadmoor Hotel and headed to USADA headquarters, feeling as though he were consorting with the enemy.

He sat with Terry Madden, the chief executive of the organization, and Travis Tygart, the agency's general counsel. As Madden questioned him, Tygart scribbled notes.

"I just wanted to tell you that you're on the right path with Tyler," Vaughters said.

"Did you ever dope?" Madden asked. Tygart glanced up from his notepad. Vaughters didn't answer.

"Well, I guess you're not going to tell us," Madden said.

More silence.

"OK, then, what can you tell us?"

Vaughters told them about microdosing EPO—how riders got away with using the drug by injecting small amounts over a long period of time. To have the best chance to catch riders doping, he advised the agency to test them the first thing in the morning and the last thing at night. He also told them riders used testosterone patches to administer tiny amounts of the steroid over many days.

Madden listened. Tygart scribbled.

Madden said the agency would be interested in helping clean up the sport. Vaughters said he was, too, but the agency would need to keep their meetings with him a secret. He had seen what happened to riders—the Bassonses and Simeonis—who spoke out against doping. He didn't want to be publicly annihilated by Armstrong. He had a cycling team of young guys to run.

Armstrong had already attracted the antidoping agency's attention. But one incident in particular had raised USADA's suspicions. Earlier that year, around the time of Hamilton's positive test at the Vuelta, Armstrong's agent, Bill Stapleton, had called to tell USADA that Armstrong wanted to donate $250,000 to the agency's antidoping work.

After Tygart hung up, he walked to Madden's office. They looked at each other and smiled. "Did that just happen?" Tygart asked. "What the hell's going on here?"

PART FIVE

CHAPTER 15

Until that fall of 2004 when Vaughters spilled his sport's secrets to USADA, Tygart hadn't given much serious thought to cycling or its long history of doping. He was a stick-and-ball-sport type of guy, a son of a lawyer in a family of lawyers who lived in Jacksonville, Florida. His great-grandparents lived one of the millions of great American immigrant stories: They arrived in northern Florida from Lebanon with nothing but ambition. They taught their children what those children taught theirs: There are no shortcuts. Success comes to those who believe in Christian values and hard work.

Travis Thompson Tygart went to the Bolles School, a local college preparatory high school that had nationally recognized sports programs. There, he played on state championship baseball and basketball teams. One of his baseball teammates was Larry Jones, destined to be a major league star with the Atlanta Braves and a likely Hall of Famer whom the world would come to know by a nickname, "Chipper." Tygart and Jones had seen steroids at work, like one opposing team's catcher whose muscles had blown up so big and grown so tight that he could hardly throw anymore.

While training for his senior-year season, Tygart had his first run-in with drugs that boost performance. He and his cousin were working out at a gym together one night. The place was a hole-in-the-wall with all manner of dumbbells and free weights scattered in the corners. But it was a perfect place to get your reps in, to go until you couldn't anymore. Tygart recalls being approached by one of the gym's meathead bodybuilders, "You guys, y'all are working *hard*."

"Yeah," Tygart said. "We're just trying to get stronger."

"You do anything else?"

"The batting cages."

"Anything else?"

"What do you mean?"

"You know, there's some drug supplements out there. They're really good and can help you."

Tygart was taken aback. Sure, he wanted to be bigger and stronger. What teenage high school jock didn't want that? He was tall and thin, seventeen years old, a third baseman. He knew what the meathead had in mind. Steroids. He looked to his cousin, then back to the meathead.

"Um, no thanks, man," he said. "We're good."

A straitlaced jock and a natural leader, Tygart would become the president of his senior class in high school and the president of his fraternity at the University of North Carolina, Chapel Hill, where he majored in philosophy. When he worked as an intern at a Florida State Attorney's Office one summer in college, he quit because of what he called "government waste." Tygart discovered that the workers who were supposed to man the main file room were playing video games on the job. Their office door set off a buzzer whenever someone came in looking for a file, and whenever the buzzer rang, they would leap to their feet and pretend to be busy. He couldn't stand being a part of a government entity that paid workers to play video games all day. He said he resigned out of protest.

Even through college, Tygart knew nothing of cycling, or the Tour de France, or Lance Armstrong. He definitely had not heard of an event that came to be known by the single word "Festina." But he knew everything about baseball. He had played in a rec league while at the University of North Carolina. Then, married and teaching in 1995, he went back to coach the game at his old school, Bolles.

A few years later, he was in law school at Southern Methodist University in Dallas. Between his second and third year, he worked at a big corporate firm, Jones Day, in Houston. It was the Summer of Mark McGwire and Sammy Sosa, the big guys who hit baseballs into low orbit and who were chasing Major League Baseball's single-season home run record. Most of America was spellbound, captivated by this outcropping of sudden history.

But if, a decade earlier as a rules-are-rules high school senior, you had been offered steroids in a sweaty, stinking gym, you might have loved the summer of '98 less. If you had been a high school teammate of Chipper Jones and for years after heard his stories of big leaguers seeking every edge they could get—corked bats, for one—you might have harbored some disquieting feelings about what might lie behind all the multiple-home-run games and the gosh-wow press conferences.

So you might forgive Tygart his skepticism, even as McGwire and Sosa became America's favorite sons and as national television cut into regular programming to show the sluggers' at-bats. Tygart knew enough about baseball and enough about steroids to tell friends, "There's no way they're doing that without being on anything."

He still loved sports. He had written two law review articles on the subject: one based on a Title IX equality-in-sports case about the baseball team's versus the softball team's facilities at his high school, the other an antitrust and relocation case involving soccer fields in west Texas. At one point, he told his old buddy Chipper that he might become a sports agent, only to hear Jones tell him not to. Such work, Chipper said, was "scummy."

Still, when the Festina team was kicked out of the 1998 Tour and the Postal Service riders and team doctor flushed their doping products into the toilet for fear of being arrested for drug possession, Tygart had no idea that four years later, he'd be in the thick of it all.

One day in late 1999, with nothing better to do, the young, bored corporate lawyer Travis Tygart went to a Web site promising jobs around the country. On the site's search engine, he typed in "sports law."

Up came a law firm called Holme Roberts & Owen, which did work for something called the United States Anti-Doping Agency.

USADA was born of the Festina debacle, which exposed to the world cycling's drug problem. Before Festina, doping rules varied widely. Each Olympic sport's international federation had its own rules, conducted its own tests and handled its own cases. Few sports, if any, were more lenient in applying their rules than the International Cycling Union, the UCI.

If riders tested positive, the UCI apparently decided its punishments only after considering the riders' careers, what they had done for the sport and "whether they're paying for their grandmother's apartment and stuff," as one antidoping expert put it. "They wanted to control it. They wanted flexibility and weren't keen on transparency." The UCI was not alone among sports and national Olympic committees interested in keeping their stars unblemished, so the International Olympic Committee did something to make things more objective—or to at least seem more objective.

In 1999, after Festina, the IOC formed the World Anti-Doping Agency to standardize drug testing rules. WADA's anti-doping code went into effect in 2004. By then, Lance Armstrong had won the Tour de France five times.

USADA began operations in the fall of 2000, given its mandate by the United States Olympic Committee and Congress to oversee all antidoping in Olympic sports in the United States. It also was expected to implement the WADA code.

USADA was not a government agency, though most of its funding came from the White House Office of Drug Control Policy. Its budget is authorized by Congress and is thereby susceptible to the lobbying of high-powered organizations and individuals who don't like its work. In time, even Lance Armstrong himself would argue that USADA's funding should be cut, maybe even eliminated.

Based on the ad he had seen on the Web that day in 2000, Tygart applied to Holme Roberts & Owen. He got the job, and would end up doing work for the United States Olympic Committee, the Pro Rodeo Cowboys' Association and the national federations of basketball, volleyball and swimming. What interested him most, though, was his antidoping work for USADA. About two and a half years later, he found himself taking a job there as director of legal affairs.

In the fall of 2002, he arrived at his new office to find a framed poster showing Lance Armstrong riding his bike on a cobblestone street somewhere in Europe. The poster carried the famous

Armstrong quote, dripping with incredulity: "What am I on? I'm on my bike, busting my ass six hours a day. What are you on?"

Though he hadn't been the one to hang the poster above his desk there, Tygart kept it. He liked how straightforward the sentiment was. His wife's family had been touched by cancer, and here was Armstrong, a young American coming straight out of a cancer ward to win his sport's biggest event, the Tour de France. Tygart thought it was one of the greatest sports stories of all time.

His life first intersected with Armstrong's a few weeks later, when Armstrong called USADA with a complaint. Until then, Tygart and Armstrong had led parallel lives with nothing much in common beyond their age, thirty-one. One man was the product of a prestigious prep school, the other a virtual high school dropout. One was churchgoing, the other agnostic. One was embraced by a close-knit family, the other scarred by an upbringing of alcoholism, philandering and divorce.

Tygart had studied up on cycling. He'd also heard about the sport's doping woes from Madden, USADA's CEO, and Rich Young, a partner at Holme Roberts & Owen who basically had written WADA's antidoping code. They told him that drug use was common in an endurance sport like cycling, but that USADA's new policy for out-of-competition testing should help catch some of the sport's dopers.

In order to do those unannounced tests, USADA required all Olympic athletes to report their whereabouts at all times. This set off Armstrong and his handlers, who complained: It's impossible for Armstrong to tell USADA his whereabouts all year long when his travel and training schedules are constantly changing. It's unreasonable. It's setting athletes up for failure, because missed tests could mean a doping offense.

Just weeks after Tygart had joined USADA, Armstrong himself was on the phone to him. "This is bullshit, we're not doing this," Armstrong said. "Showing up at our house to drug-test us is not right. It's not fair."

Tygart turned in his desk chair and said, "Listen, man, you're getting every benefit of the doubt. I'm sitting here looking at your picture on the office wall, and what you should understand is we need to give your fans the guarantee that you're doing it right. Out-of-competition is a good thing. It's the best way to catch people. If you're clean—like this poster says—you have nothing to worry about."

Tygart knew just how far other elite athletes would go to succeed. He was heavily involved in the doping cases that stemmed from the Bay Area Laboratory Co-Operative steroids investigation, in which the company claimed to have supplied elite athletes with legal supplements and vitamins when it was actually dealing performance-enhancing drugs to them.

The slugger Barry Bonds and the sprinter Marion Jones were two of the athletes who received drugs from BALCO. Another athlete caught in that scandal was track cyclist Tammy Thomas, once a silver medalist at the world championships. She had been barred from competition for life after testing positive for steroids in 2002.

In one of the most bizarre doping cases ever, she had insisted on her innocence, but one glance at her suggested otherwise. Broad-shouldered and buff, she had a five o'clock shadow, a receding hairline and a deep gravelly voice.

Just thinking about Thomas's case made it obvious to Tygart that cycling had major doping problems, and that Armstrong might not be clean after all. What made him particularly suspicious about the Postal Service team was that several of its former riders had tested positive. Some of the tests were administered by USADA, some by the UCI.

In 2002, Kirk O'Bee failed a test for testosterone. In 2004, Hamilton failed a test for a blood transfusion and fought like mad to get out of it, a process that took nearly two years and ate up a significant amount of Tygart's time. And there would be others.

No matter how much Tygart wanted to believe in Armstrong's courageous comeback from cancer to win the Tours, he couldn't ignore the mounting pile of clues that Armstrong had probably doped. Every time a former Postal Service rider was caught doping, Tygart tried his hardest to convince that cyclist to talk about the culture of drugs in professional cycling. He wanted someone to squeal on the sport and on his former teammates, for the good of the younger riders who might someday be faced with the same decision of whether to dope or not.

He tried to convince Hamilton to talk about the doping that may have occurred on his teams by saying, "We understand that you aren't alone in this." While Hamilton suspected that Tygart wanted him to turn on Armstrong, Tygart never uttered Armstrong's name. He was fishing for a lead, but riders like Hamilton—who were loyal to the sport's code of silence—wouldn't bite.

Chris Carmichael, Armstrong's coach (at least on paper), gave Tygart even more reason to doubt cycling's hero incarnate. Tygart and Carmichael were friends from Colorado Springs because their children had attended the same school. At a kids' birthday party one day, Carmichael supposedly brought up Betsy Andreu's claim that Armstrong had confessed to doping. Tygart claims that Carmichael then "vilified her" at great length. The alleged insults were so "over the top and so nasty" that Tygart thought it was obvious Carmichael was overcompensating. "You just knew there was more to it, because he wouldn't have reacted the way he did. I went home and said to my wife, 'What is he trying to keep me away from?'"

None of these events proved anything, but all of them piqued Tygart's interest. He didn't buy the popular theory among Armstrong fans that no cancer survivor would risk the danger of using drugs simply to ride a bike faster.

"If I personally was on the brink of death and went through a terrible situation and came out of that as an atheist," he said, "I'm going to do everything in life that benefits me because I might not be here tomorrow.

"Treating people fairly or being decent or putting myself aside for other people—those basic moral values that most of us practice regardless of what religion we are—wouldn't matter. I'd have no moral constraints.

"The logical extension of that would be: 'I don't give a fuck about anything. I'm gonna get it when I can get it.'"

Tygart reminded himself of that as the years went on and the evidence against Armstrong mounted.

CHAPTER 16

Tyler Hamilton had created a good life for himself. He and his wife, Haven, lived in a palatial house set on the edge of a canyon in Boulder, Colorado. The home's rear windows framed a breathtaking landscape of rolling hills covered with evergreens reaching to the snow-capped mountains of the Continental Divide.

In the living room, his Olympic gold medal hung around the neck of a wooden moose with a grin on its face. Near the moose, there was a box containing the ashes of his dog, Tugboat, a lock of the retriever's pale tail affixed to the lid. Two months after Hamilton tested positive for blood doping with someone else's blood, he said, "This is the lowest point of my whole life. I could lose all of this."

While the Postal Service team geared up for Armstrong's push to win a record seventh Tour before retiring, Hamilton fought to get his good name back. He insisted he would never have transfused someone else's blood. He told me it was a ridiculous notion because he was afraid of getting AIDS and spreading the disease to his wife.

Haven Hamilton, in a blog posted on the Web site www. believetyler.org shortly after her husband's positive test, called the result a mistake. She said both of them had an aversion to transfusions after Tugboat's experience before the Olympics that summer. Internal bleeding caused the dog to lose more than half of his blood, and the second of two transfusions left Tugboat paralyzed on one side of his face before he finally died.

"With the dangers of transfusing blood so fresh in our minds, it is ridiculous to think Tyler would consider taking another person's blood," she wrote.

Part of what Tyler Hamilton said was true. He hadn't used someone's blood, he'd used his own, but Fuentes or someone in the doctor's office had mixed up the blood bags. Compared with the Postal Service program, it seemed like an organization run by the Keystone Cops.

Armstrong demanded the best and, with the amount of money the Postal Service was pouring into the team, he had the ability to organize whatever he wanted to reach his goals. Riders were monitored by doctors who were experts in doping, beginning with del Moral and Ferrari. The team's cyclists for years apparently flew to Belgium to see a trained doping control officer so he could remove their blood and store it.

The team had lucrative sponsorship contracts, and, according to Landis, generated the necessary cash to pay for the doping regimens by selling bikes.

He learned about the bikes-for-cash deal in 2004. In March that year, his bike frame snapped just as he was in position to win a stage of an eight-day race in France. When he asked Bruyneel for a new bike, Bruyneel told him the team didn't have enough money to outfit riders with new equipment. Landis wondered why riders didn't get new equipment on a consistent basis, when Armstrong was able to ride on a private jet.

Incredulous, Landis called several sponsors, asking how much equipment they provided because the equipment they used was either not enough to go around to all the riders, or was badly worn. When he called Trek, the bicycle company told him that the team should have enough bikes and components for 120 new bikes a year. In 2004 alone, then, Landis figured that 60 bikes had gone missing. At maybe $3,000 each, that would generate $180,000 in cash. He had an epiphany: *So, that's how the team pays for its doping.* He discovered that the sponsors were, in a very roundabout manner, unknowingly paying for the team's drugs.

Bruyneel allegedly was furious when he learned of Landis's calls. Landis had gone over the manager's head. He had asked too many questions. By making sponsors wonder where their equipment was going if not to the team, Landis had come very close to breaching the unspoken code of silence that protected cycling's doping programs from the outside world.

To punish him for not being a good, quiet soldier, at that year's Tour Bruyneel and Armstrong supposedly dumped one of Landis's blood bags down the toilet. Despite that, Landis helped Armstrong win his sixth Tour de France. But he never rode for Postal Service again.

While Hamilton was entrenched in a two-year legal battle with USADA, Landis took his spot with the Phonak team. He had finally become the lead rider he thought he deserved to be.

But Phonak did not have a safe, team-run doping program; Hamilton's use of the Spanish doping doctor Fuentes had proven that. Landis, however, didn't care. He thought he could be the exception to the many expatriate Postal riders who had left Armstrong's side only to become mired in mediocrity or, worse, test positive. Landis thought he could win the Tour clean.

An early backer was the Saris Cycling Group, the company that manufactured the electronic device many riders used on their bikes to measure their power output. To help Landis navigate the cycling world without the riches and savvy of the Postal Service team, Saris hired Allen Lim, a Ph.D. student in exercise science at the University of Colorado in Boulder, to work with him as a physiologist.

Lim, a former competitive bike racer, had used Saris's power meter in his doctoral research and was eager to transfer his academic work into on-the-road experience. Now he could analyze the power profiles and energy expenditure of one of the world's great cyclists throughout the three weeks of the Tour. To his knowledge, no one had ever done that before.

Lim, a self-described "nerdy, scrawny Chinese kid from the Philippines," had immigrated to Los Angeles with his parents just before he turned two. As he pursued the education that the U.S. provided, he endured two tragedies. His father died after choking during a meal. A very close friend, while visiting Brazil, was raped, and returned to Boulder with a cocaine addiction.

Lim first spoke to Landis in depth about racing in January 2005 when they met at Landis's home in Temecula, California.

Landis asked Lim a question.

"What do you think about my chances in the Tour this year?" he said.

"Um, well, you know, based on what you did last year and your performance, and now you're the captain . . ." Caught off-guard by the question, Lim paused to collect his thoughts. He felt Landis staring through him. "It would be really amazing if you got top five at the Tour. That would be a good goal to shoot for."

Landis snapped at him. "Fuck, dude, if you don't fucking believe I'm going to win the fucking Tour de France, then just get the fuck out of here. Because I'm going to fucking win the Tour."

Lim was shocked into silence. But Landis calmed down as quickly as he had exploded, one of the dramatic, out-of-left-field mood swings Lim would see many times. More calmly, Landis added, "Cuz, look, if we don't train and work like we're going to win the Tour, then we're never going to learn how to win the Tour."

"OK, OK," Lim said, "I think you can win the Tour."

"Good, dude, that's what I wanted to hear."

The Mennonite church had asked the young Landis to accept the church's teachings on faith alone, and he had refused. But now, unwittingly, Landis had practiced what his church had preached so long ago. He'd asked Allen Lim to *just fucking believe*.

The first week of May 2005—two months before the Tour de France—Lim flew to Girona to begin working with Landis. They lived together and became a tight-knit team. Early on, though, Landis asked Lim, "Do you think altitude training can work as well as blood doping?"

Lim thought Landis had always ridden clean. But the question made him curious. *Why would Landis care about finding a method that would be "as good as blood doping"? Had he blood-doped before?*

In time, Landis admitted to Lim that he took part in Postal Service's doping program. Landis told him how Armstrong had persuaded him. On a training ride, Landis could barely keep up with Armstrong, prompting Armstrong to say, "You don't have to suffer like you do. I can help take your pain away."

After telling the story, Landis turned to Lim.

"Lance has all these guys looking after his program," he said. "All I have is you."

Until then, Lim had no real idea of doping's presence in cycling. Now he'd heard Landis say that anyone who succeeded was probably dirty.

"There's a system that's in place, but I don't need any of it," Landis said. "I'm better than that, I don't need the stuff. I can win clean."

Landis told Lim about an irate Bruyneel flushing his blood down a toilet at the 2004 Tour to get back at Landis for his constant insubordination. Landis had still finished a respectable 23rd. Lim was encouraged that Landis had done so well without doping.

Landis also told Lim about the time the team doctor gave him a special pill. After ingesting it, he had a great ride. So when the doctor gave him another one of those pills the next day, Landis kept it without ingesting it. He had a brilliant idea. He would bring the pill home and have its ingredients identified. He would then make the pills himself. He would sell the powerful stuff. He would make millions of dollars and probably win the Tour every year for the rest of his life.

But the testing turned up only one ingredient. Sugar. The pill was a placebo.

Landis told Lim he wasn't sure what had made him more upset—that he had been given a sugar pill when a real doping product could have helped him win more money, or that he couldn't reproduce the pill and become even richer.

In Landis's crazy stories, Lim tried to find a positive lining. He was encouraged that Landis had been truthful about his experience on Armstrong's team. He also was happy to hear Landis asking questions about legal, natural methods that could improve his performance, even if he always seemed to return to doping.

On May 26, Landis asked "the Chinaman"—his crude nickname for the physiologist—to drive him the 275 miles from Girona to Valencia for an appointment. Lim was gung ho. "Oh, great, we're going to Valencia!" he said. "Valencia, I've never been to Valencia before. Do they really have oranges down there? Ha, ha!"

In Valencia, Lim saw only a small sports clinic. Landis had him park in an adjacent lot and wait. In less than an hour, Landis reappeared with a Band-Aid in the crook of an arm. Lim didn't like the looks of it.

"What's that, what the hell is going on?" Lim asked.

A nervous and fearful Landis paused. Lim could tell he felt guilty about something.

A minute later, Landis admitted that he had visited del Moral, the former Postal Service doctor, and had his blood withdrawn and stored in del Moral's clinic for future use at the Tour.

The plan was for Landis to pick up the blood just before the Tour and take it to Grenoble, France, where his father-in-law, David Witt, would store it until the Tour went through town. There, the blood would be reinfused into Landis, the day before the race headed into the Alps. The extra blood would give him a huge boost.

Landis told Lim the blood doping was a last-minute idea. He had planned to ride that Tour without drugs or extra blood, but there was too much at stake to race without doping. He blamed it on Armstrong.

He followed up with a three-hour explanation of why he needed to dope to beat Armstrong.

Armstrong's doping had begun an arms race among top-level riders in Europe, Landis said. Every team knew Armstrong took a cornucopia of drugs to boost his endurance and dull his pain. They also knew he was blood-doping. Landis said he had a responsibility to himself and to the team to level the playing field, to wipe out Armstrong's medical edge.

Still, Lim and Landis debated whether doping was necessary. Lim said Landis's physiology was so superior that, with his talent, he could win clean and shouldn't stoop to the Postal Service team's level and cheat.

The problem with Lim's argument was the word "cheat." Professional cyclists believed that doping was not cheating as long as everyone did it. And everyone did it, in part because Lance Armstrong did it so well.

To back up his argument, Landis told Lim the history of Armstrong's doping for Postal Service, as he knew it. Armstrong had doped in 1999 to win the Tour for the first time, and he'd never stopped. Landis said it was unfair to riders like him who were exceptional naturally.

Maybe because of all the sermons Landis had heard in his church—twice on Sundays, once during the week—he often came off as a charismatic preacher. He likened his need to dope to a religious battle waged against Armstrong. While he was the Christian saint, Armstrong and Bruyneel apparently were devils tempting riders into evil.

"Sometimes to beat the devil, you have to drink his blood," Landis said.

With tears in his eyes, Landis told Lim how his father made him stand for hours in the sludge of their home's septic tank, in sneakers, and shovel the stuff out. He said he had trained on his bike in the dead of night so his parents wouldn't find out. Later, when he'd train or race in the daytime, he wore baggy sweatpants, because Mennonites thought it immoral for a man to show his legs.

Landis believed that such a rider, someone who had grown up so simply, with so little, deserved a chance to beat the great cheater, Armstrong. He claimed that cycling's pandemic of doping could be traced to the Postal Service team's band of what he called Mafia-esque enablers—teammates, officials and corporate sponsors who played dumb while doping occurred right under their noses.

"Hey, Al, you're not changing this, and I'm not changing this," Landis said on the car ride from Valencia back to Girona. He believed it was his moral duty to do the immoral thing and cheat if cheating was what it took to beat the really immoral guys whom Armstrong led.

Lim walked away with his head spinning. He wanted to fly home immediately, but was worried about what would happen if he left Landis alone. He believed that Landis had been talking so irrationally about doping that he might try something dangerous to gain an edge.

For advice on what to do next, Lim e-mailed Prentice Steffen, a former Postal Service doctor who had worked with Landis on the Mercury team from 1998 to 2001. He knew Steffen had claimed that the Postal Service team had replaced him with a Spanish doctor because the team wanted to start a doping program. Lim thought that Landis and Steffen could work together to out Armstrong as a doper. He also looked for help from the doctor on how to deal with Landis's erratic behavior.

Steffen told Lim that Landis didn't have to dope to level the playing field. He had another option: File suit against Armstrong in federal court. The doctor had tried to convince others connected to the team—Hamilton, O'Reilly—to join him as plaintiffs in a federal whistle-blower lawsuit. He had contacted a San Francisco lawyer who specializes in those suits, which are filed under the False Claims Act, giving citizens the right and financial incentive to bring suits on the government's behalf.

Steffen said the suit would claim that Armstrong and the team's management company, Tailwind Sports, were aware of the doping when they entered into a sponsorship agreement with the United States Postal Service. That knowledge of the doping constituted fraud, the suit would say. But Steffen needed someone with firsthand knowledge to join him.

When Lim spoke to Landis about the whistle-blower lawsuit, Landis said, "That's the stupidest thing I ever heard."

Lim also asked Steffen about Landis's emotional well-being. Landis was still depressed, as he was in 2002 when he joined the Postal Service team and was living with David Zabriskie. His instability made Lim nervous.

He worried that Landis, who seemed to be struggling with an inexplicable sadness, might hurt himself. "Dude, I think Floyd's crazy," Lim said. "I think he needs real professional help." To Steffen, that was old news. He told Lim that other Mercury staffers once had a rolling pool as to when Landis might kill himself.

Landis woke up after 4 p.m. following the Valencia-Girona blood doping trip, still groggy from the daylong nap. At Lim's urging, he talked about his depression. He showed Lim a neurophysiology textbook and told him that reading about the brain was helpful in understanding his extreme emotional highs and lows.

"Basically, you're here to keep me alive," Landis said. It was a joke, but Lim was terrified.

The next day, Landis trained on his bike while Lim monitored his power output. Less than twenty-four hours after having had a bag of blood withdrawn, Landis should have been weak. Instead, he put up fantastic numbers that, in Lim's estimation, showed he was a strong enough rider that he didn't need those extra red blood cells anyway.

Several days later, though, Lim walked into their apartment, opened the kitchen door and saw Landis injecting himself with EPO. Lim had never seen the act performed.

"I'm sorry," Lim said. "I can't be a part of this. I'm leaving."

"No, stay," Landis said. "Look, if I'm deciding to dope, what you do for me is still the most important thing. I still cannot do this without you."

He wanted Lim to believe that a rider's training meant more than his doping, that doping was a small part of the preparation. The difference was, Landis said, Armstrong had ten times as many people helping him get ready for the Tour.

"If you leave, it would mean that I have nothing," he said.

Despite Landis's plea, Lim flew home the next day. It was all too weird and creepy. He wanted to tell USADA the story, about Landis, Armstrong and the whole sport. But Landis scared him, and he suspected that no one at the antidoping agency would be brave enough to investigate doping allegations involving one of the nation's most revered athletes. He had seen Armstrong publicly crush people—Bassons, Simeoni, O'Reilly, Walsh—who dared speak out about his doping.

So Lim told no one what he had learned.

Back in Boulder, Lim was angry at Landis, distraught over his father's death and his mother's resulting depression and heartbroken by his close friend's cocaine addiction. Though he had earned his Ph.D., Lim was forced to borrow money from family and friends for rent, not exactly the proper ending to the job of his dreams.

Then a check for $7,000 arrived in the mail. It came from Amber Landis, the rider's wife. Lim felt torn. It wasn't much money; just a good-faith gesture by Landis. But it got Lim thinking.

The chance to train a world-class cyclist didn't come along often for an immigrant kid like Lim. He also felt guilty about leaving Landis. *What if something bad happened to him because I wasn't there to watch over him?* Already, Lim felt terrible that his close friend who was raped had turned to drugs in his absence.

So he cashed the check, paid some bills and bought an airplane ticket to Europe. Less than two weeks after he'd left, he returned to Girona. It was mid-June, with just a few weeks to go before the 2005 Tour. Landis was stranger than ever. One moment he was edgy and upset, the next charismatic, sincere and cracking jokes.

"He was now clearly exhibiting signs of someone with bipolar disorder," Lim told me. "Suddenly, my concerns had little to do with doping." It was as if Landis needed to win the Tour to stay alive.

This time, instead of running away, Lim burrowed in. He wanted to know everything that Landis was up to. Landis told him: While Lim was in Colorado, Landis had decided to become a blood doping expert. He joked that "Dr. Landis" would withdraw blood from himself and do it better than any MD ever had.

Landis said he needed to become an expert because he had doubts about using the blood he had stored with del Moral.

"I can't believe I just made a deal with this guy who is still probably working for Lance," he told Lim. "Stupid, stupid."

He worried that del Moral might tell Armstrong about his plan and that Armstrong would do something to subvert it. So he decided that he would return to del Moral's clinic and have the doctor reinfuse him right then and there. After learning that Levi Leipheimer, another American who had ridden on the Postal Service team, also had deposited a bag of blood with del Moral, Landis convinced him to retrieve his blood bag as well.

Before making the trip to del Moral, Landis removed an entire bag of blood from his body without anybody's help. He would need it to replace the blood he'd stored with del Moral.

Lim walked in while Landis was finishing up the transfusion, and watched him panic as he tried to figure out where to store the blood he had just removed. He couldn't keep his blood bag in the refrigerator. Landis's wife and young stepdaughter were arriving from the United States the next day. So Landis bought a cooler, an electronic thermometer, ice and a box of orange juice. He cut the top off the juice carton, slipped the bag of blood inside, then placed the carton into the cooler with ice. He also put the thermometer inside a Ziploc bag and into the cooler. Now his replacement bag for the del Moral blood bag was good and ready.

The presence of Landis's family only added to the household stress. Days and nights were filled with his shouting matches with his wife. At those moments, Lim took their elementary-school-age daughter, little Ryan Landis, for walks in town. Lim's mantra became "Keep my mouth shut, don't piss Floyd off, get through the Tour and be done with it."

Landis soon took on a new project: He would help Leipheimer, who was riding for the German Gerolsteiner team, blood-dope for the Tour. The two of them would undergo blood transfusions together when the Tour passed through Montpellier, France. Instead of blood-doping in Grenoble for a boost in the Alps with the blood from del Moral, Landis had opted for

Montpellier and a boost in the Pyrenees using the blood he had taken from himself.

So Landis and Leipheimer became partners in blood doping, but without anywhere near the Armstrong level of sophistication.

About ten days before the Tour started, Lim drove them to Montpellier. They were greeted by Landis's in-laws, David and Rose Witt, and David was part of the team that would carry out the plan. While Lim went for a walk with Landis's mother-in-law, the other men went to work. "Dr. Landis" took 500 ccs of blood—a single bag—from Leipheimer. When Lim returned, Landis placed Leipheimer's blood bag inside an orange juice container, then put the container in a cooler packed with ice. Leipheimer's blood bag would then be stored in the hotel room's mini-fridge. David Witt would drive to Girona to pick up the blood that Landis had removed from himself and drive back to Montpellier to store it alongside Leipheimer's. Landis's grand plan to dope at the Tour was finally falling into place.

But Landis had forgotten one important item: a Ziploc bag for a thermometer. They needed it because the thermometer was electronic and not waterproof, and it needed to stay dry. Lim drove his two friends to store after store as Landis and Leipheimer asked for Ziploc bags in bad French accents that sounded like *The Pink Panther*'s Inspector Clouseau.

"*Est-ce que vous avez un sachet du Ziploc? Ziploc sac? Sac du Ziploc? Avez-vous?*" They became so desperate that once, stuck in traffic, Leipheimer rolled down the car window to stop a passerby. "*Excusez-moi, où est une supermarché? Je cherche pour un sachet Ziploc.*" As Lim giggled, he realized that, like his companions, he was veering into madness. They found the Ziploc and drove back to Girona that night.

Three days later, Landis flew to Valencia to reclaim the blood that he had deposited with del Moral. His plan went awry. Lim saw him afterward and quickly noticed that Landis looked pale and sickly. Landis's temperature soared. He was nauseated. He and Lim suspected that the blood transfusion was the culprit and that the blood had gone bad. They both knew the worst-case scenario: Landis could die.

"We need you to get to an ER," Lim said. "A doctor needs to look at you—and now!"

Landis refused. He didn't want anything to thwart his Tour chances, and especially didn't want the news coming out that blood doping had possibly made him ill. The race was one week away.

After two long days had passed, Landis recovered. But he knew he was in trouble. With the bad blood in him, his hematocrit level had plummeted, meaning he would start the Tour at a deficit. He had one choice—and that was to boost his level back to normal by using the blood that was supposed to dope him for the Tour. His father-in-law, David Witt, hadn't taken it to Montpellier yet.

Landis took that blood bag and disappeared into his room alone. He left the door ajar. Lim walked past the room to see Landis crouched in a corner with the blood bag taped to a wall and a needle in his arm. His blood was going back where it came from.

Now, though, he had zero bags of blood to use at the Tour. Dr. Landis was having a tough time—both of his plans to blood-dope at the Tour had failed.

The first aborted attempt had been with del Moral, when Landis balked because of the doctor's relationship with Armstrong. He had reinfused that blood and gotten sick. The second attempt backfired because Landis needed new blood in him after the bad del Moral blood bag had made him so weak. Landis used that second bag of blood to boost his red blood cell count even before the Tour began.

Oddly, Landis seemed happier. Later that morning after his transfusion, he pounded out his workout in the mud and rain, and came to a stop alongside a deep canyon overlooking farms and vineyards. As Lim watched, Landis took off his clothes, piece by piece, and wadded them all into a ball that he tossed into the canyon.

There he stood, naked, and let out a series of screams so primal they raised the hair on Lim's arms.

"How'd Grenoble work out for you?" Armstrong said.

During the 2005 Tour's first mountain stage—after the Tour had passed through Grenoble—Armstrong rode alongside Landis to drop a hint that, yes, he knew of Landis's initial plan to blood-dope in Grenoble. Landis surmised that del Moral had told him.

Now it all fit together. Landis was so paranoid that he thought Armstrong might have convinced del Moral to mishandle Landis's blood.

"Holy shit, remember when I got sick?" he told Lim at a stage finish. "What if I got sick because Lance fucked with my blood?"

Would Armstrong do anything to physically harm Landis? Lim didn't know, but believed Landis believed it. In late 2013, Landis told me he had reacted badly just once after receiving blood from del Moral, but that he didn't know why. For Lim, though, the possibility of Armstrong's having a hand in that incident confirmed his opinion of him: Landis considered Armstrong the enemy.

A few days later, Lim bumped into Vaughters, who was working as a guide for a bike tour company. Landis had been talking to

Vaughters about taking a job with Vaughters's new development team, called TIAA-CREF. Lim was relieved to see a familiar face, someone he could talk to.

"Jonathan, this sport is a fucking mess," he said. "Let me just tell you what happened to me in the last two weeks."

Vaughters wanted to know if the sport had cleaned up since 2002, when he retired from racing in Europe. Lim told him, "Not a chance—it's even worse."

"It's horrible; it's like a nuclear arms race, but the two superpowers can't control it anymore. Doping is so commonplace that individual riders are like kids making their own atomic bombs. They are like little terrorists, with no formal training, but with access to plutonium."

Lim told Vaughters many stories that Landis had told him about doping on the Postal team—how the doping had grown complex during Landis's time there.

He said that Armstrong's team used a motorcycle courier to transport blood to riders. The blood was kept cold by the motorcycle's refrigerated panniers, and Landis had photos of them.

Lim said the doping culture was so competitive that Landis believed Armstrong's line—"How'd Grenoble work out for you?"—meant Armstrong knew Landis had received tainted blood.

Vaughters thought, "This is crazy."

Two days after the Tour, Vaughters ("Cyclevaughters") sent an AOL instant message to Frankie Andreu ("Fdreu"). Vaughters was relaying to Andreu what Lim had told him.

It began a string of eighty-three messages, mostly about Armstrong and the Postal Service squad, some specifically addressing the doping.

CYCLEVAUGHTERS: anyhow, i never can quite figure out why I don't just play along with the lance crowd—i mean shit it would make my life easier, eh? it's not like I never played with the hotsauce, eh?

FDREU: I play along, my wife does not, and Lance hates us both

FDREU: it's a no win situation, you know how he is. Once you leave the team or do something wrong, you are forever banned

Vaughters wrote that when he went to the Crédit Agricole team, he saw that not "all the teams got 25 injections every day" and said he "felt guilty" for what he had done on Postal Service. On Crédit Agricole, he said, riders received no injections. He wrote, "So, I realized lance was full of shit when he'd say everyone was doing it."

Vaughters and Andreu commented on Hincapie's unexpected success in the mountains at that 2005 Tour. He was a specialist at one-day classic races. Yet he had won the Tour's hardest stage. It was a six-mountain odyssey that only the best climbers handled at great speeds. Hincapie's victory was the perfect example of how blood-doping changed the sport. That victory was as improbable as a 100-meter sprinter winning a marathon.

FDREU: explain that, classics to climber

CYCLEVAUGHTERS: i don't know—i want to trust George

CYCLEVAUGHTERS: but the thing is on that team, you think it's normal

Vaughters told Andreu about the allegation that Armstrong and Bruyneel apparently "dumped Floyd's rest day blood refill down the toilet in front of him in last yrs tour to make him ride bad," and that Landis had photos of the refrigerated panniers on the motorcycle that transported riders' blood to the Tour.

> **FDREU:** crazy! It's just keep going to new levels
> **CYCLEVAUGHTERS:** yeah, its complicated, but with enough money you can do it.

Vaughters told Andreu that he could "explain the whole way lance dupes everyone, that it's very complex how they avoid all the controls now, but it's not any new drug or anything, just the resources and planning to pull off a well devised plan." He repeated what Lim had told him: that riders on Armstrong's team in 2004 had their blood removed before the Dauphiné, which is held in June. A man on a motorcycle would bring them the blood on the Tour's rest day. They would refuel and take off together on the next mountain stage.

> **FDREU:** I know, I get tired of hearing how great Lance is, what a super person, etc. It's crazy and it's hard to not just tell people he is a cheat and asshole

Landis finished ninth in that 2005 Tour without blood-doping—an amazing feat. Leipheimer, who had transfused blood with Landis's help during the race, finished sixth. Collectively, American riders had their best showing in years.

But, as always, Armstrong was the main attraction. He had won a record seventh Tour de France in the fastest average time in history—26.8 miles an hour. He had a rock star girlfriend in Sheryl Crow. His cell phone's contact list included Bill Clinton and U2's Bono.

His foundation, which would become known as Livestrong, was booming. What started out as just a bicycle ride in Austin for nearly three thousand people had become a brilliant story of philanthropic branding. From 2002 to 2005, the foundation's revenue grew nearly eight times, propelled to over $63 million. By the time Armstrong won that final Tour, the foundation had sold nearly 53 million little yellow Livestrong wristbands at a dollar each. Donations rose by about $10 million in the year after the bracelets were introduced.

Many people said the bracelet meant more than a connection with Armstrong. Buddy Boren, a sixty-one-year-old Dallas cyclist and cancer survivor, wore his bracelet in 2005 as he cycled the perimeter of Texas to raise money for cancer. "People say, I see you're wearing your Lance Armstrong bracelet," he told the *Dallas Morning News*. "I say, 'It's not just a Lance Armstrong bracelet.' I tell them it's a Livestrong bracelet—and I'm going to live my life strong."

Each year, Nike gave the foundation $7.5 million, which included $2.5 million that went specifically to Armstrong for his endorsement of its products. In 2005, Nike branched out from marketing just the Livestrong bracelets to selling a line of Livestrong gear—jerseys, shorts, vests and other items marking the date Armstrong was diagnosed with cancer, 10/2. Nike called it "his carpe diem day, a day to overcome adversity and reaffirm life."

Stores were requesting so much Livestrong gear from Nike that the company was worried that its other departments—like Nike basketball and Nike running—would suffer because stores wanted to sell Armstrong's gear rather than merchandise from Nike's other lines.

In its first eight years, Livestrong raised $85 million for cancer research, cancer awareness and programs to help people with the disease navigate the cancer-treatment bureaucracy. It had supplied more than $15 million in grants.

At the 2004 Ride for the Roses, 6,500 cyclists raised $6 million for the foundation in a day. Other Livestrong athletic events—more bike races, run/walk events and triathlons—popped up across the nation. The watchdog group Charity Navigator gave the organization its highest rating, four stars.

For many people, the money raised was the least of Armstrong's impact on the cancer community. Cancer once came with a stigma. It was the "C-word" because people were afraid to even say it out loud. Armstrong and Livestrong helped change that. He made it fashionable to wear a yellow wristband identifying you as part of a club of cancer survivors or those affected by a loved one's battle. Presidential candidate John Kerry even wore one on his campaign trail, and photos spread of that little yellow bracelet hanging from his wrist. Armstrong was the leader of the "Livestrong Army," bringing together people from all over the world.

He was a member of the President's Cancer Panel. Though he'd hated public speaking at first and was raw at it, he agreed to be trained by the best—including high-powered political consultant Mark McKinnon, a board member of Armstrong's foundation. Armstrong became a polished orator. When he spoke, even powerful people listened. And, McKinnon said, "When he wanted to turn it on, he could be very good." Armstrong toyed with running for governor of Texas.

Senators John Kerry and John McCain, both cancer survivors and influential lawmakers in Washington, listened to Armstrong's impassioned speeches. The summer of Armstrong's seventh Tour victory, the senators shared their survivor stories on Livestrong's Web site.

"Lance Armstrong has been instrumental in demonstrating to people affected by cancer that fighting not just the disease but the fear and isolation is paramount," McCain said. "When people realize they are not alone, they gain the strength to handle obstacles they face when their lives are affected by cancer. That sense of unity is a powerful tool."

People in the cancer community read Armstrong's autobiography, *It's Not About the Bike*, and for some it became their bible, a handbook of hope and perseverance.

"I don't think there's anybody involved who would say the foundation would be what it is today if it wasn't for Lance Armstrong," McKinnon said. "But not just because Lance Armstrong gave us the equity and the interest. He put sweat equity into it. He put a lot of time and energy and thinking. And what Lance does well is drive an organization. He drove an organization like he drove the bike team."

Armstrong's involvement came with a personal touch as well. He visited cancer wards and children's hospitals to hear people's stories. He often was eager to call or e-mail a cancer patient if someone asked him to. "There's not a whole lot of things more powerful than life," McKinnon said. "He was telling people, you can live."

One note sent to the foundation in 2005 came from a ten-year-old girl who had survived cancer. She said, "Thank you Lance for being strong. I was strong, too."

His impact on cycling was unparalleled. The number of riders with official USA Cycling licenses rose 21 percent from 2001 to

2005. Trek Bicycle Corporation's sales had doubled since 1998, the year it signed him. "If not for Lance, we wouldn't be expanding our factory and we wouldn't have new offices with carpeting and windows and a gym," said Zap Espinoza, a company spokesman. Everything Armstrong had touched in the sport seemed to flourish. People called it the "Lance Effect."

By the time he won his seventh Tour, he was one of the world's megastars. To reach that status, he had survived not only cancer but years of scrutiny about the legitimacy of his athletic achievements.

The French government had failed to prove he used performance-enhancing drugs. He'd brushed off accusations by his former *soigneur* Emma O'Reilly. He'd emerged relatively unscathed from an investigative book by David Walsh and Pierre Ballester. Journalists had asked him repeatedly if he doped, and he'd always rebutted them with such conviction that it seemed impossible he was lying.

As Armstrong became more successful, he became even more defiant. On a July day in 2005, he stood atop the podium at the Tour de France after winning the race for an unimaginable seventh straight year. There he heard the cheers from the thousands of people lining both sides of Paris's grand boulevard, the Champs-Élysées. Smiling alongside him were his children—five-year-old Luke and the three-year-old twins, Grace and Isabelle. The girls wore sunflower yellow dresses that matched the iridescently bright leader's jersey worn by their father.

As he looked out onto the crowd, Armstrong said, "Finally, the last thing I'll say to the people who don't believe in cycling, the cynics and the skeptics, I'm sorry for you, I'm sorry that you can't dream big. I'm sorry you don't believe in miracles.

"But this is one hell of a race. This is a great sporting event and you should stand around and believe it. You should believe in these athletes, and you should believe in these people. I'll be a fan of the Tour de France for as long as I live. And there are no secrets—this is a hard sporting event and hard work wins it. Vive Le Tour."

It was over for Armstrong. He would retire from racing. There was nothing more to do. He had beaten the Eurobastards, the gendarmes, the trolls, the Alps, the Pyrenees. He had beaten them all.

Or so he thought.

CHAPTER 17

At a glance, nothing about Bob Hamman suggested he would become one of Armstrong's greatest enemies. He wasn't an incredible, volatile athlete—a Floyd Landis—driven by vengeance and envy. Nor was he a single-minded spitfire—a Betsy Andreu—motivated to expose what he saw as moral turpitude.

When Armstrong won his seventh and final Tour de France, Hamman was sixty-six years old, a portly, white-haired bridge champion. But he did have one thing in common with Landis and Andreu: He didn't want to be cheated. In his case, he didn't want Armstrong to cheat him out of millions of dollars.

Hamman and his Dallas-based insurance company, SCA Promotions, had entered into a contract in 2001 with Armstrong and Tailwind Sports, the company that managed the Postal Service/Discovery Channel cycling teams. SCA would pay Armstrong a bonus for winning his fourth, fifth and sixth Tours. The company paid $1.5 million for his fourth and $3 million for his fifth. But it balked at paying $5 million for his sixth.

SCA balked after Hamman read David Walsh's book *L.A. Confidentiel*. He decided SCA wasn't paying Armstrong a penny until he personally investigated Walsh's claims. If Armstrong really did dope, Hamman felt that he didn't need to pay him. News of Hamman's withholding the bonus got out in the fall of 2004.

Armstrong retaliated by doing what had become a habit: He filed a lawsuit.

Armstrong was outraged that someone would challenge him in front of the American public. Such attacks usually came from the French, or maybe from reporters like Walsh, who wrote for a British newspaper, but certainly not from a fellow Texan. Hamman's office was in Dallas, just down the street from Armstrong's boyhood home.

Bill Stapleton, Armstrong's agent, went right to work. First, he hammered at Hamman's credibility with a full-page ad in *Sports Business Journal*. It touted Armstrong's Tour wins as an achievement that, "along with his inspirational story of cancer survivorship, has made his story transcend sport and culture." The ad claimed that SCA didn't live up to its contract and was trying to change "the rules when it is time to fulfill its obligation."

Stapleton's ad signaled to SCA that the fight would be dirty. Hamman's son, Chris, told Hamman to back down, saying, "Their PR machine is too big." But Bob Hamman wouldn't quit. He wanted to keep his company's $5 million, but he also wanted to stand up for his company's integrity. Armstrong and Stapleton should have known Hamman was a fierce competitor—he was arguably the best bridge player in history, a twelve-time world champion, the Michael Jordan of a complex, challenging game mastered only by players who, in Hamman's words, "hate their opponents and who want to win, win, win."

SCA Promotions underwrote the risk companies took when they held special promotions and events, such as a million-dollar prize for a half-court basketball shot or a new car for a hole-in-one. SCA had accepted propositions of all kinds. Would a frog do a world-record jump? (The eventual outcome was no.) Could a farmer grow a pumpkin that weighed more than 1,000 pounds? (Outcome: yes. It grew to the size of a Volkswagen.) Could someone find a cockroach set loose in Houston bearing a numbered tag? (The roach disappeared forever.)

SCA also took on risks in sports. Could Ernie Els win the British Open when the bookmakers had the odds at 470-1? (SCA lost that one.) Could Armstrong win a fourth, fifth and sixth Tour in a row? (Hamman thought no. Wrong again.)

Though Hamman had heard the doping accusations that followed Armstrong, he sold Tailwind Sports the $420,000 insurance contract—a legal way of gambling, really—because he believed no cancer survivor would use drugs after nearly dying. It was an educated guess by a man who spent much of his life calculating other people's moves.

Hamman had dropped out of college to compete in professional bridge, a game he had played since the age of six or seven. He has won more than fifty North American championships and was the top-ranked player in the world for twenty straight years, until 2004.

He told me it angered him that he had made the Armstrong deal based on the fundamental premise that cycling would enforce its rules. He said he would have passed on the deal if he had known about what he called Armstrong's close relationship with the sport's ruling body, the UCI.

Throughout Armstrong's reign, Stapleton frequently made trips to the UCI's headquarters in Switzerland to visit Hein Verbruggen, the UCI president from 1991 to 2005. Part of Stapleton's dealings with Verbruggen focused on money. In 2006, Stapleton told me that Armstrong had donated $100,000 to the UCI's antidoping program. Later, he said he'd gotten the numbers mixed up, that the donation was only $25,000. Pat McQuaid, Verbrug-

gen's successor, said in 2006 that he couldn't remember any donation from Armstrong.

It all mystified Sylvia Schenk. Once president of the German
Cycling Federation and a former member of the UCI management
committee, Schenk told me in 2005 that the Armstrong donation
was more like $500,000 and that it smacked of impropriety. She
claims that neither Verbruggen nor McQuaid ever explained to
Schenk or the rest of the management committee the purpose for
that donation, or how the UCI used that money. "It was kept secret," she told me, adding that she assumed that Armstrong had
gotten special treatment from the UCI, but didn't have hard evidence to back up that belief. "How much, we will never know because Hein Verbruggen and Pat McQuaid wouldn't address it."

Years later, McQuaid said that in 2002 Armstrong and his
wife had given a personal check for $25,000 to the UCI and that
Stapleton's company sent $100,000 to the cycling union in 2005.
The money was used to purchase the UCI's blood analysis machine to help in the fight against doping.

Those donations—whenever they were made and however
much they were for—were only a part of the financial ties Armstrong and USA Cycling had with Verbruggen, who had been the
longtime president of the UCI. For example, from 2001 to 2004
part of Verbruggen's personal financial assets were managed by
the investment bank founded by Thomas Weisel, the same man
who owned Armstrong's cycling team. The broker handling Verbruggen's accounts was Jim Ochowicz, Armstrong's former team
manager and close friend, and the president of USA Cycling's
board of directors from 2002 to 2006. Travis Tygart of USADA
said those ties "stink to high heaven" because of the conflicts of
interest and the obvious risk of abuse that those ties created.

For his part, Hamman learned about those donations only during the arbitration of Armstrong's lawsuit.

Hamman's first problem had been finding a lawyer. Dallas loves its sports heroes: its Cowboys, its high school football players and, yes, Lance Armstrong, a Texan once considered an outsider by classmates who called him "a sissy who wears tights." Hamman said several law firms turned him down because they didn't want to be seen attacking the hometown hero Armstrong.

So Hamman ended up at Jeff Tillotson's door. Tillotson, a partner at Lynn Tillotson Pinker & Cox, was initially reluctant, but felt obliged to take the case because no one else wanted it. His mother had survived lymphoma and was part of Armstrong's cheering section. When she learned her son was representing Hamman, she said, "I'm so embarrassed. I read his book and it motivated me to survive." It got worse for Tillotson.

"As soon as we were publicly identified," the lawyer told me, "I probably got a hundred fifty e-mails within the first few days, saying you're a shithead, you're a liar, I hope your firm goes under."

As part of his case strategy, Tillotson wanted the public to know the doping accusations in the Walsh-Ballester book. He sent the book to U.S. publishers and offered his legal services for free if Armstrong sued for libel after the book was published in the United States. But there were no takers.

Then came a huge break. On August 23, 2005—three days after Armstrong spent the day riding bikes with George W. Bush on the president's Texas ranch—the influential French sports newspaper *L'Equipe* ran a big headline across its front page: "LE MENSONGE ARMSTRONG" ("THE ARMSTRONG LIE").

The story claimed that Armstrong's remaining backup urine samples from the 1999 Tour had been retroactively tested for

EPO. Six came back positive for the banned endurance-boosting drug. "The extraordinary champion, the escape from cancer, has become a legend by means of a lie," wrote Damien Ressiot, the *L'Equipe* reporter.

Ressiot landed his scoop by figuring out which of the tested urine samples were Armstrong's. (Samples are identified only by numbers.) By antidoping rules, however, the six positives for EPO were not official because the tests had been conducted for research purposes only.

Quickly, Armstrong claimed that the scientists had not followed proper testing procedures and, because of that, the test results could not be trusted. No, he had not tested positive six times, he said, though *L'Equipe* and the lab insisted that he did. Armstrong said he was innocent.

Several cycling and Olympic officials defended Armstrong. Gerard Bisceglia, USA Cycling's chief executive, called *L'Equipe*'s accusations "preposterous" because only Armstrong's backup samples had been tested. For a test to be officially positive, both the athlete's initial and backup sample must test positive. Sergey Bubka, chairman of the athletes' commission of the International Olympic Committee, called for the French lab to be suspended because it had breached antidoping rules.

Broken rules or not, the damage to Armstrong was already done. Dick Pound, the head of the World Anti-Doping Agency, publicly said the case was finally "not a he said-she said scenario" and that scientific research proved something was awry with Armstrong's urine samples. "Unless the documents are forgeries or manipulations of them, it's a case that has to be answered."

Pound said he heard from Armstrong first in a series of e-mails, one with the word *Livestrong* written three times in capital letters and underlined, in the signature section of the note. Then

Pound said he received what he called a "Kafkaesque phone call" from Armstrong, in which Armstrong told him again and again, "I love my sport." The WADA boss took that to mean Armstrong would fight his innocence to the end, no matter what the cost, so Pound had better lay off him. After that call, without any warning, Armstrong sent a letter to the president of the IOC asking that Pound be expelled from the organization because he was "a recidivist violator of ethical standards."

Some other officials took the EPO positives as proof that Armstrong had cheated. Tour director Jean-Marie Leblanc, the same man who said Armstrong had saved the sport by winning the 1999 Tour of Redemption, said *L'Equipe*'s allegations were the first "proven scientific facts" that Armstrong had doped.

"He owes explanations to us, to everyone who followed the Tour," Leblanc said. "Today what *L'Equipe* revealed shows me that I was fooled and we were all fooled."

Leblanc wanted an explanation from Armstrong, and he got it. The day of the *L'Equipe* story, Armstrong called Bob Costas, the sportscaster then working as a cohost on the television talk show *Larry King Live*. He asked to go on the show for a full hour to refute the allegations. Of course, Costas said.

Armstrong tried to blame *L'Equipe*'s accusations on the tense USA-France relationship. (France refused to join the U.S. invasion of Iraq in 2003.) He also said that the day before the 2005 Tour, the French minister of sport took two urine samples and two blood samples from him, but from no other riders.

"I can't say 'witch hunt' loud enough," Armstrong said. "This thing stinks. I've said it for longer than seven years: I have never doped. I can say it again. But I've said it for seven years. It doesn't help. But the fact of the matter is I haven't."

He told Costas, "If you consider my situation, a guy who comes back from arguably, you know, a death sentence, why would I then enter into a sport and dope myself up and risk my life again? That's crazy. I would never do that. No. No way."

Costas said, "There's no way they could have found EPO in your urine because you're flatly saying you never used it?"

"When I peed in that bottle, there wasn't EPO in it. No way."

Costas asked if Armstrong planned to sue over the accusations. Armstrong said yes, possibly, but he didn't know where to start. The French lab? *L'Equipe*? The French sports minister? The World Anti-Doping Agency? "All of these people violated a serious code of ethics," Armstrong said.

Costas then said to Armstrong what millions of the rider's fans likely thought: "Here in the United States you are one of the most admired athletes of—of all time. People do not want to believe this of Lance Armstrong."

Armstrong: "Right."

Armstrong ended the interview by reminding viewers why they would want to believe that he was clean: because he was a celebrity hero. He talked about his cancer work with Livestrong. Larry King asked if he was going to marry Sheryl Crow, causing Costas to pipe up, "You know, that's why Larry's here, Lance. I wouldn't have asked that." He seemed irritated that King had veered from the very serious subject of Armstrong's possible doping.

Armstrong provided no real answer to the question about his love life, either, and the show ended awkwardly, with plastic smiles all around.

Within two weeks of *L'Equipe*'s story, and soon after the damage control accomplished with the help of Costas and King, Armstrong shared with the American public his personal happy news.

Two and a half years after he told Kristin Armstrong that he'd had enough of their perfect-on-the-outside marriage, he had, in fact, proposed marriage to Crow. The tabloids ate it up.

Hamman and his lawyers knew they needed an airtight case to beat this Houdini who'd escaped from every perilous situation in his career. Now, on national television with Costas and King, Armstrong had wriggled out of an accusation that he had tested positive for EPO *six times*.

"You're swinging for the fences with these guys, because they have celebrity wattage," Tillotson said. "All Lance had to do was pick up the phone and he was on a talk show bashing us, denying the allegations on TV."

Hamman, the master bridge player, reckoned he had a losing hand. So he came up with a Plan B that was devilish in its conception.

If SCA lost the suit—nearly a certainty; a contract is a contract—Hamman believed the evidence gathered under oath would convince open-minded people that Armstrong had, in fact, doped. In turn, he hoped, sports entities that had the power to do something about Armstrong's cheating would open an official investigation into the allegations raised by the SCA case. Hamman thought that an official investigation might uncover the truth and even result in Armstrong's losing his Tour de France victories. In that roundabout way, SCA might get its $5 million back.

"Bob was insistent that he wanted all the facts out there," Tillotson said. "He was playing the long game. Even if he never got his money back, one day the truth would be known about Lance, and he would've had his measure of peace."

Walsh, Ballester and New Zealand cyclist Stephen Swart

agreed to be witnesses in the SCA suit, as did Betsy Andreu, who supplied background information and texted/e-mailed/called Hamman nearly continuously. Tillotson had to tell Hamman, "Back off from Betsy. She's not on our team in the legal sense. She's a witness." Tillotson told me Armstrong's lawyers had requested copies of her communications to prove she was a prejudiced witness. "It played into Lance's hand that she was a crazy bitch," Tillotson said.

Tillotson and his fellow SCA lawyers used sworn testimony to paint a vivid picture of Armstrong the doper. Swart said Armstrong had pushed the Motorola team in 1995 to use EPO. A blood doping expert, Michael Ashenden, said Armstrong's urine samples from the 1999 Tour showed evidence "beyond a reasonable doubt" that Armstrong had used EPO. He pointed out that Armstrong's hematocrit levels rose at certain points in the Tour where EPO shots would have helped his performance. Emma O'Reilly, the former *soigneur*, said she helped cover up Armstrong's drug use.

The most riveting testimony came from Betsy and Frankie Andreu. They were served subpoenas to testify in Detroit, and took turns testifying. While Frankie stayed in Dearborn to watch the kids, Betsy drove to a hotel for her deposition.

She walked into the hotel to see Armstrong in the hallway with his Austin cycling buddy and Stapleton's business partner, Bart Knaggs. She walked back out and called her husband.

"He's here! Lance is here, Frankie, what do I do?"

"You've got to be shittin' me."

"Nope. And you know what? He's got to be stupid if he thinks he's going to scare me."

She took his presence as a compliment, as proof that he thought her testimony would be consequential. It emboldened her to tell the truth, more so than she already was. She was still upset that he had called Frankie just three days before to remind him that Armstrong's cancer doctor, Craig Nichols, had agreed to submit a sworn affidavit in the case. In that testimony, Nichols would say that he had no record of Armstrong's hospital room confession.

Armstrong told Frankie, "How's it going to look if you say it happened and the doctor says it didn't? I'm just looking out for you." The Andreus weren't fooled by his faux thoughtfulness. He hadn't called them for a year and now he cared about how people would perceive them?

Despite her toughness, Betsy was nervous when she came face-to-face with Armstrong in the conference room where the deposition was about to take place. She was shocked when he greeted her with a wide smile and oozed kindness as they shook hands. She recalled how they used to say hello with a kiss on the cheek.

He whipped out a stack of photos and started showing her photos of him with Crow and photos of his children. Her oldest son, Frankie Jr., and Armstrong's son, Luke, were the same age. Now look how much Luke had grown! Betsy sensed that it was Armstrong's way of saying, "C'mon, old buddy, old pal. You and I are friends. You wouldn't do this to a friend, would you?"

Tillotson was also surprised to learn that Armstrong and Knaggs had flown in. Armstrong was on his way from Texas to New York, where he was to host *Saturday Night Live* and where Crow would be the musical guest. Tillotson thought it was a tip-off that SCA was onto something. Tillotson thought, "OK, this is the most famous athlete on the planet and he supposedly thinks we're all liars and crazy, so why would he bother to show up?"

Armstrong, the man who had sent the Andreus an e-mail

with one word in the subject line, "Cuidado"—Spanish for "Be careful"—now sat at a conference room table hearing Betsy Andreu testify under oath.

Tillotson asked if she had knowledge of Armstrong's doping. She said yes, and described the day, October 28, 1996, that she and Frankie visited Armstrong in the Indiana hospital. She named those who were there: Frankie; Chris Carmichael; Carmichael's then-girlfriend, Paige; Armstrong's old girlfriend Lisa Shiels; and his Oakley representative, Stephanie McIlvain. Andreu described the doctor: young, thin, glasses, black hair.

She repeated the doctor's question to Armstrong: "Have you ever taken performance-enhancing drugs?"

And Armstrong's answer: "Growth hormone, cortisone, EPO, steroids and testosterone."

Betsy Andreu told Tillotson everything she knew about Armstrong. She recounted how many people she had told about Armstrong's confession: friends, cousins, reporters, wives of friends—twenty-three people in all. Then she said, "I'm sorry. Two more names." Later, she added three more, including a neighbor and Kristin Armstrong's mother, Ethel Richard.

She talked about the mysterious package, the "liquid gold," that trainer Pepe Martí allegedly delivered to Armstrong after dinner that night in France. She recalled Armstrong meeting Ferrari at a gas station en route to the Milan-San Remo race. She testified that Kristin Armstrong knew about Lance's doping, that Kristin said it was "a necessary evil." She described Bill Stapleton asking Frankie—who was secretly taping the talk—to keep Betsy quiet about Armstrong's hospital room admission because it "will blow the whole sport."

For years, she could say nothing publicly. She believed that breaking the code of silence would destroy her husband's cycling career. But now, for three hours, she unburdened herself.

By the time she was done, Armstrong was long gone. He'd taken off during a lunch break, bound for Manhattan. It was a relief for Frankie. He shared none of his wife's confidence.

In his turn under oath, Frankie took Betsy's place at the table in the conference room and confirmed her version of the events that had occurred in Armstrong's hospital room. But when asked if he had known Armstrong used performance-enhancing drugs, he said no. Asked if he ever had a discussion with Armstrong about using EPO or had knowledge of Armstrong's using drugs, again he said no.

Unlike his wife, Frankie Andreu remained so afraid of Armstrong that he perjured himself, several of his former teammates said.

Stephen Swart, a former Motorola teammate, couldn't explain why Frankie would have denied under oath that he knew about Armstrong's doping—or that he ever talked to Armstrong about doping—because he said the whole Motorola team in 1995 talked about using EPO. He said Frankie was just another participant in the drug culture of cycling and of the Motorola team, just like Armstrong was, just like many top riders at the time were. He recalled that Frankie's hematocrit at the 1995 Tour was nearly 50.

Armstrong said there were "no secrets" on the team back then, and that many riders on the squad—including Andreu—were open about their drug use, which included taking cortisone or cortisone-type substances and later EPO, which he claims was overseen by team doctor Max Testa. Andreu denies that he and his teammates ever talked about their drug use so nonchalantly among them.

After providing his testimony, Tillotson said Andreu corrected his written deposition and in doing so, Andreu seemed to backtrack. He now testified he "wasn't sure" if Armstrong had used performance-enhancing drugs, and that he wasn't sure if he ever spoke to him about EPO one-on-one. He also said, "While he [Armstrong] was racing postcancer, I can't recall at this time any use of drugs firsthand."

Instead of going with his initial comment that he never heard Armstrong say he had used PEDs, Andreu changed his testimony to something that was borderline comical: "This was the first time I heard him admit all the drugs he admitted to taking."

No matter what Andreu said under oath—or, really, didn't say—Armstrong still felt threatened by the Andreus' testimony. He was so frightened that his skillful public relations people went to work to push positive press about him. First, they announced that the Lance Armstrong Foundation had given $1.5 million to the Indiana University School of Medicine. The donation established an endowment for a chair in oncology for Lawrence Einhorn, Armstrong's primary oncologist.

Later, Nichols, one of Armstrong's doctors and a board member of Livestrong, submitted an affidavit to the arbitrators, just as Armstrong had warned the Andreus he would. Nichols said he had monitored Armstrong's blood levels on a regular basis from January 1997 to October 2001, and that he had seen nothing to suggest drug use. He said, "Had Lance Armstrong been using EPO to enhance his cycling performance, I would have likely identified differences in his blood levels." He told me in 2013 that Armstrong had duped him, then hung up on me when I asked him to elaborate.

Four days after the Andreus' testimony in Michigan, Armstrong hosted *Saturday Night Live*. In his monologue, he says: "I've been working really hard on the show, trying to do a good job, but just not too good. Because the last time I did something too good, the French started testing my urine every fifteen minutes."

A fake audience member then got up and asks in an exaggerated French accent if he can have a urine sample. Armstrong says no. The man points at him and yells: "It's our race! Stop winning it! J'accuse!"

After months of depositions and three weeks of the arbitration hearing, Tillotson thought he'd learned the inner workings of cycling and how far people would go to protect its secrets. Armstrong had called Emma O'Reilly "a whore" and said Betsy Andreu lied about him because she hated him and that Frankie Andreu lied about him because "he's just trying to back up his old lady." He said he'd never dope because it would cause him to lose "the faith of all cancer survivors around the world . . . hundreds of millions of people."

Tillotson saw Stapleton, the agent, deny that there was a possibility that Armstrong had doped without him knowing it. "It is inconceivable," Stapleton said in his testimony. He said he even met secretly in 2000 with executives of Coca-Cola, one of Armstrong's worried sponsors, "looked them in the eyes" and gave them his word that Armstrong was clean.

He saw the Oakley rep, Stephanie McIlvain, testify—in direct contradiction of Betsy Andreu's testimony—that she knew nothing of an Armstrong drug confession in his Indiana University hospital room. (Later, a phone conversation between McIlvain and Tour winner Greg LeMond was given to the arbitrators. In it, McIlvain said she did hear the confession. "I was in the room. I heard it," she said.)

Still, by February 2006, Tillotson knew Hamman's case was going nowhere.

The arbitration panel had said that SCA would likely have to pay Armstrong the $5 million because, as the original contract stated, the money was due to him for the simple reason that he had officially won the Tour de France. So SCA wrote a check for $7.5 million—the $5 million plus fees—to end the parade of witnesses who may or may not have been telling the truth.

Armstrong added it to his string of legal victories. He also had won the libel suit against Walsh and the *Sunday Times* of London, with the newspaper paying him about $500,000. (But he ended up dropping all of his libel cases in France, saying they were a waste of time and money.)

When the SCA case ended, Armstrong declared it another victory. "I recently won a major arbitration, defeating allegations of performance-enhancing drugs after a three-week trial," he said in a statement.

"It's over," Armstrong said. "We won. They lost. I was yet again completely vindicated."

That was not exactly true. The two parties had settled the case, but the arbitrators had not determined whether he had doped or not. Still, when I spoke to Armstrong, I couldn't get him to admit that he hadn't won the case outright.

"I was totally vindicated," he told me in 2006.

"But they didn't rule on whether you doped or not, so technically you didn't clear your name at all," I said.

"No, I won the case, hands down."

The same week, Armstrong was in the news again when he broke off his five-month engagement with Crow. Later, he said it was because she wanted to have a child and he didn't. But Crow would go on to announce darker news: She was fighting breast cancer.

CHAPTER 18

As Hamman had hoped, evidence against Armstrong spread. News organizations around the country reported leaks of the SCA testimony. Even before the press got ahold of it, USADA was on the phone to Tillotson. *Could their lawyers come to review the evidence?*

Less than a week after the case was settled, Tygart and an associate, Bill Bock, flew to Dallas to debrief SCA's lawyer.

Tygart and Bock were especially interested in Frankie Andreu's testimony. They believed that if a rider that close to Armstrong had provided information on his doping, they could build a strong case. They returned to Colorado Springs with copies of everything—depositions, hearing transcripts, exhibits from both sides.

Hamman had lost once, but now the bridge master had dealt himself a second hand. And this time, USADA was in the game.

In the deepening love affair between the American public and Lance Armstrong, however, the SCA settlement meant little. No one much cared about an obscure company called SCA—they only cared about Armstrong, an international celebrity who had transcended sports by raising hundreds of millions of dollars for the Livestrong Foundation. He had built a formidable bank of goodwill. The rest was mind-numbing legalese and creeping litigation.

What helped the public believe him when he insisted that he never doped was a report released in the spring of 2006 that addressed *L'Equipe*'s accusation that six of Armstrong's urine samples from 1999 had tested positive for EPO.

Less than two months after *L'Equipe* broke the story, the UCI had commissioned what it called "an independent report" to examine how the French lab conducted its analysis of the urine samples and how the news of the results were leaked to the press.

Dutch lawyer Emile Vrijman, the former head of the national antidoping agency in the Netherlands who later represented athletes in doping cases, was paid by the UCI to compile the report. He said his investigation would be unbiased and that neither the UCI nor Armstrong would have a role in it.

"In no way will they be able to see the report in advance or influence the results," Vrijman said.

Behind the scenes, according to two people with direct knowledge of how the report came together, it was the complete opposite. The whole idea allegedly started as a way the UCI could make Armstrong—its star—and the entire sport appear clean when in fact the doping problem that had hovered over cycling for a hundred years still existed. Armstrong, his agent and his lawyers supposedly were upset that *L'Equipe* had been able to figure out which urine samples from the 1999 Tour were his—and they blamed the UCI for it. The cycling union needed to help fix the mess it and *L'Equipe* had caused, they allegedly said.

Pat McQuaid, the UCI president, apparently hired Vrijman at the urging of Verbruggen, who was the UCI's honorary president after stepping down from the head role in 2005. Verbruggen, a Dutchman who was a powerful player in the Olympic movement and an honorary IOC member, was supposedly friends with both Armstrong and Vrijman.

Instead of acting independently as he said he would, Vrijman allegedly received feedback from the UCI in compiling the report, according to the two people with knowledge of how the report was created. Vrijman supposedly also received input from Armstrong, through his representatives, as suggested by the wording in the report. The language in the final document ended up very similar to the arguments Armstrong had used to defend himself in the past.

The 132-page "Vrijman Report" was released in the spring of 2006. It blamed the French lab for violating athlete confidentiality and said the lab did not follow international standards when its scientists examined Armstrong's samples. The Vrijman Report also chastised the World Anti-Doping Agency for its conduct regarding the so-called positives. But it neglected to address two very important points: whether EPO was, in fact, found in those samples or the possibility that Armstrong had used EPO to win his first Tour.

Vrijman said his report "exonerates Lance Armstrong completely with respect to alleged use of doping in the 1999 Tour de France."

The American media bought right in. The Associated Press said Armstrong had all along called *L'Equipe*'s story about the six positives "a witch hunt," and that "he may have been right." The *Fort Worth Star-Telegram* in Texas ran an editorial titled, "Sweet Vindication," that addressed the report. It said, "Count the report as Armstrong's eighth Tour de France victory."

Dick Pound, the head of the World Anti-Doping Agency, was one of the few outspoken naysayers. He said the report was "so lacking in professionalism and objectivity that it borders on the farcical." But Armstrong and the UCI had won that crucial round.

In the spring and summer of 2006, when he normally would have been training for the Tour, Armstrong, in retirement, enjoyed his status as an American icon.

There were no more surprise drug tests. No more clandestine prerace injections. No more reasons to even come close to France. Between his trips to Livestrong functions or to advocate in other arenas for cancer awareness, he moved into his dream estate in Austin.

At the Indianapolis 500, he drove the pace car, a 505-horsepower Corvette. At Tufts University in Boston, upon receiving an honorary doctorate, he told graduates: "Somebody send the photos to the principal at Plano East Senior High and let them know that I, in fact, graduated from Tufts and that he has to call me Dr. Armstrong now." In Washington, D.C., he lobbied Congress for an increase in cancer funding and some lawmakers clamored to meet with him. At least one powerful politician, Jim Oberstar, a long-serving Democratic congressman from Minnesota, had one of Armstrong's yellow jerseys framed and mounted on his office wall. At a gathering of Livestrong supporters in front of the Capitol, Armstrong talked to the crowd and was met with cries of "Lance for President!" The Arby's fast food chain proclaimed him the "Greatest Natural Athlete of All Time," ahead of Jim Thorpe and Muhammad Ali.

Armstrong soaked in fame, while some of his former teammates mounted their bikes and chased after it. After seven straight years as the Tour de France winner, Armstrong saw his former teammate-turned-nemesis, Floyd Landis, win the race in 2006.

Landis's victory was achieved primarily with a breathtaking performance that overshadowed even the best of Armstrong's rides. It came on Stage 17. A day after falling eight minutes behind the leader, Landis rode solo over three Alpine passes to win the stage. He crossed the finish line in Paris as only the third American to win the world's most famous cycling race.

That 2006 Tour had begun with nearly a dozen riders—including those who finished second, third, fourth and fifth behind Armstrong the year before—being banned or withdrawn from the race because they or their teams had been linked to a blood doping ring in Spain. At Tour's end, Landis was touted as a clean rider who could take American cycling into a new post-Armstrong era. His old friend Allen Lim wasn't sure what to think of that.

Lim had visited Landis in his plush Paris hotel suite the morning after Landis won the Tour. He had not worked directly for Landis during that race, but was still part of his entourage while recording and publishing his power numbers as part of a marketing push for Saris Cycling. In appreciation for his support, Landis gave Lim both of his wheels from his Tour bike.

As Lim turned to leave, Landis said, "Al, do you know why guys cheat?"

"No, Floyd, why do guys cheat?"

Landis pulled off his shirt. Then, as if he were a ripped and strutting linebacker rather than a whippet-lean cyclist with a farmer's tan, Landis struck a pose.

"Because they're pussies, Al," he said. "Because they are all fucking pussies!"

Lim left the room dazed. He wanted nothing more to do with Landis, with doping, with the moral relativism that said cheating was OK as long as everyone did it. He left Paris that afternoon determined to use his unique experience with Landis to change cycling for the better. If only he knew how.

Only four days after Floyd Landis stood on the podium on the Champs-Élysées with the American flag flapping in the wind behind him, his Phonak team announced that their champion had failed a drug test.

The positive test came from urine supplied during his amazing and improbable Stage 17 solo ride over the Alps. His ratio of testosterone-to-epitestosterone was 11-to-1, nearly three times the acceptable limit.

In a hastily organized teleconference, Landis took the Armstrong approach: Deny, deny and then deny more loudly, preferably on national television. He said the positive test could have come from the Jack Daniel's and beer he drank the night before. That, or from his naturally high testosterone level. It seemed as if the only excuse he didn't use was Tyler Hamilton's vanishing twin story.

On a teleconference with dozens of reporters around the world, I asked him if he had ever used performance-enhancing drugs or doping methods. He paused, awkwardly: "I'll say no."

In Ephrata, Pennsylvania, his parents staked a big yellow sign on their lawn with an array of spiritual proverbs: "The glory of young men is their strength" and "To God be the glory." Even after the report of his positive test, Landis's family remained hopeful of his innocence. His mother, Arlene, appeared on WGAL, a local news station, in her modest brown dress and Christian head covering. She said, "They stirred up trouble for Lance, too" and "I think God is allowing us to go through this so Floyd's glory is even greater." Floyd's sister Charity said, "I am proud of my brother. It humbles me to know that my brother can claim his victory with integrity."

A few days later I learned that his urine had tested positive for synthetic testosterone.

More than a month after Frankie and Betsy Andreu testified, Betsy was getting restless. She wanted the public to know that she and her husband didn't offer to testify against Armstrong—they were impelled to by subpoenas.

"If I had to, I'd do it all again because I did what I thought was right," she said. "But next time, I'd brace myself emotionally. Just because it's the truth, people aren't going to embrace it . . . America wants to believe this fairy tale about Lance, that he's this great guy who's a hero, but I know who he really is. He's just a fraud."

The Andreus were worlds away from the life they had once enjoyed in Europe. Betsy took care of the couple's three children, all of them younger than eight years old, and volunteered each week as a lunch monitor at their Catholic school. Frankie had directed a small U.S.-based cycling team, Toyota-United, until he was fired shortly after his SCA testimony broke in the news. His team owner had a previous relationship with Armstrong, which they figured was all they needed to know.

"Once you're out of Lance's inner circle, you're way out," Frankie Andreu said. "He holds grudges and wants to crush you, and that's exactly what he's trying to do to us." With the subpoena, Frankie said he and Betsy were "put into a difficult position, a position that we gained nothing from, and, if anything, it was going to hurt me. I chose to tell the truth."

They felt as though they had risked their livelihood by complying with the law. Betsy was concerned for her family's safety. While the SCA case moved forward, she filed a police report saying someone had accessed her AOL e-mail account without her permission. She had a hunch it was Armstrong or one of the henchmen in what she called "the Lance Mafia."

Her father once complained of her obsession: "Why do you have to keep talking about Lance? Can't you just stop and forget about it? It would be so much easier . . ."

She cut him off. "Lance Armstrong is trying to destroy this family. I'm not going to shut up about it."

Even her postman knew what occupied Betsy's every idle thought. He waved to her one day as he brought the mail. She was on the porch having a bite to eat.

"Got a picnic there, Betsy?" he asked.

"Yes, Joe," she said. "Want some tea and cookies?"

"Wish I could," he said. "But I don't have time to talk about Lance!"

It might seem weird that everybody in town seemed to know about her preoccupation with Armstrong. But to her, exposing Armstrong was a serious mission. After the SCA case, she began giving away all of the family's Nike gear—sweatshirts, sneakers and hats—because she had convinced herself that the company must have turned a blind eye to the doping. On the Nike gear she kept, she placed a dark piece of tape over the iconic swoosh. Betsy felt that her family was being threatened for taking a stand against Armstrong. She had good reason.

One night in 2005, Stephanie McIlvain, Armstrong's former Oakley representative, left a message for Betsy on the Andreus' answering machine, saying, "I hope somebody breaks a baseball bat over your head. I also hope that one day you have adversity in your life and you have some type of tragedy that will definitely make an impact on you."

Frankie Jr., her seven-year-old, immortalized the family's feelings in a crayon drawing. It showed gun-wielding G.I. Joes running toward a man behind bars. Next to the jailed man was a name: "LANCE."

Her friends in cycling—women with whom she had lounged on the French Riviera—no longer spoke to her. Angela Julich, the first cycling wife Betsy had talked to about Armstrong's hospital room confession, "didn't want to get involved" when I asked her to comment for a story I was writing about the Andreus. Leipheimer's wife, Odessa Gunn, was also indifferent. Two other wives I spoke to worried that Armstrong might ostracize their husbands if they dared to pick up the phone to talk to Betsy—or even about her.

Frankie Andreu told me that having talked about Armstrong's hospital room confession, even under oath in a supposedly confidential legal proceeding, made it difficult for him to work in cycling. "I would love to see this pass over and go away, but Betsy very much believes in the truth and believes that there is a right and a wrong," he said.

During the week I visited them in August 2006, Betsy and Frankie argued about my presence. From the next room, I heard them bickering in the kitchen.

"Why is she here?" Frankie said.

"We need to talk to her, Frankie. C'mon, *please*!"

It was a surprise, then, when Frankie talked with me for two hours, and answered one question I never thought he would: "Did you ever dope?"

He sighed, bowed his head and said, "No one has ever asked me that. I don't want to answer."

"Does that mean yes?" I said.

He said, "I tried my best never to use performance-enhancing drugs. I did make a couple of bad choices, but that was a long, long time ago. It's not something to be proud of. I did use EPO, but only for a couple of races."

I was stunned.

"Sorry, did you say that you used EPO?" I asked.

"Yes, I'm not gonna lie. That's what I said."

He then made a distinction I had never heard before. "There are two levels of guys. You got the guys that cheat [to win] and the guys that are just trying to survive [by cheating]."

But he said he felt guilty and couldn't keep his secret any longer. If riders kept lying about doping, he said, sponsors and fans would be scared away from the sport for good.

Later, when Frankie was out of the room, Betsy said, "It was all for Lance. Everything those teammates did was for the glory of Lance."

I called all seven other riders who supported Armstrong on that 1999 Postal Service team and asked if they, too, had doped, and if they had seen any doping on the team. Both Europeans on the squad—Peter Meinert-Nielsen and Pascal Deramé—said they did not dope, would never dope and had never seen doping in the sport.

Only one of the riders, Jonathan Vaughters, said something different. We had talked many times since the SCA testimony was leaked to reporters. I tried to get him to go on the record with what he knew about Armstrong. I told him that one rider—I didn't name Andreu yet—on the 1999 Tour team had said he had doped. I was looking for others to confirm that there had been doping on Armstrong's squad that year. *Did you dope for that Tour?* Vaughters said to answer would be to commit career suicide. Initially, he warned me not to quote him: "Just so you know, my father is a lawyer." But days later, when I told him that none of his 1999 American teammates would even call me back, he agreed to go on the record, albeit anonymously.

I then told him the other rider was Andreu.

"I'm not going to leave Frankie out there by himself, just hanging there," Vaughters said. "Somebody has to back him up."

Both he and Andreu echoed Betsy. They said they felt pressure to use EPO if they wanted to make that 1999 Tour team. "The environment was certainly one of, to be accepted, you had to use doping products," Vaughters said. "There was very high pressure to be one of the cool kids."

Neither Andreu nor Vaughters would say they had seen Armstrong dope. Both said they had no firsthand knowledge of his ever doing so.

The story ran on the front page of the *New York Times* on September 12, 2006. At last, Armstrong's teammates—two brave ones—had told the truth about doping on the Postal Service squad.

Though the story didn't accuse Armstrong of doping, his "mafia" saw it as an attack. His agent, Stapleton, called me "the worst journalist in history" and threatened a lawsuit. "You must have fucking failed journalism school."

Armstrong told the Associated Press that the story was "a hatchet job . . . to link me to doping through somebody else's admission." He told *USA Today* that the *Times* had displayed "a severe lack of journalistic ethics by linking an admission by Frankie Andreu to me." He was just as angry with the Andreus. He and team manager Johan Bruyneel called upon the Postal Service/Discovery Channel team and cycling authorities to look into stripping Frankie of his race results and asking him to pay back prize money. (There is irony in that proposal, as time would tell.)

Armstrong also e-mailed a statement calling the article "categorically false and distorted sensationalism . . . My cycling victories are untainted. I didn't take performance-enhancing drugs, I didn't ask anyone else to take them and I didn't condone or encourage anyone else to take them. I won clean."

In what was now old hat, he concluded his statement with a plea to his base: "I want the millions of cancer patients and survivors with whom I battle cancer to know that these allegations are still untrue and to be assured that my victories were untainted and that they, too, have reason to hope for a full, healthy and productive future."

After Travis Tygart read my *New York Times* story on Frankie Andreu, he called the Andreus at home in Michigan.

He asked Betsy, "Could Frankie come to the phone?"

Betsy thought to have fun with Tygart. "What are you gonna do, sanction Frankie or something?"

He told her that Frankie had, after all, admitted to using EPO for the '99 Tour and a confession was a confession. And at seven years and two months, it was a confession that fell within the World Anti-Doping Code's eight-year statute of limitations.

So, to Betsy's question of sanctions, Tygart said, "Well, that's what we've had to consider."

"Are you fucking kidding me?" she said to Tygart. "You have Lance, the biggest fraud, the biggest cheat in the history of sport still out there, and you're coming after us? Frankie was fired. You're telling me you're going to go after a small guy like him because he refused to go on a doping program with Lance? Fuck you and fuck off!"

The next sound Tygart heard was the infinite hum of the dead line at the other end. It was the beginning of a beautiful friendship.

David Zabriskie, Landis's closest buddy, said he cried for hours, unable to leave his bathtub, after hearing that Landis had tested positive. He had last seen him in a sublime Parisian hotel suite, the Tour winner living large.

Zabriskie knew Landis had it coming: He had doped with Landis in the off-season before that Tour. Landis also had supplied Zabriskie with growth hormone, testosterone patches and EPO that made up his training regimen. Without Landis's access to drugs, Zabriskie said he would have had no way to obtain those pharmaceuticals. Both men felt pressure to perform well at the Tour, the only race most Americans paid attention to—if they paid attention at all.

To hard-core cycling fans who knew about the sport's history with doping, Landis had become just the latest cheater in a sport of cheaters. Zabriskie had gone from feeling happy for his friend's success to sympathizing with his downfall. He knew the pain Landis had endured—and it was more than just the ritual disgrace of the failed test.

On August 15, 2006, a month after the Tour, Landis's father-in-law—and best friend—committed suicide. David Witt was found dead in a parking garage in San Diego. He'd shot himself in the head.

Landis had told Zabriskie that Witt was his source for testosterone patches—they had come by way of a rejuvenation clinic Witt visited in Southern California—and that Witt had sometimes watched over his blood during the Tour.

It all left Zabriskie confused. Soon after the Andreu/Vaughters admissions, he claims, he once again explained his feelings about the Postal Service team's doping to Steve Johnson, who recently had been named chief executive of USA Cycling. He wanted help from one of the most powerful men in American cycling—a man who once had been his mentor. Instead, Johnson allegedly said Andreu never should have gone public. Then he supposedly told Zabriskie, "If you ever do drugs, I'll kill you."

Already depressed by Landis's positive test, Zabriskie was dismayed to hear Johnson's criticism of Andreu. Nor did he understand Johnson's admonition.

"Uh, Steve," he said, "I already told you that I have used drugs, that the guys on Postal were injecting me with all sorts of stuff. Remember at worlds two years ago? I told you that they were doing drugs on that team."

Zabriskie's best guess was that Johnson simply didn't want to hear it. As he did at the world championships two years earlier, the cycling boss looked at Zabriskie like he was speaking in tongues. Johnson just sat there, saying nothing until his wife walked into the room and gave him a chance to change the subject.

Zabriskie thought, "I already told him *twice* that the Postal team was doping. He didn't do anything about it then, and he's not going to do anything about it now . . . Ugh, he must know everything."

Confrontation was not Zabriskie's thing. He'd never had the courage to take on his alcoholic father. Now, rather than risk his riding career, he would not join Andreu and Vaughters in their public confession. He was embarrassed by his weakness.

Allen Lim's good-bye to Floyd Landis in Paris in 2006 was just one of their many farewells.

The first had come a year before.

After the 2005 Tour de France, Lim promised to babysit a bag of blood in Landis's apartment during the Vuelta a España and deliver it on a rest day.

At the time, Lim was contemplating working with young men riding clean for Vaughters, on a development team for riders under twenty-three that Vaughters had started in 2003. "Those young kids are not like Floyd, they are not like Lance, they are good kids," Lim told me later. "I don't ever want to see them go through this."

He spent an afternoon with those kids in Girona. Then, instead of delivering the blood bag to Landis, he took it out of the refrigerator, placed it in the kitchen sink and stabbed it with a knife again and again.

Days later, Landis called. "How's everything going?"

"It's not going so well," Lim said. "You don't have a bag of blood anymore. It went down the drain."

Lim expected Landis's rage.

Instead, the rider said, "Shit, well, I guess it's time to go home then, isn't it?"

Lim thought he heard in Landis's voice a tone of regret that he had dragged his friend back into doping.

"Yeah, Floyd, it's time to go home," Lim said. "It's over."

CHAPTER 19

Lance Armstrong's power had long ago transcended what it meant to be a famous cyclist. In 2007, he was the public face of a political effort in Texas to secure $3 billion for cancer research. He traveled the state on something of a campaign bus to speak to voters. Speaking for an hour to various members of the Texas House of Representatives, he won 65 votes out of the 100 necessary for a proposed constitutional amendment to be placed on a ballot. Waiting for the final tally, Armstrong said, "It's only fun if you win." It passed.

In a *Vanity Fair* profile written by the historian and journalist Douglas Brinkley that dealt with both the prospect of Armstrong's future career in politics and his cancer work, Brinkley called him "a regular 365-days-a-year walking-talking Jerry Lewis Telethon." As for the gubernatorial run, Armstrong answered, "Probably." Then he dropped a bombshell: He wanted to win an eighth Tour de France.

In the months that followed, many friends argued against it. They were happy he had escaped intact from years of doping allegations.

"Man, I don't know about this," John Korioth, his closest friend, said. "Pigs get fat, hogs get slaughtered."

Armstrong wasn't hearing anyone's sermons. His nightlife

already had become tabloid fodder. He was out and about with the actor Matthew McConaughey so much that they were dubbed Siamese twins. After leaving Sheryl Crow, he spent time on both coasts with other blondes: the clothing designer Tory Burch, the young, elfin actress Ashley Olsen and the movie star Kate Hudson.

Korioth warned the thirty-six-year-old father of three that his May-December romance with Olsen could damage his cancer work. "Whoa, dude, bad idea," Korioth said. "You've got to put a stop to this right now. "

"She's twenty-one," Armstrong answered. "Fuck you."

Armstrong had watched the 2008 Tour in a state of jealousy and anger. Carlos Sastre, the tiny, quiet Spanish climber, had won the race, to Armstrong's dismay. Sastre, really? Christian Vande Velde, his former *domestique*, the kid who once had fetched him water bottles and cortisone pills, finished fifth.

"The Tour was a bit of a joke this year," Armstrong told a British reporter, John Wilcockson. "I've got nothing against Sastre . . . or Christian Vande Velde. Christian's a nice guy, but finishing fifth in the Tour de France? Come on!"

He hated it, too, that the '08 Tour had been called the cleanest ever. If so, all other Tours—including the seven he won—were deemed to be dirty. Even in retirement, Armstrong felt the sting of doping accusations. His answer, as always, was to ride.

Vaughters and Lim, meanwhile, were working together and had become antidoping crusaders while leading Vaughters's TIAA-CREF under-twenty-three development team. Lim never wanted to see another rider tortured as he'd seen Floyd Landis punish himself. Searching for a way to scare athletes straight, Lim found an answer while reading *Outside* magazine.

Don Catlin had proposed a new antidoping system. He was the scientist who investigated cycling's EPO-related deaths in the late 1980s and helped break the BALCO steroids scandal. "Athletes still get away with stuff," Catlin told *Outside*, "and I maintain you can get away with stuff with everybody looking right at you."

He proposed that athletes submit urine and blood samples to create biological profiles. Biomarkers, like each rider's hematocrit, hemoglobin and testosterone levels, would be monitored. Any variations would suggest doping.

Lim took Catlin's idea to Vaughters. "We should do something like this with the young guys," he said. Catlin told Lim the effort would be "brave."

With Catlin's help, Lim and Vaughters worked out the details for their development team, then for the professionals who would join their team in 2008. The new team initially was called Slipstream Sports. The 2008 Tour accepted Vaughters's "Clean Team" as a wild-card entry into the race partly for its drug-free image.

Armstrong disliked both the idea of the team and its creator, Vaughters. He said as much to Vande Velde, who took it as a warning to Vaughters and asked Vaughters's co-owner, Doug Ellis, to sweet-talk Armstrong. Vande Velde was afraid of what Armstrong could do to the team if he continued to despise it.

Ellis was a private investor from New York City. He went to Armstrong's penthouse apartment on Central Park South. Engaging and bright, as he could be, Armstrong impressed Ellis with his knowledge of the inner workings of the Slipstream squad. He certainly knew that Ellis had invested millions in Vaughters's fledgling team. For the 2008 season, Slipstream had hired top-notch riders—the ex-dopers Vande Velde and Zabriskie (who said they stopped doping in 2006, scared straight after Landis's positive test), and the Brit David Millar, another convert. Millar had served a two-year EPO suspension. The team became a safe haven for reformed cheaters and former Postal Service riders.

Armstrong got down to business.

"You don't have the right guys on the bus," Armstrong told Ellis.

"What do you mean?"

"You're spending all this money on the team, and it's not exactly working out, is it? JV, he's not the kind of guy you want to bet on."

Slipstream, he suggested, was a team of losers, including its manager, Johnny Weltz, whom Armstrong had long ago replaced with Bruyneel. Ellis, though, didn't care about the winning and losing like Thomas Weisel did; he was not a guy who went on training rides with the pros as if he were one. Ellis funded Slipstream because he, like Vaughters, wanted to save cycling from itself. He'd expected Armstrong to disagree with him. That's how he'd know he was doing something right.

Armstrong once said he came back to "raise awareness of the global cancer burden," a sentiment that makes Korioth roll his eyes. "Please," he said to me, "he came back because he thought he could still kick everybody's ass."

Armstrong made a deal to reunite with Bruyneel on the Kazakh cycling team Astana. He'd be riding in a new world. Though Armstrong had been gone only three and a half years, doping tests were more advanced and done more frequently.

The French national antidoping lab that had declared six of his 1999 urine samples to be positive for EPO was eager to have another crack at him. Pierre Bordry, the head of the lab, told colleagues that he couldn't wait for Armstrong to be tested again on French soil. Tygart and other USADA officials were anxious to see if Armstrong could withstand the new system of antidoping. The circumstantial evidence against Armstrong had grown and grown, but a black-and-white positive was something that would be much harder for him to wriggle out of.

Armstrong did what he had to do to make it seem like he was clean: He hired Don Catlin to basically act as a PR man to build his reputation as an antidoping advocate. The scientist who once said "to ride the Tour, you have to be doping" would now run a program consisting of Armstrong alone. He would test Armstrong as often as he wanted. He would take urine and blood samples to compile a biological baseline and would analyze those levels to see if Armstrong was breaking the rules. The terms of the agreement were still being discussed, but Catlin wanted to get approval to publish the results.

Armstrong held the first news conference regarding his comeback in September 2008, in conjunction with the Clinton Global Initiative, a group of world leaders, philanthropists, entrepreneurs and corporate types gathered to talk about the world's problems. Armstrong was one of the main speakers at the event, held at the Sheraton New York Hotel near Times Square in Manhattan.

Just after Armstrong finished sharing a main stage with New York City mayor Michael Bloomberg and former president Bill Clinton—whom he called "two of the most powerful men in the world"—he climbed onto a small makeshift stage in one of the adjacent ballrooms. Catlin, wearing a Livestrong bracelet, took his place on Armstrong's right. Taylor Phinney, a future star whom Armstrong had poached from Jonathan Vaughters's under-twenty-three team, stood at Armstrong's left. He also was wearing a Livestrong wristband.

Vaughters had groomed the prodigy for years, and Phinney had promised to return to JV's team the next season. But within weeks of Armstrong's comeback announcement, Phinney's parents—Olympians Connie Carpenter and Davis Phinney—stopped returning Vaughters's calls. Vaughters soon heard that Phinney was training with Armstrong in Aspen, Colorado. Next thing he knew, Armstrong was starting an under-twenty-three team to showcase Phinney. Vaughters wanted to tell him, "You stole him just to fuck with us."

Landis, who knew about Armstrong's new development team, was even more incredulous. After losing his long, acrimonious and very public fight with USADA, Landis had been serving a two-year doping ban for testing positive at the 2006 Tour, and that ban was set to expire on January 30, 2009. He and Armstrong had talked about Landis's possibly becoming the director of Armstrong's new team for young riders—an offer that never materialized. Instead, Armstrong hired the Belgian and former Motorola rider Axel Merckx for the yet-to-be development team. He told Landis that his team couldn't be involved with someone with a doping past.

Hiring Landis would have kept him quiet. Armstrong had hushed up his former Postal Service lieutenant, Kevin Livingston, by letting him base his personal training business out of his Mellow Johnny's bike shop in Austin. But when Armstrong refused Landis a job as a team manager, then as a bike racer on Armstrong's pro teams, it was the biggest mistake he'd ever make.

Nike was all in. Scott MacEachern, Armstrong's longtime Nike representative, was giddy when he had heard the comeback news. With Armstrong, his career had soared. His wife, Ashley, had even written a children's book about Armstrong in 2008.

Nike executives were thrilled because Armstrong's return was bound to be a marketing boon for the company as he rode back into the public consciousness as a cancer-fighting cycling super-hero. They'd seen it before: His name alone could bring consumers to the Nike section of a sports store and could spark a lifelong loyalty to the company.

So Armstrong's team at Nike hunkered down to generate ideas to bring the Livestrong brand—and the Nike swoosh—into living rooms all over the world, more than ever before. In advance of the Tour, the company announced that it was launching a Livestrong "Hope Rides Again" line of apparel and footwear to commemorate Armstrong's return to the sport. (All proceeds, after expenses, went to the Lance Armstrong Foundation, as did all the proceeds from the Livestrong collection.) There was also a Nike-sponsored touring art exhibition, headlined by big names like Shepard Fairey and Damien Hirst, which also made money for Livestrong. The tour featured its own exclusive collection of Nike/Livestrong gear.

Nike, as it had done before, capitalized on Armstrong's in-famy. A TV spot showed Armstrong training alone on his bike, the ride intercut with scenes of recovering cancer patients. Over dramatic music, Armstrong says, "The critics say I'm arrogant. A doper. Washed up. A fraud. That I couldn't let it go. They can say whatever they want. I'm not back on my bike for them."

In October 2008, while sitting at a west Texas café with his newest girlfriend, a mountain biker named Anna Hansen,

Armstrong read a story by the French news service Agence France-Presse that addressed his comeback. The article referenced an editorial written by Jean-Marie Leblanc, the former Tour de France race director. Why, Leblanc asked, would Armstrong subject cycling to the questions certain to come with his return?

"Us former riders generally have respect for winners, but that's not always the case with the public, above all the media, who have heavy suspicions about you . . . The hounds will be let loose, column inches will be written, images repeated and debate sparked about the one word which has petrified our passion over the past ten years: doping."

Armstrong's heart fell. Leblanc was basically telling him that a comeback would be a disastrous move. Armstrong thought: "*Do I want to face all the scrutiny again? Do I want to test fate?*" Sure, he had thought of those downsides before, but Leblanc's words for some reason had gotten through to him. Since announcing his comeback, he had only been tested once by USADA, but his instincts told him to be careful, that he might really be pushing his luck, like Korioth had warned him. It dawned on him: "There are people who will not rest until I am cooked."

He turned to Hansen: "I got to get out of this."

They had just started dating. She hadn't a clue what he was talking about.

"Get out of what?"

Armstrong explained the situation to her and stewed about it. He began thinking up excuses to back out, like, "I blew out my knee." Or "My knee hurts." Or "I woke up this morning and my kids said, 'Don't do it.'"

But Nike's exclusive Livestrong apparel and footwear lines were already moving forward, and his charity was jazzed that millions of dollars more than usual were likely going to roll in. Fans from all over the world were sending him notes that praised him for his comeback and his publicly stated goal of taking his message of cancer awareness to a global stage. He wouldn't just race in France. He'd race in Australia, South Africa, Ireland.

He told me later that this new chapter of his life was rolling and gaining speed, and that he just couldn't make himself jump off the ride, because everyone was watching.

"I didn't have the courage," he said.

At a news conference attended by hundreds of journalists before the 2009 Tour of California—the first American race of Armstrong's comeback—he was as defiant as he'd been on the Champs-Élysées in 2005 when he said he felt sorry for anyone who didn't believe in cycling.

He had been chastised by reporters for failing to participate in USADA's out-of-competition testing program for six months before he could race. When he had competed at the Tour Down Under that January, he had been less than a month short, but the UCI let him compete anyway.

He was criticized for touting the virtues of his independent testing program, the one run by the antidoping scientist Catlin, when that program hadn't even gotten off the ground. Catlin told me that Armstrong had balked at the logistics and cost of it.

At the Tour of California's news conference, one question stopped him. Paul Kimmage, once a pro cyclist himself and now an award-winning reporter for the *Sunday Times* of London, asked why Armstrong said Landis and Italian rider Ivan Basso should be welcomed back into the sport after serving doping bans.

"What is it about these dopers that you seem to admire so much?" Kimmage asked.

Armstrong recognized Kimmage, an outspoken antidoping advocate who had written a book, *Rough Ride*, about the sport's doping culture. Stapleton and Mark Higgins, Armstrong's personal PR man, had seen Kimmage take a seat in the front row of the news conference, and had given Armstrong the heads-up.

Armstrong responded to Kimmage as if he had rehearsed his answer.

"When I decided to come back for what I think is a very noble reason, you said, 'The cancer has been in remission for four years, but our cancer has now returned,' meaning me. I am here to fight this disease. I am here so that I don't have to deal with it, you don't have to deal with it, my children don't have to deal with it."

He then said to Kimmage, "You are not worth the chair that you're sitting on with a statement like that."

The season had just begun.

When Landis's suspension ended, he couldn't find a job. Even Vaughters, who had remained friendly with him, said no. "I would trust Floyd to babysit my son, which I would say about very few bike racers," Vaughters said. "If he needs money, I will loan him cash. But I couldn't hire him as a bike racer."

Landis finally signed with a lower-level cycling team, the U.S.-based OUCH squad. While he rode in small-time races, Armstrong was back at the Tour, welcomed heartily by thousands. One farmer propped a sign in front of his cornfield: "Armstrong: Pourquoi pas?" ("Armstrong: Why not?")

Even with nearly four years off, Armstrong rode brilliantly, battling his own teammate, the Spanish rider Alberto Contador, to be Astana's team leader. Eleven years his junior, Contador would win that battle, but Armstrong still showed his strength by whipping dozens of younger riders. On one stage that ended atop the legendary Mont Ventoux, he finished fifth.

While Contador proved to be better, Armstrong was a serious challenger, once missing out on the leader's yellow jersey by two-tenths of a second. At the end of the 2,150-mile race, he finished third behind Contador, who had won. Armstrong became the second-oldest rider to finish in the top three in the Tour's long history.

L'Equipe, the newspaper that had broken so many doping stories about him, ran a headline, "Chapeau, Le Texan," which means "Hats Off to the Texan." French President Nicolas Sarkozy raved about him, saying he "did more in five minutes [at the Tour] than his public relations team did in ten years." At Tour's end, Armstrong announced that he'd be starting his own team, sponsored by RadioShack, and would be its lead rider for the 2010 season.

Landis envied Armstrong. Ever since serving his doping ban, he had threatened Armstrong with blackmail if Armstrong didn't find a job for him in cycling. When that job didn't materialize, it is claimed that he was so bitter that he began threatening other former Postal Service riders, saying he was going to expose them as dopers. If he had to suffer because he had doped, others were going to suffer with him.

In 2008, he told Zabriskie he intended to expose the universally admired George Hincapie. Zabriskie called Hincapie the night before the legendary Paris-Roubaix race.

"Floyd says he's going to call the police on you and that they'll be waiting for you at the finish line," Zabriskie said. "I wouldn't have said anything, but I think he might be serious this time . . ."

Hincapie was so unnerved that he finished ninth, more than five minutes back in a race he was favored to win.

Landis also talked about making a video about the doping that occurred on the Postal Service team, and then posting it on YouTube. That threat caught the attention of David "Tiger" Williams, one of the Wall Street financiers who was an early backer of the Postal Service squad.

Williams was a former captain of Yale's hockey team, a competitive cyclist and an investor in Tailwind Sports, the management company that owned the Postal Service team. He was also a top donor to the Lance Armstrong Foundation and one of the big-time donors to the Floyd Fairness Fund—a pool of money that helped Landis pay the $2 million in legal fees he had incurred while fighting his antidoping case.

Williams did not have confirmation that Armstrong had doped. He had asked Vaughters again and again if there had been doping on the team, but Vaughters never gave him a straight answer.

In 2009, Williams felt bad that Landis was out of work so the company Williams co-owned—eSoles, which sold athletic shoe insoles—paid $200,000 to sponsor Landis's OUCH team.

At the same time, Williams had been close to Armstrong, at least in a business sense. He once had pledged $1 million to Armstrong's foundation in exchange for using the "Livestrong" logo on his company's shoe liners. But in April 2009, Williams learned the deal was off. He was told that Nike, the foundation's primary sponsor, had nixed it.

When Williams asked what happened, Armstrong responded

by e-mail: "To be honest, and I say this as a good friend of yours, I don't feel like dealing with this right now. I'm afraid it's up to you guys to sort out. For what it's worth, and maybe a good solution, is to return you all of your money and let's all get on down the road."

Williams had paid only a portion of the pledge. Still, the foundation refused to give that money back, Armstrong said, informing Williams that donations had to be made with no strings attached. Williams was supposedly livid and vowed to do something about Armstrong's backing out of the eSoles deal. George Hincapie had known Williams for years and figured the sky was about to fall: "I'd never, ever want to get on Tiger Williams's bad side."

Soon enough, Williams allegedly told a friend, "Get ready: Big Texas is going down."

Armstrong had no idea what was in store for him. He was too busy enjoying the fanfare of his comeback year. In October 2009, at the annual Ride for the Roses in Austin, throngs of fans came to ride with him, support Livestrong and celebrate his return to cycling.

Terry Armstrong, his adoptive father, was among them. In the years since divorcing Armstrong's mother, he had become a staunch Christian. Feeling an inconsolable regret about how his relationship with his son had evaporated, he drove from his Dallas suburb to Austin to ask his son for forgiveness for the pain he had caused him and his mother in another life.

At the Ride for the Roses, he came within a foot of his son at the finish line, close enough to touch his arm and call out, "Lance Edward."

Armstrong asked Stapleton to have police take him away.

* * *

In the fall of 2009, Landis confided in Zabriskie before the Tour of Missouri. He was emotional. He said he had turned into a terrible person and didn't know what to do with his life. His marriage had fallen apart. He had moved out of his spacious house in Temecula, California, and into a small, bare-bones cabin in Idyllwild, a remote town tucked into the San Jacinto mountains. He loved bike racing, but it had become a dead end. He wanted to race again in Europe. He deserved that chance, right? He was the winner of the freakin' Tour de France, right? He had maintained cycling's code of silence for so many years—and for what?

"Remember the conversation we had in our apartment in Girona?" Zabriskie said. "If we ever get caught, let's not bullshit around, let's just stop and come clean? So man, maybe you should admit it?"

Zabriskie wasn't surprised, then, when he received a text message from Landis in the spring of 2010. Landis was apologizing for what he was about to do. He was going to come clean about everything and everyone. He said he was going to tell USADA that he, Armstrong and other top Americans in the sport had used performance-enhancing drugs and blood transfusions.

"Man, can't you just leave me out of it?" Zabriskie said. "Isn't this just between you and Lance?"

"No, I'm sorry, man, I'm sorry."

Landis felt safe enough to come forward because he had Tiger Williams's support. Landis didn't have to worry about money or a roof over his head. Williams had a place on Central Park South in Manhattan and a guesthouse in Connecticut.

For Williams, helping Landis was a win-win. He allegedly

could exact a measure of revenge against Armstrong for reneging on the agreement Williams thought he and eSoles had with the Lance Armstrong Foundation. (Williams had previously denied that revenge played a role.)

By then, Landis had e-mailed a puzzling array of Led Zeppelin lyrics to Vaughters, words heavy with misery and confusion. He said he was about to let go of everything he'd held inside so long. "I can't live with this," he told Vaughters. "I can't live with this secret."

Vaughters heard the darkness in Landis's voice.

"I felt like he was going to commit suicide," he said, "or tell all."

CHAPTER 20

Night after night in the spring of 2010, Landis sent e-mails to Armstrong, taunting him with what he was about to do, goading him into trying to do something to stop it. Landis would send them past midnight during the Tour of the Gila, a multistage race in New Mexico in which they both were competing. But Landis never said a word to Armstrong at the race itself. It creeped Armstrong out.

The week before, Armstrong had eavesdropped on a phone conversation between Zabriskie and the former Postal Service team manager Johan Bruyneel, in which Zabriskie had called to warn Bruyneel about Landis's plans to come clean.

Armstrong had never been so jumpy. Landis had long said he was going to go public with his doping claims, but this time he seemed prepared to follow through. While he needled Armstrong, he dared Steve Johnson, the chief executive and president of USA Cycling, to act. On Friday, April 30, 2010, at 5:19 p.m., after the third stage of the five-stage Tour of the Gila, Landis wrote to Johnson under the subject line: "nobody is copied on this one so it's up to you to demonstrate your true colors . . ."

In that single e-mail laying out the highlights of his allegations of the doping that occurred on the Postal Service and other pro teams, Landis implicated nearly every top American rider and several cycling officials. It read like a description of a drug ring.

He claimed that in 2002 Bruyneel had instructed him on how to use testosterone patches. He said that Armstrong had handed him a box of patches in view of Armstrong's wife; that Ferrari extracted blood from him to be reinfused at the Tour. He also alleged that Armstrong told him he had made a financial agreement with the former UCI president Hein Verbruggen to hide a positive test for EPO.

More charges: In 2003, Armstrong had asked him to keep an eye on Armstrong's blood while he was out of town. Landis's job was to ensure that the temperature inside Armstrong's refrigerator didn't fluctuate so that the blood stored there would remain fresh.

During the 2003 Tour, Landis received a blood transfusion alongside riders that included Hincapie and Armstrong. The team doctor gave him and Hincapie testosterone oil. Landis also claimed that later that season, Bruyneel told him to get EPO from Armstrong, who complied when asked for it. Another claim was that Bruyneel explained to Landis how to use growth hormone, and that Landis bought it from the trainer Pepe Martí. Landis's Postal teammates Matthew White, an Australian, and Michael Barry, a Canadian, shared their testosterone and EPO.

In the e-mail, Landis also wrote that in the 2004 Tour, he and teammates received a transfusion along a mountain road on their way to the team hotel. In 2005, he hired Allen Lim to prepare transfusions and keep the blood cold when Landis performed the transfusions on himself and Levi Leipheimer.

Landis claimed that he told the Phonak team owner, Andy Riis, in 2006 that he needed money to dope, and Riis supposedly granted it. (Riis denies it.)

After all that, Landis told Johnson he had "many, many more

details" in diaries. He signed off with an ominous line: "Look forward to much more detail as soon as you can demonstrate that you can be trusted to do the right thing."

To the others, Landis warned that he was about to drop a bomb. And soon. He wrote to Andrew Messick, the race director of the Tour of California; Bill Stapleton, the agent who'd said the Postal Service team could help him "with further doping"; and UCI president Pat McQuaid, as well as a handful of cycling sponsors. Then he wrote to Armstrong again: "I'll just come out and say directly that I'm going to accuse you and our former teammates of using blood doping and performance-enhancing drugs to help you to win the three Tours de France in which we raced together. So make no mistake about that."

He called the doping on those teams "a fraud perpetrated on the public" and said Armstrong could not intimidate him.

"My only goal in enlightening the public and the press regarding these matters is to clear my conscience and thereafter be able to sleep at night," Landis wrote. "I'm certainly not oblivious to the fact that the thought of this would cause you and many others considerable anxiety and am sympathetic to your reaction but need to remind you that I don't react well to threats or bullying and see no good outcome if that continues."

In April 2010, Floyd Landis arranged a lunch meeting with the race director Messick in downtown Los Angeles, at an upscale restaurant called the Farm of Beverly Hills. More than a year had passed since the end of Landis's suspension.

He liked Messick and wanted to warn him that the sport was about to implode, perhaps within a month, maybe during Messick's Tour of California in May. He placed a tape recorder on the table and pressed "Record." He wanted proof that he had told the truth about his doping to someone who was an authority in the sport.

"I used performance-enhancing drugs pretty much throughout my whole pro career," he said. "I can't keep the truth inside anymore. It's going to come out, and soon."

Messick was dumbfounded. The man who had written a book called *Positively False: The Real Story of How I Won the Tour de France*—a story about Landis's winning clean, despite his positive drug test—was now admitting that he had lied to the public *for four whole years*? The man who had shouted his innocence and solicited money from donors for his defense was now saying his version of his story was, actually, positively false?

"How do you expect people to believe you when you lied for so long?" Messick said. "Have you told your mother? Have you told Travis Tygart?"

He had not. Telling his mother required more courage than Landis could summon. And Tygart, who had slapped him in 2007 with a two-year ban, was not someone Landis could tolerate helping. (Landis said he spent $2 million, including at least $478,354 in public donations from 1,765 people, and nearly two years fighting his case.)

Though he gave up nothing about Armstrong, Landis told Messick that all the veteran riders referred to their code of silence as "the omertà."

"When you're in the Mafia, and you get caught and go to jail, you keep your mouth shut, and the organization takes care of your family," Landis said. But in cycling, he said, there was no honor among thieves. "You're expected to keep your mouth shut when you test positive, but you become an outcast. Everyone just turns their back on you."

Cyclists had violated the omertà in the past, but none had been as high-profile a rider as Landis. Even Frankie Andreu, who had tattled on the sport four years before, had been a mere *domestique*.

In the spring of 2010, Austria's Bernhard Kohl admitted to a lifetime of doping, saying "it's impossible to win without doping." He had finished third at the 2008 Tour, but was stripped of that result because he had tested positive at the race. He said it was easy to get around the drug testing: "I was tested two hundred times during my career, and a hundred times I had drugs in my body," he told me in 2010. "I was caught, but ninety-nine other times I wasn't."

In 2004, Spain's Jesús Manzano exposed the systematic doping that occurred on the Kelme team and later admitted that a team doctor at the 2003 Tour had given him the veterinary drug Oxyglobin—bovine hemoglobin, used to treat anemia in dogs. After taking the drug, Manzano collapsed during a stage and had to be airlifted to a hospital.

The revelations of cycling's dark side weren't just spokes on the dubious wheel of Lance Armstrong. But the sport in America was about to receive a potent injection of truth-telling, maybe for the first time ever. And Landis was the tip of the needle. He had been abandoned by everyone and everything that had meant something to him: his sport, his wife, his father-in-law, most of his former teammates. The truth, he told Messick, was all he had left.

About a week before the Tour of California, Landis called Tygart, and they planned to meet at the Marriott at the Los Angeles airport a few days later. Tygart knew what to expect. He had heard the basics of Landis's doping stories from a USADA scientist named Daniel Eichner who two weeks before had heard the details of Landis's drug use through an anti-doping expert Landis had recruited to be his intermediary. After his lunch meeting with Messick in Los Angeles, Landis had been eager to talk to USADA—yet he didn't want to confess to Tygart right away because they'd had such a contentious relationship during Landis's doping case. Telling Eichner his dirty deeds was his first step toward full disclosure.

Sitting across from each other in a conference room at the airport Marriott, both Landis and Tygart were cautious. Learning to trust each other would take time.

"If I'm willing to come forward and be truthful, are you going to do what everyone else would do, or are you going to do your job?" Landis said.

Tygart was surprised at his skepticism. He made a point of looking him straight in the eyes. "We are going to do our job and follow up with whatever evidence is presented. That's if you tell the truth."

So Landis told the truth. They sat for hours, with Landis reeling off details of his doping, Armstrong's doping and other riders' doping. Tygart tried to keep his jaw from hitting the floor.

"We were all doing it—Lance, me, all the other guys on the team; everybody was doping," Landis claimed. "It was just part of the sport."

"Well, we're going to try to change that," Tygart said. "You have a lot of courage for coming forward. I know how tough it is for a single person to speak the truth. You get vilified in the press."

Landis didn't name any of the other riders who doped—just Armstrong. For the moment, Zabriskie was in the clear. Landis was trying his best to convince Tygart that his friends—"the guys that want to clear their conscience" about doping—should receive no punishment for their confessions. He didn't put Armstrong in that category.

After the meeting, Tygart contacted an old friend—Jeff Novitzky, a bald-headed, 6-foot-6 criminal investigator for the Food and Drug Administration who had made a name for himself as the country's top antidoping cop. Tygart told him that Landis had explosive information about Armstrong's doping and the doping on Armstrong's Postal Service team, and suggested that the two of them team up to interview Landis on the record.

Novitzky had been the lead agent in the BALCO steroids case that implicated elite athletes like the slugger Barry Bonds and the sprinter Marion Jones. (Both were convicted of felony crimes stemming from their doping.) He and Tygart had worked closely together on that case, and had since been in touch about the doping problem in cycling and other sports.

Novitzky was already investigating PED use in cycling when Tygart reached out to him about Landis. His investigation had been spurred by the doping case of a rider named Kayle Leogrande, a medium-level cyclist who'd left some EPO behind when he moved out of his Southern California apartment, causing his landlady to call the FDA. Novitzky was working on that case, so he jumped at the opportunity to hear what Landis had to say.

The three of them met in early May at the Marriott in Marina del Rey, not far from the Los Angeles airport. Landis also brought his doctor, Brent Kay, to the meeting because Kay had felt threatened by Armstrong when they had corresponded through e-mails.

Landis recalled detail after detail, and even gave them his diary, in which he had written his doping schedules in code. He wanted to be thorough. What he didn't want was to lie anymore.

As the Tour of California, the most prestigious road cycling race in the U.S., grew closer, Armstrong became increasingly edgy. He asked Landis's doctor, Kay, to persuade Landis to reconsider his vendetta. But Landis was stubborn, even when he heard that Stapleton was preparing to sue the cycling shorts off of him. Power had shifted. Now Landis was the bully.

"See all these security guys around here?" Armstrong supposedly asked his former teammates Hincapie, Leipheimer and Zabriskie as they gathered for a press event before the Tour of California. "I called these guys in. I'm scared. I'm scared of Floyd. He's, like, texting me with pictures of him and a gun. That motherfucker's going to shoot me." Landis told me in late 2013 that he didn't remember sending Armstrong such a text.

Four days later, Landis's doping confession and his accusations that others had doped with him went public. Thanks in part to Tiger Williams, Landis's mentor, who apparently held a grudge against Armstrong, the contents of several of Landis's e-mails to Armstrong and top cycling officials—including the naming-all-names note to Johnson—showed up on the *Wall Street Journal*'s Web site several hours before midnight on May 19, the eve of the race's fifth stage.

Armstrong texted Hincapie: "Check out the *Wall Street Journal*. It's going to be rough tomorrow." Vaughters saw the story and called Zabriskie about it right away.

Zabriskie called Bruyneel, who supposedly told him, "We have it covered." Zabriskie then ran to Hincapie's hotel room.

Hincapie was frazzled. "The FDA is calling me—this Novitzky guy who dealt with Marion Jones and stuff," he said. "He left a message saying, 'Please call me.'"

Vaughters had heard the rumor that Novitzky was investigating drug use in cycling, and knew it was only a matter of time before he would reach out to his Garmin-Chipotle-sponsored team. Many of the squad's riders had doped in the past. Vaughters had purposely hired them and given them jobs where there would be no pressure to cheat.

He brought Zabriskie into his hotel room and told him he had his support, that if Novitzky came calling, Zabriskie shouldn't be afraid to tell the truth about his experience with performance-enhancing drugs. *You will have a job with us, no matter what you say.*

Vaughters also spoke to Tom Danielson, another American rider who'd been Armstrong's teammate, and echoed what he'd said to Zabriskie: *If Novitzky comes calling, don't be scared to tell him what you know. We will back you up.*

Then he gathered his team and instructed everyone, no matter how upset with Landis, to decline comment about the situation.

"Do not call Floyd a drunk. Do not cause a media explosion at the race," he said. "Let's just finish the race and figure out what we're going to say."

Armstrong's counterattack had already begun. First, he taped a short video that was posted on YouTube.

"I had a fairly uneventful day," he said, explaining that it was "an honor" to ride for MCA, the rapper Adam Yauch from the Beastie Boys, who was battling cancer. Then he spoke about his own struggle. He said that in the next stage, he would be riding for LaTrice Haney, the nurse at Indiana University Cancer Center who had helped him through his cancer treatment. He called her and other nurses "unsung heroes."

"LaTrice was a very special woman," he said. "She was somebody that really made the leap for me from the nurse-patient relationship; she crossed the line and we became friends."

The next morning, barely twelve hours after Landis's e-mails first appeared on the Internet, Armstrong walked off the Radio-Shack team bus near the stage start in Visalia, California. He looked coolly out into a roiling sea of reporters.

"So obviously everybody has a question about Floyd Landis and his allegations, and I would say that I'm a little bit surprised, but I'm not," he said. "The harassment and the threats from Floyd started really a couple of years ago and at that time we largely ignored him. Finally, a year or so ago, I told him, do what you have to do."

Reporters thrust tape recorders toward him. Television boom microphones hovered over his head. Not one, not two, but three public relations people (Armstrong's, the team's and the Tour of California's) stood within five feet of him, each wearing Livestrong bracelets.

Armstrong looked confident. He thrived in combative situations. As if for the thousandth time, he said Landis had "no proof; it's his word versus ours. We like our word. We like where we stand. We like our credibility."

He called Landis's accusations ridiculous and said Landis was simply seeking attention because his cycling team had not been given an entry in the race. Landis cannot be trusted, he said—remember, Landis wrote a book that mentioned none of his latest accusations. Keep in mind, he added, that Landis took "what some would say was close to a million dollars from innocent people" who contributed to his defense fund after he tested positive at the 2006 Tour.

One reporter asked if he would take legal action against Landis. "I don't need to do that anymore," Armstrong said. "My energy needs to be devoted to my team, to Livestrong, my kids."

Another reporter asked, "So, Lance, you never paid the UCI any money?" He answered, "Absolutely not." He chuckled, but caught himself.

"If you said, give me one word to sum it all up, I'd say 'credibility,'" Armstrong said. "Floyd lost his credibility a long time ago. I'm not breaking any news here to you guys." Armstrong brought up the long-standing rumor that Landis had a photo of the alleged refrigerated panniers Armstrong's team used to transport blood bags from one Tour stage to the next. "Where's *that*? Where's *that*? It's all a bunch of bullshit. It never existed," Armstrong said.

As the impromptu press briefing went on, Armstrong tightened. "From our perspective, from what's gone on at U.S. Postal and Discovery, all those Tours, we have nothing to hide. We have nothing to run from," he said. Then he folded his tanned, muscled arms across his chest so his veins bulged.

"Are you gonna tell the truth to federal prosecutors who are investigating this?" one reporter asked.

"Absolutely," he said. He tried to smile and failed.

When asked about Novitzky, Armstrong cracked a little. Though he usually spoke with authority, he seemed to have trouble organizing his thoughts.

"If—what—why would Jeff Novitzky have anything to do with, which is fine, if that's the case, we'll be, because we'll be more than happy to participate as well," he said. "But that would, why would Novitzky have anything to do with what an athlete does in Europe?"

On the team bus that morning and later with reporters, Bruyneel attacked Landis without reservation.

"What an idiot! Floyd, what a douche," Bruyneel said. Then he told reporters that Landis had "threatened, blackmailed" him ever since testing positive. He said Landis had asked him for "a lot of money" and a job in exchange for his silence about Postal Service's doping—an accusation, Bruyneel added, that was completely untrue. He also said he thought Landis was mentally ill: "Floyd should seek professional help, and by that I don't mean lawyers."

The RadioShack team posted on its Web site a string of e-mails that it said showed Landis's accusations were "a troubling, angry and misplaced effort at retribution for his perceived slights," including that RadioShack would not hire him. A statement from the team's lawyer said Landis had been threatening Armstrong for two years.

"Getting no satisfaction and not receiving a position on the RadioShack team, Landis then carried through with his threat and provided the press with false accusations," the statement said.

The individual riders struck a more sober tune:

"I don't know what is in the head of Floyd Landis, what his motivations are," Vaughters said.

Hincapie released a statement through his team, BMC Racing, saying he was "very disappointed" by Landis's accusations.

Leipheimer said he had no idea why Landis would accuse him of anything: "I can't believe it. He said we were teammates and we did stuff together, launched all these allegations. We were never even teammates. . . . All I'll say is it is absolutely false, and I just hope that Floyd gets some help. I think he needs it."

During the first few warm-up miles of the Tour of California's next stage, riders talked about the Landis affair.

Zabriskie rode next to Armstrong. "So now what?" he asked, to no reply. "Now what!"

"They're going to ask me stuff, so you won't have to worry about it," Armstrong said. "It's all going to be on me."

Armstrong chastised Hincapie for not giving stronger statements against Landis.

"Why don't you just deny it?" Armstrong asked.

"I just don't think that's the way to go," Hincapie said. "Why don't you just admit it? You could say it, get it over with and people would forgive you after a while and that would be that."

Armstrong stared at him. "Admit what?"

Five miles into that stage of the Tour of California, the *peloton* came to a town called Farmersville. On a road that cut through fragrant orange groves, a rider skidded on gravel and crashed. Several riders in his wake were unable to avoid him. They, too, fell. One was Armstrong.

In an instant, an official on the race radio called out, "Armstrong's down! Armstrong's down!" The sport's greatest star was on the street with his legs splayed out and quarter-sized rips in the back of his red-and-gray RadioShack jersey. Blood flowed down his face from a cut beneath his left eye.

Bruyneel and another team employee dragged Armstrong to his feet. They led him to his bike, and Armstrong spent the next eight miles riding next to the team car, with Bruyneel driving.

"How do you feel?" the team manager asked. "You have a headache, or is it just the eye?"

"It fucking kills, my face," Armstrong said. He fought to catch his breath.

Bruyneel said the race doctor could control the bleeding. He suggested that Armstrong take an anti-inflammatory pill or a painkiller. Armstrong said he thought his elbow might be broken, that it would be hard to go on.

"I don't think it's broken," Bruyneel said.

"I can't stand on the bike," Armstrong said. "I don't want to . . . We got to decide. I don't want to be a pussy about this, but I can't get up. The slightest of pressure, it makes it worse, it's almost nauseating."

"Let's give it a try first, Lance, to see if we should stop or not," Bruyneel said. "Let's see how it goes." Bruyneel again suggested that Armstrong take medication. Armstrong said it wouldn't do much good.

Injured and with Landis's accusations ringing in his head, Armstrong almost pleaded with Bruyneel.

He said, "I don't know what to do!"

"OK, let's stop," Bruyneel said.

"What do I do? What do I, how do I, I don't think, I don't, I don't know the last time I stopped in a race. What do I do?"

"Just pull to the side of the road," said Bruyneel. Soon, Armstrong was on the team bus with a doctor tending the wounds before they drove to a hospital. Allen Lim, whom Armstrong had poached away from Vaughters at nearly six times his salary for the 2010 season, sat next to him, and saw a glint of tears in Armstrong's eyes.

"Why am I doing this?" Armstrong said.

Lim had seen dozens of riders after crashes. Their emotions were always raw. For the first time, he saw a sadness swell in Armstrong.

"Why the fuck am I doing this?" Armstrong said again. "What the hell? I have more money than I would ever know what to do with. I have these kids who adore me, who are constantly asking me why I do this. And I have no explanation for this. Why am I doing this?"

"I don't really know," Lim said. "But, Lance, here's the deal, buddy. The happiest I've ever seen you, really the happiest I've ever seen anybody, is when we were training in Hawaii earlier this year and you were with your family, and all you were doing was riding your bicycle. So if you're asking me why you are doing this and if you want advice from me on what to do, I would say, 'Go get your family, fly them all to Hawaii and just go for a bike ride. Just go for a bike ride and don't worry about this.' All this? This is stupid."

PART SIX

THE TRUTH

CHAPTER 21

W hat forever had been whispered about the Tour became a public outcry. For a long time, Americans didn't care what cyclists did to themselves or their sport. It was a curious enterprise: men in Technicolored spandex racing bicycles past oblivious cows and through narrow village streets in France, of all places. Lance Armstrong changed that with every Tour he won. Texas vouched for the Tour de France, so the nation's sports pages did, too. Before Landis's accusations went public, Armstrong was a symbol of survivorship and dominance. It took only hours for him to transform into the most infamous example of the Tour's cheating ways.

Frankie Andreu's admission to having used EPO in order to ride on Armstrong's team appeared on the front page of the *New York Times*, and it wasn't a lone voice: Another Armstrong rider, Vaughters, though he went unnamed in the article, said he too doped. The former Motorola rider Stephen Swart said Armstrong had convinced his teammates to use EPO.

But the hardest blow Armstrong received from a former teammate, hands down, was dealt by Floyd Landis. He had been a loyal soldier to Armstrong, had won the first Tour after Armstrong's retirement and had that title stripped before stepping into the spotlight to basically say the whole sport was a sham.

Armstrong called him a liar. So did Armstrong's team manager, Bruyneel. So did other former teammates of Armstrong: Leipheimer and Michael Barry, the Canadian who took EPO with Zabriskie that first time in 2003. The international cycling organization's boss, Pat McQuaid, invoked the loaded words "scandalous," "mischievous" and "traitor" before telling me he felt sorry for the guy. He called the revelations "the last roll of a desperate man" and said, "It's unfortunate. He's turned on us." Fans wearing Armstrong's Team RadioShack shirts confronted Landis with posters bearing his name alongside the image of a menacing black rat.

Jonathan Vaughters knew the truth, and when he saw the vilification of Floyd Landis, he realized it was time to come clean, finally and officially. But he also knew he needed other riders to join him in admitting that they had doped, and that they knew Armstrong and others on the Postal Service team had doped. He framed it less as an attack on Armstrong than as a defense of Landis, a good friend.

Vaughters said, "It's almost like you've got to say, 'Sorry, Lance, but Floyd's telling the truth—so is Betsy, so is Simeoni— and you're wrecking these people. The federal government and USADA are investigating this. We can't lie for you. We can't lie. It's wrong.' It's as simple as that."

Cycling could no longer keep the world at bay. Its secrets once were safe because of the sport's obscurity, and then later because of the code of omertà when the Tour became a cash cow. But now? The United States government, in the form of the towering and initimidating Jeff Novitzky, honored no one's code of silence. So Vaughters got Novitzky's number from Tygart and called the agent to learn that the rumors were true, that the federal government had started an inquiry into doping-related crimes and cycling.

"When the time is right," Vaughters told him, "and if you decide to speak to anyone [on his Garmin team], I'm going to ask them to cooperate. I can't force them, but I can ask them."

Zabriskie didn't want to be the only witness for the prosecution. He eventually knew that Vaughters, Danielson and Vande Velde (who had been racing in Italy during that Tour of California) were also going to testify. But even the idea that it would be only him and three others gave him doubts when he considered the size of Armstrong's army. To spur Zabriskie forward, though, Vaughters needed only one word to persuade him: "Bruyneel." Zabriskie recalled the pain he claims the team manager had caused him, of how Bruyneel was supposedly the person who convinced him to dope and, in turn, apparently caused Zabriskie to become just like his drug-using father who had drunk himself to death.

Zabriskie claims that he had trusted Bruyneel and had been betrayed. He said he believed Bruyneel targeted him because he was vulnerable in the wake of his father's death, and then led him into the culture of doping.

No, Zabriskie thought, what happened to me should not happen to anyone else.

No, Landis was neither an alcoholic liar, nor a vindictive madman.

No, too many people knew the truth to let his be the only voice in the courtroom.

"OK, fuck it," he said. "Here we go."

After meeting with Danielson and Vande Velde, Vaughters issued a statement saying the members of the Garmin squad, if asked, would talk to investigators. It was a warning directed at

Armstrong, and talk they did. Though only Vaughters told investigators he had actually seen Armstrong dope, all four described systematic drug use by the Postal Service team.

Danielson, once dubbed the Next Lance Armstrong because of his talents, talked about a panic attack after a blood transfusion. It was so bad that Bruyneel and the team doctor thought he was having cardiac arrest.

Vande Velde told how Armstrong had summoned him to his apartment and subtly threatened him to follow Ferrari's doping program or be fired. "Lance called the shots on the team," Vande Velde said. "What Lance said went."

Hincapie didn't return Novitzky's calls. He wanted to get legal advice first.

He was concerned that testifying would hurt his sportswear company, Hincapie Sports, which employed a lot of his family. He was upset that the doping allegations would tarnish his legacy as one of the country's best cyclists. Maybe cost him his career.

It wasn't fair, he thought. He had just cruised along and done what everyone else did—dope.

At the final press conference at the 2010 Tour of California, Hincapie's eyes filled with tears upon being asked about Landis's confession, which implicated Hincapie as one of the Postal Service riders who had received blood transfusions and used drugs like testosterone.

"I would like to say there isn't anybody out there—the press, the fans, USADA—who wants a clean sport more than me," he said. "I'm out there suffering day in, day out. I don't get to see my kids that much even when I'm home because I'm training five, six, seven hours a day. We're the ones busting our asses on the road."

He sounded a little like Armstrong's defiant Nike ad. Though he hid his real feelings, Hincapie was unhappy that Landis had turned him into a doper, dragging him back to his Postal Service days after he had ridden clean for years. He told me that he stopped doping in 2006, the first Tour in seven years that he didn't have to do Armstrong's bidding. He said it was also the first Tour in maybe five years in which he hadn't had a blood transfusion.

He was sick of doping. Sick of the needles, the potions, the fear of getting caught, the secrecy and the lies. He had a wife and kids; he needed to support his family and not embarrass them. In 2005, after he had won the hardest mountain stage of the Tour, he had heard the whispers: Hincapie, a sprinter, must have doped to finish first that day.

Enough, Hincapie thought, enough. The days of protecting the sport and protecting Armstrong were about to end.

Landis showed up at the Tour of California on the final day. He wore a T-shirt, jeans and dark sunglasses. Flanked by private security guards wearing bulletproof vests and carrying guns and nightsticks, he was escorted to a private hospitality area to watch the finish. Earlier that week, Landis had been interviewed by ESPN.com's Bonnie Ford. He said he didn't feel remorse about his doping because everyone was doing it, but that it was time for him to tell the truth. "I want to clear my conscience," he said. "I don't want to be part of the problem anymore."

Landis said that he first used drugs on the Postal Service team in June 2002. That meant the World Anti-Doping Code's eight-year statute of limitations on some of the team's doping was about to expire and he wanted to confess before that. "If I don't say something now, then it's pointless to ever say it," he said.

It was also true that Landis had another statute of limitations in mind. It had nothing to do with antidoping rules. It was part of the United States government's whistle-blower law.

On June 10, 2010, less than three weeks after his accusations against Armstrong and basically the entire sport, Landis filed a federal lawsuit under the False Claims Act. Such suits give citizens the right and financial incentive to bring suits on the government's behalf.

Landis's lawsuit named Armstrong, Bruyneel and the Postal Service team owner, Thomas Weisel, as well as Armstrong's agent, Bill Stapleton, and Stapleton's business partner, Bart Knaggs. It also named the business entities tied to the Postal Service team, like Tailwind Sports, the management company, and Capital Sports & Entertainment, Stapleton's company.

The suit claimed that each defendant knew—as everyone in the sport seemed to know—that the Postal Service team was doping. In doping, the suit claimed, the team had defrauded the U.S. Postal Service.

The team's sponsorship contracts with the U.S. Postal Service were worth about $40 million. Under the law, defendants who lost a False Claims Act case could be forced to pay three times that amount in penalties—in this case, possibly $120 million. The whistle-blower in such a case could be awarded as much as 30 percent of the penalty—in this case, $36 million.

As Landis sat in the hospitality tent, his former Postal Service teammates approached the finish line, and the race announcer belted out their names:

George Hincapie, the United States road racing champion!

Three-time defending Tour of California winner Levi Leipheimer, "Mr. California!"

Dave Zabriskie, the five-time national champion in the road race time trial!

Of those possible witnesses in the case against Armstrong, Landis was the only one who could come out of it a double-digit millionaire.

Two days after the Tour of California, Zabriskie walked into the Marriott Hotel in Marina del Rey, into the same conference room Landis had occupied weeks before. He sat with Novitzky and prosecutors from the U.S. Attorney's Office in Los Angeles. For five hours, Zabriskie told his story. He described his first EPO experiences. He backed up many of Landis's claims, including the one about Armstrong and Bruyneel's alleged sabotaging of Landis at the 2004 Tour by dumping a bag of his blood. He said that Landis gave him doping products and showed him how to inject human growth hormone. He repeated Landis's claim that the growth hormone would make him "fucking strong." Zabriskie used the drug, even though he'd asked Landis, "Isn't that how Lance's cancer got out of control and stuff?"

Zabriskie told the feds about life with his drug-dealing father—how a SWAT team burst into his house when he was fourteen; how his father drank himself to death; how he had promised himself he would never do drugs, never be like his dad. Twice, he had to take a break to regain his composure.

For the first time, the federal investigators realized that they had a real case. Zabriskie was Landis's friend, yes, but he was not Landis. He was not seeking vengeance. He was not screaming to be heard.

He was believable.

Tygart sat in on Zabriskie's interview. As he listened to the testimony, his duty crystallized in his mind. He understood there to be a difference among dopers. Some, like Zabriskie, regretted it and wished they could take back their bad decisions to use PEDs. Others, like Armstrong and Landis, would do it all over again if they could.

Even after all Landis had been through, all the money he had lost and all the embarrassment he had brought to his family, Landis said he didn't "feel guilty at all about having doped." "I would do everything the same and I would just admit it [doping] afterwards." But at least he believed he had cheated. Armstrong just thought he was competing.

At the heart of it, Tygart was fighting for the clean athletes—like the Postal Service team's Scott Mercier and Darren Baker—who never chose to dope and never had the opportunity to test themselves against a clean Armstrong. And he was fighting for guys like Zabriskie, the ones who felt forced to dope and who fell victim to the peer pressure of the sport.

Thinking about all that, Tygart had told the federal investigators and prosecutors that they needed to push forward against Armstrong—they needed to nail him. "For guys like Zabriskie, you have to win," he said. "We have to stop this."

Headed back to Europe, Zabriskie was content to have finally told the truth to someone who might make a difference. And he was preoccupied by the hope that others would join him before news leaked that he had squealed. Flying to Barcelona, Zabriskie sat one seat over from Hincapie, who asked, "Everything OK?"

"Just great," Zabriskie said.

"Really? Because you're kind of looking at me funny."

"Nope. All good."

By then, May 2010, a grand jury had already convened in Los Angeles to investigate Armstrong and his alleged crimes—crimes that amounted to fraud, money laundering and drug trafficking. Investigators also looked into charges under the Racketeer Influenced and Corrupt Organizations Act, which historically had been brought against Mafia organizations.

As a witness for the prosecution, Zabriskie had been told to say nothing of his session with Novitzky and the prosecutors. But he confessed to Hincapie that he'd told the federal investigators everything. "I think you should, too. I didn't know anything about you, so I didn't say anything about you. But I think this is the right time to talk."

Hincapie said nothing.

"Oh, man, I wasn't supposed to say anything," Zabriskie said. "Now I'm in trouble."

In Girona, Zabriskie and Hincapie met Leipheimer, who complained that Landis had created a mess. "You know, don't tell anybody, but you don't have to talk to those people," Leipheimer said, meaning the federal agents.

Zabriskie glanced at Hincapie, then said, "Uh, yep, I know."

From then on, he kept his mouth shut. Even when Danielson hinted that he had spoken with "the bald guy"—Novitzky—Zabriskie feigned ignorance of just who "the bald guy" was. He didn't comment at all when Vande Velde called him and said, "I'm in L.A., and I had to do what you did, man." No one knew what Armstrong would do if he ever found out.

Novitzky and federal prosecutors worked toward the center of the wheel, toward Armstrong. They had Zabriskie, Danielson and Vande Velde on record, and now they sought eyewitness proof from other riders. They wanted George Hincapie, Tyler Hamilton and Kevin Livingston.

Along with Landis, they had been the closest Americans to Armstrong. They trained together in the mountains and rode together in Armstrong's Tour victories, Hamilton in the first three, Livingston in two, and Hincapie in all seven. Like Armstrong, they were Ferrari clients. They knew Armstrong's secrets.

Livingston wouldn't volunteer his testimony and would later testify to the grand jury in Armstrong's case. Hamilton ignored the first missed call to his cell phone from Novitzky. He also didn't want to talk. So Novitzky called Hamilton's lawyer, Chris Manderson, and tried to convince him to set up a meeting. The lawyer declined. Finally, Novitzky gave Hamilton no choice. He served him with a subpoena to appear before a grand jury in Los Angeles on July 21, 2010. Now Hamilton *had* to talk. There was no backing out.

Hamilton considered his options. If he testified, he would stand alone in front of a grand jury at the United States Attorney's Office. No lawyer. No Armstrong public relations man whispering in his ear. He could stay true to big-time cycling's omertà and say he knew nothing, or that he simply couldn't recall those long-ago years. After all, it was only perjury.

In the meantime, Armstrong lied.

In Rotterdam, he faced reporters before the prologue of the 2010 Tour de France and again answered to Landis's allegations.

"C'mon, it's been ten years, ten years, it's nothing new," he said.

No, he had never doped. He disputed Landis's claims that the Postal Service team had sold bikes from its sponsor, Trek, to fund a doping program. In a statement he had sent to the media mob that morning, Armstrong likened Landis's credibility to a carton of sour milk: "Once you take the first sip, you don't have to drink the rest to know it has all gone bad."

Armstrong had left the Tour of California battered and be-leaguered. He took Lim's advice and rode his beach-cruiser bike and just tried to relax with his girlfriend, Anna Hansen. Only he couldn't.

"No one is taking this away from me," he told Lim, who had joined Armstrong's team for the Tour de France. "Al, I'm all in, buddy, we're doing the Tour. I'm going to do this. I'm going to win that bloody, fucking, goddamn whatever race."

Lim kept a close eye on Armstrong. Unlike his hands-off pol-icy with Landis's doping, he wanted to prove to himself that he could "kick Lance in the 'nads" if he caught him doping. After learning from his mistakes with Landis, Lim wanted to prove that Armstrong couldn't cheat on his watch. But to his surprise, he came to think that Armstrong wanted to ride clean for the first time and had sincerely wanted Lim's help.

"It hurt his sense of pride and ego so much that these other guys were riding clean and he had not," Lim said. "He wanted to end his career with honor, with some legacy intact."

It underscored Lim's decision to join the team. "If I could change Lance, then the whole sport could change, because he had that much power," he told me.

In training Armstrong for the Tour, Lim came to the opinion that Floyd Landis had been far superior to Armstrong in terms of the power he could generate on the bike. "I've seen them both, and Floyd is way better. He's a way better athlete, bottom line." If there had been no doping in cycling, Lim contends, Landis would have won ten Tour de France titles, maybe more.

Lim considered it funny that stories about Armstrong always touted his superior physiology. I mentioned a story in the *New Yorker* from 2002 that described Armstrong's physical superlatives, like his unusually long thighbones. Lim laughed.

"All top riders have thighbones that are unusually long," he said.

His heart is unusually large, a third larger than the average man's?

"So is Christian Vande Velde's, so is Bradley Wiggins's," he said, mentioning two top Tour riders with whom he had worked.

He has a resting heart rate of 32?

"So does Christian Vande Velde, so does Floyd Landis."

But none of them were trying to win an eighth Tour de France, at the ripe age of thirty-eight. And certainly none of them were trying to focus on that task with a federal criminal investigation and the prospect of prison time hanging over their head.

During the Tour of Switzerland, a warm-up race for the Tour, a sleep-deprived Armstrong paced around hotel rooms. Before a time trial, he put on and took off his tight-fitting uniform again and again. His eyes stared out over puffy bags. Finally, he shouted it out loud.

"I'm not scared of USADA," Armstrong said. "USADA, I'm not scared of those guys, yeah, I'm not fucking scared of them. But the feds? The feds? Oh, dude, dude, I'm scared of the feds."

Lim was stunned.

"They can take everything I have," Armstrong said. "But they'd better not touch Livestrong. Fuck, dude, *fuck*! Livestrong—it's the only pure thing I've ever done."

What would Tyler Hamilton tell the grand jury?

Hamilton's lawyer, Manderson, learned the full scope of his client's knowledge only on the eve of his testimony. On July 20, 2010, the same day Armstrong rode over four mountain passes in the Pyrenees, Hamilton told the lawyer about transfusions he had performed with Armstrong—told him all about the EPO and the bad blood bags stored in a freezer called Siberia, recounted the story of Armstrong's 2001 failed test and how Armstrong had boasted that the UCI covered it up, related how blood feels when it slides from a chilled IV bag into your veins.

To Manderson, Hamilton's story did not sound like a sports story. It sounded like a well-organized criminal operation. The lawyer knew the federal investigators likely would go after Armstrong for drug distribution. He made Hamilton repeat the story of Armstrong's dripping testosterone onto his tongue, and how Armstrong sent EPO from Texas through the mail to Hamilton in Massachusetts.

Hamilton occasionally stopped for breaks and played with Manderson's kids, lightly pulling Manderson's four-year-old daughter's curly hair and goofily going, "Bo-*ing*!" Then he would return to the patio and describe his furtive traveling in Europe with secret cell phones that could not be traced back to the Armstrong team.

So who, exactly, was Tyler Hamilton? The good Tyler persuaded people he could never have been one of Armstrong's key henchmen on a team obsessed with pushing the limits of doping. But if Armstrong was the all-time champ at leading a double life, easily morphing from doping kingpin to cancer hero, Hamilton was a close second.

"You're the first person I've really told this to except for my wife," Hamilton said to Manderson. "Chris, you must really have a low opinion of me. You must really think I'm a bad guy."

"No," Manderson said. "I think you did what a lot of other people did."

Armstrong finished fourth in the Tour prologue in Rotterdam, a decent showing for so old a guy. But under the threat of criminal prosecution, Armstrong was not the spry, tough Texan who had garnered so much fame over so many years.

After Stage 3, with a thin coat of dust covering his body, and with his eyes locked in a thousand-yard stare, Armstrong might have been a zombie. He had been caught behind a crash and suffered a flat tire on a cobblestone road, misfortunes that dropped him from 5th to 18th.

He came more undone each day. Winning was out of the question—it was all he could do to stay upright. On Stage 8, the rider known for avoiding crashes in his Tour career became entangled in not one, not two, but three crashes. He clipped a pedal on the curb of a roundabout, causing his front tire to roll off and throwing him against the pavement at nearly 40 miles an hour.

To avoid a second crash, he was forced to stop on a grassy road-side. And, in the day's last misadventure, ten miles from the finish of the 117.4-mile route, a Spanish rider crashed ahead of him and Armstrong again came to a full stop. But this time his leg became stuck in a wheel and Armstrong toppled over. He stood up, put his hands on his hips and snarled at his bike, as if to say, "*How could you let this happen?*" He finished 61st in that stage, nearly twelve minutes off the pace.

Reporters wondered if the federal investigation was a distraction. No, he told Neal Rogers of *VeloNews*: "I might be distracted, but I'm not distracted on the things people are speculating I'm distracted on. I don't have any fear about any of that. I know what's gone on in my life. I rest at night perfectly well. But if I was distracted by the other stuff, I wouldn't sleep at night. And I sleep like a baby."

Armstrong's PR team begged him not to talk to reporters about the criminal investigation that was ensuing in California, but he couldn't help himself. Before Stage 10, he stomped down the stairs of his team bus and planted himself in front of a small crowd gathered there, myself included.

My colleague Michael Schmidt and I had broken a story the previous day saying the grand jury had served subpoenas to witnesses in the Armstrong case and that those subpoenas represented a significant step in the investigation. The grand jury was especially interested in people, including Armstrong, who had financed the Postal Service team.

"You've got to stop writing this stuff," he said. He claimed he had nothing to do with the operation of Tailwind Sports, the Postal Service team's management company. He wasn't an owner and he had no idea about the ownership structure. He was a rider, an employee, like any other guy on the team.

"It wasn't my company," he said. "I can't make it clear enough to you. I don't know. I didn't know the company. I didn't have a position. I didn't have an equity stake. I didn't have a profit stake. I didn't have a seat on the board. I was a rider on the team. I can't be any clearer than that."

Those statements stood in contrast to Armstrong's testimony in the SCA Promotions case when he said he gained a financial interest in Tailwind in 2004. His agent, Stapleton, also testified that Armstrong was granted an 11.5 percent interest in the team sometime that year. When asked at that Tour why he hadn't cleared up misconceptions about his role, Armstrong said, "I'm correcting that now."

Armstrong said that neither he nor Stapleton's company, Capital Sports & Entertainment, gained equity in Tailwind Sports until 2007. Tailwind's cycling team folded the next year, after the Discovery Channel did not renew its sponsorship. So Armstrong was given stock that soon would be worthless.

How odd: Armstrong, in 31st place, debating ownership of a defunct team in the middle of a Tour. He didn't even know who signed his paychecks, he said, so why would he have any knowledge of Tailwind's fraudulent sponsorship contracts—especially when none of the riders did? He wanted people to know he was a nobody, just a low-level *domestique*, when it came to his team's business side.

On accusations that he had doped, he remained consistent in telling me, "As long as I live, I will deny it. There was absolutely no way I forced people, encouraged people, told people, helped people, facilitated. Absolutely not. One hundred percent."

As a leader of a Tour team, he said, he was the equivalent of an NFL quarterback. He would have no idea if teammates—say

Landis or Andreu—were doping. "I can't speak to what they did themselves," he said. "It would be like me asking you, 'Listen, do you think there's any abuse of performance-enhancing drugs in the NFL in the offensive line?' Most people would probably say yes. Does that mean Peyton Manning is guilty? I mean, I can't control what other riders do."

He questioned whether the American people would consider a criminal investigation of him a good use of tax dollars. It would be "a shame for a lot of people," he said, if Livestrong crumbled because the government came after him. "I'm not going to participate in any kind of witch hunt. I've done too many good things for too many people," he said.

On his bike three days later, Armstrong crashed again. It happened even before the start of the race's Stage 13. In the warm-up zone, he collided with a teammate and fell, scraping his left elbow. The next morning, I had a single question for him. He ignored me, hopped on his bike, pushed me out of the way and rode off. I jogged after him and asked, "Why do you keep crashing?"

Armstrong only glared.

Five thousand miles from France, on July 21, Hamilton entered a federal building in Los Angeles. Hoping no one would see him, he took an elevator to the floor above the grand jury room and took an interior staircase back down.

Hamilton's testimony, halting and circuitous, lasted for several hours in front of the grand jury. Doug Miller, the main prosecutor on the case, was frustrated. He just couldn't seem to get Hamilton to give him clear-cut answers that would help build the government's case against Armstrong. Miller emerged from the grand jury room and asked for the help of Hamilton's lawyer. *Could he convince Hamilton to leave the grand jury and talk directly to the investigators?* It would be so much easier for both parties, he said. That way, the government's entire team—not just Miller alone—could question Hamilton. Also, Hamilton wouldn't be forced to participate in the grand jury's very formal Q&A.

Hamilton's lawyer said yes, but only if they first had a deal for immunity, which was granted. With limited immunity secured, Hamilton spoke to investigators as they sat around a table in a nearby conference room. The federal investigators asked if Hamilton knew anything about Armstrong being an owner of the Tailwind team? "No."

Where were the drugs coming from? He claimed, "Different places, including Bruyneel and Armstrong."

Did Armstrong ever give you any drugs? "Once, he mailed EPO from Texas to me in Massachusetts. Another time, he dropped testosterone oil onto my tongue."

For three hours, Hamilton spoke to investigators as he gripped one of his legs with both hands. He gripped that leg so hard and for so long that blood from a large wound on the leg—suffered when Hamilton fell jogging—seeped through his pants.

The day Hamilton spoke with the federal investigators, Armstrong tried to make a final mark on the Tour de France. His hopes of winning an eighth time were long gone. But he might still win a stage—he had won twenty-five previously—and Stage 16 was his last, best chance to experience a Tour victory.

He had come to the stage in 38th place. He had taken it easy in previous days, several times slowing up before a stage finish to thank fans for coming. *L'Equipe* poked fun at his lack of effort, saying that he started the Tour as a professional cyclist, then became a tourist on a bike, then was simply a tourist.

But while Hamilton testified, Armstrong made it into an early breakaway on the 124-mile route with four grueling climbs and remained out front until the Frenchman Pierrick Fedrigo—seven years younger—outsprinted him to the finish.

It enraged him. Armstrong barreled through the crowd on his bike. At one point, for no apparent reason, he lowered a shoulder and body-checked a gray-haired man, nearly knocking him down. At the team bus, Armstrong twice pushed a fan trying to take a photo, finally snapping, "Get off me, get off!"

Armstrong knew he needed help. Not on his bike; it was too late for that. He needed to control the narrative of his story. So in the middle of the Tour, he and his personal lawyer, Tim Herman, decided to try to dig up dirt on Novitzky. Herman would pay $50,000 to the lobbying firm the Ben Barnes Group to "raise concerns" about Novitzky in Congress.

Armstrong also spent some of his downtime at the Tour meeting and hiring Mark Fabiani, a political spin doctor who represented President Bill Clinton during the Whitewater scandal.

Fabiani would help with the public relations aspect of Armstrong's federal case. First, he told Armstrong to stop talking to reporters until a countering narrative was in place. It would go like this: Armstrong would say the government should not waste taxpayer dollars on the investigation of a cyclist who'd supposedly doped in Europe a decade before. He would attack the credibility of accusers. The effort also would stress Armstrong's persona as a heroic cancer survivor.

As it happened, Armstrong had a PR team of sorts already at work. Dozens of Livestrong workers and volunteers were at the Tour, spreading the pro-Armstrong and pro-Livestrong message. Along the Tour's course and in the start and finish towns of stages, they sold Livestrong bracelets for a euro, about $1.30 each, to raise money for cancer survivors in France. They handed out chalk so fans could write messages on the road.

Nike also sent a gigantic machine called the Chalkbot to stencil bright yellow chalk messages on roads. Those messages reminded fans of Armstrong's cancer and his philanthropy. They also were reminders that Armstrong was the most popular rider at the Tour and one of the most popular athletes in the world.

The Chalkbot stencils usually were messages from people touched by cancer. Many others were directed to Armstrong: "Love, Laugh & Livestrong. Go Lance!" "Your passion is my inspiration." "You are unbreakable." In some towns, the messages spanned hundreds of feet. In one instance, they ran for nearly eleven miles. On a Web site dedicated to the Chalkbot messages, Armstrong wrote: "Your messages show that we are stronger together." Betsy Andreu, watching the Tour from her home outside Detroit, saw it and said mockingly, "Cancer shields, up!"

Armstrong and his RadioShack teammates arrived at the starting line for the final stage of that Tour wearing all-black uniforms with a yellow "28" on their backs. The Livestrong people said the number stood for the 28 million people around the globe living with cancer. Race officials, however, ruled that the "28" jerseys were unauthorized and ordered Armstrong and his team's riders to change into their approved red-and-gray RadioShack uniforms, delaying the start of the stage by twenty minutes.

No one much cared. It was Lance Armstrong's last Tour de France, and what would a Tour de France be without a Lance

Armstrong brouhaha? He finished 23rd in the Tour, 39 minutes, 20 seconds behind winner Alberto Contador. It was his worst finish since 1995.

When Hincapie sat with investigators after that Tour, he quoted Armstrong from 1995. "This is bullshit," Armstrong told him. "People are using stuff."

Hincapie said he had understood that to mean Armstrong wanted the Motorola team to use EPO. So Armstrong went to Ferrari, and Hincapie eventually followed. He recounted Frankie Andreu telling him where to buy EPO and how to use it, and recalled that Hamilton and Livingston used it, too.

Reluctantly, Hincapie also told investigators about the team doctor, Pedro Celaya, whom he claims was involved, but whom he also considered to be caring and gentle. It was emotionally easier, he said, to name other Postal Service employees—Bruyneel, for one—who he claims had supplied him with testosterone and growth hormone. He said the doping was systematic and surprisingly casual. During the 2001 Tour, he blood-doped and saw others, including Landis, blood-doping in front of other team members. He said Armstrong twice had supplied him with EPO after his own stash ran out.

He couldn't remember it all, and with good reason. "They were asking me about Lance's doping, but doping then was like going to the bathroom," he told me. "I can't tell you how many times I saw Lance go to the bathroom."

He had been Armstrong's right-hand man, his best worker bee, through all seven of the Tour victories. They had become friends, and now Hincapie had been impelled to testify against him. He only hoped Armstrong would never know.

Everywhere Armstrong turned, he caught a glimpse of his shattering world. Novitzky and his investigators looked for witnesses who could prove he used drugs, provided drugs to his teammates and forced them to dope. They interviewed Sheryl Crow, who allegedly told them she knew about his doping and had even accompanied him on a trip to Belgium for one of his blood transfusions. They tracked down Armstrong's old *soigneur*, John Hendershot, who had opened up a successful dog-training business in Colorado. He said he wouldn't talk unless they forced him to because almost everybody doped back in the 1990s, when he had worked with Armstrong. It wasn't fair that they were singling out Armstrong for it, he said. "Cycling is a drug sport, that's it," he says. "It will always be a drug sport."

Landis's whistle-blower case brought in investigators from the Office of the Inspector General of the United States Postal Service. Those investigators were looking for evidence that Armstrong and the management of Tailwind Sports had defrauded the government by entering into a sponsorship contract knowing the team's riders were doping.

Then, there was USADA. Tygart eventually had stepped aside to let the federal investigators lead the inquiry into Armstrong's doping, but he was trying his best on his own to gather evidence for USADA's case.

Armstrong reacted fiercely. He demanded that Fabiani, on the payroll at $15,000 to $20,000 a month, reach out to Democratic senators, to President Clinton, to the former president's aides—to anyone, really, with influence to wield. He ordered Mark McKinnon, the political strategist and board member at Livestrong, to appeal to Senator John McCain, a 2008 presidential candidate for whom McKinnon had been an advisor.

McKinnon recalled Armstrong's order for me: "It was like, 'McKinnon you blah, blah, blah, get your ass over there and talk to McCain, you pussy. If you're a man, you'd go talk to McCain.' " McKinnon said he never spoke to McCain because he didn't want to put the senator's reputation at risk if it turned out that Armstrong was, in fact, a doper.

Armstrong's lawyers scrambled, reaching out to riders like Vande Velde and Hamilton to try to arrange joint defense agreements, or to offer free criminal lawyers. His legal team allegedly tried to find former teammates who could say that they never saw any doping on the Postal Service team.

While Armstrong and his team were on the offensive, his pursuers interviewed officials from the French national antidoping agency that had discovered Armstrong's six EPO positives at the 1999 Tour, and collected the incriminating documentation. Italian officials also gave the Americans documents, from doping investigations of their own.

Armstrong taunted Novitzky during one of the agent's trips to Europe. He had opened a Twitter account with his nickname, Juan Pelota. (Juan sounds like "one," and cancer had cost Armstrong one testicle. *Pelota* is Spanish for "ball.") He then tweeted:

"Jeff, como estan los hoteles de quatro estrellas y el classe de business in el aeroplano? Que mas necesitan?" The Spanish was crude, but pointed. The translation: "Jeff, how are the four-star hotels and the business class in the airplane? What more do you need?"

As shown by the government's failed case against Roger Clemens or the lame outcome of its case against Barry Bonds, the American public has no heart for chasing down its sports heroes, however 'roided up they may be.

Armstrong had that working for him. Prosecutors in San Francisco had spent nearly seven years chasing Bonds for lying to a grand jury about his doping. They won one conviction on five charges, and that conviction was on a weak charge of being evasive during his testimony to a grand jury.

In the summer of 2010, prosecutors in Washington brought a similar perjury case against Clemens. They claimed he had lied to Congress about using steroids. In 2011, the judge declared a mistrial. Retried, Clemens was acquitted.

As the Armstrong investigation dragged on with no indictment, word went around that Hamilton had told his story to *60 Minutes*.

"Somebody in the government wanted *60 Minutes* to do that piece, and made it happen," the lawyer Manderson said. "The feds were investigating and getting ready to prosecute Lance. If they indicted Lance with what the public knew at the time, you could imagine what would have happened. He'd say, 'I'm Saint Lance; this is a vendetta.' But I think *60 Minutes* changed that perception. They wanted the public to see the angel could actually be a doper, and they accomplished that."

During taping of the segment, Hamilton said Armstrong did what the majority of the *peloton* did, including blood transfusions, EPO and testosterone. Several times, as Hamilton seemed about to break down, the show's producer, Michael Radutzky, encouraged him. "You are not a rat. You are a truth teller. What you're doing is heroic. You're a truth teller."

As soon as Armstrong saw the show in May 2011, his lawyers fired off a letter to CBS News chairman Jeffrey Fager, demanding the network make an on-air apology for its assertion that Armstrong had used EPO. They called the report "a vicious hit-and-run job." CBS did not apologize.

Three weeks later, at 2 a.m. in Aspen, Colorado, Hamilton texted Manderson, claiming that he ran into Armstrong and that it was ugly. Hamilton later told Manderson that Armstrong had threatened him during an unfortunate reunion in a restaurant called Cache Cache in the skiing hub's quaint downtown.

According to Hamilton, as he was making his way from the bathroom back to his table, he had to pass Armstrong at the bar. Armstrong allegedly put his arm up to stop him, then got in his face. He claims that Armstrong said, "How much are they fucking paying you? . . . When you're on the witness stand, we're going to tear you apart. You are going to look like a fucking idiot. I'm going to make your life a living fucking hell."

The FBI rushed to investigate the incident for evidence of witness tampering. It wasn't the first time that federal investigators had looked into claims that Armstrong was trying to intimidate a witness in his federal case.

Armstrong had supposedly already sent Levi Leipheimer's wife, Odessa Gunn, a text message out of nowhere, saying, "Run don't walk," shortly after Leipheimer testified to the grand jury.

Armstrong, feeling ever invincible, was pushing his luck. He hired two high-powered lawyers, John Keker and Elliot Peters, whose résumés included a victory over Novitzky.

Keker and Peters's San Francisco firm, Keker & Van Nest, had represented Major League Baseball players in a case arguing that federal investigators, including Novitzky, had no right to seize baseball's drug-testing samples and results from companies that had gathered them. They won the case.

Within a week of taking Armstrong on as a client, Keker had arranged a meeting with André Birotte Jr., the United States Attorney for the Central District of California, which was the office investigating Armstrong. Keker essentially argued that Armstrong shouldn't be prosecuted because his foundation had done so much good for cancer awareness. The lawyer also reminded Birotte that many of the government's witnesses had credibility issues because they had doped and/or lied about doping.

"You're going to have a hard time prosecuting this guy," Keker said. He thought the feds should quit the dawdling and decide if they would press for an indictment. So much time had gone by since the grand jury convened, he said, that Armstrong's reputation and foundation were being unfairly damaged.

"You know you guys are going to be litigating this fiercely because we're going to be really vigorous here," Keker said, which some of the prosecutors took as a veiled threat.

It's likely that if Birotte had been moved by Keker's language, he would have shut down the investigation then and there. Instead, almost another year went by. Then the team of assistant U.S. attorneys on the case prepared a full prosecution memo that detailed the legal theories, strengths and weaknesses of the case and evidence they had gathered on Armstrong in the nearly two years of their investigation. Those attorneys recommended an indictment. They were 99 percent sure they could convict Armstrong on charges of drug distribution, mail fraud, wire fraud and witness tampering.

They submitted that memo to Birotte.

And they waited.

And they lost.

On the Friday before the Super Bowl, February 3, 2012, press release No. 12-024 appeared on the Web site of the U.S. Attorney's Office for the Central District of California. It was titled, "U.S. Attorney Closes Investigation of Professional Cycling Team."

Birotte said the investigation into federal criminal conduct by members and associates of a professional bicycle racing team owned in part by Lance Armstrong had been concluded. No explanation followed. Birotte told one investigator that the decision to close the investigation was his and his only, and that there would be no discussion on the matter.

Novitzky was inconsolable. Prosecutors Doug Miller and Mark Williams, the main lawyers on the case, were speechless. Several investigators thought Birotte dropped the case because Armstrong's powerful buddies in politics had pressured him. The Justice Department had received three letters totaling more than twenty pages from members of Congress regarding the investigation. None of the letters were released to the public.

As soon as Armstrong heard the good news, he exhaled. *Whew, close one!* He had escaped from yet another tight spot. His lawyers called to congratulate him. His friends called to tell him how happy they were for him. He and his girlfriend, Anna, popped open a bottle of wine and toasted their good luck. But their celebration was premature.

Minutes later, a press release appeared on USADA's Web site.

It was a statement from Tygart: "Unlike the U.S. Attorney, USADA's job is to protect clean sport rather than enforce specific criminal laws. Our investigation into doping in the sport of cycling is continuing and we look forward to obtaining the information developed during the federal investigation."

The federal investigation was over, but USADA's was only beginning.

CHAPTER 23

Compared with the federal case against Armstrong, US-ADA's seemed puny. The agency, which has fewer than fifty full-time employees at its headquarters, had a fraction of the people and funding that had been brought to bear in the federal case. It was David versus Goliath.

Armstrong had armed himself with a legal team of more than half a dozen high-powered litigators, many with Yale, Princeton and Harvard pedigrees. Even Armstrong's spokesman, Fabiani, came from Harvard Law.

At USADA, Tygart was working with just two other main lawyers and one who was relatively new to the agency. One was Bill Bock, the agency's general counsel. He was a father of five and earned his undergraduate degree at Oral Roberts University and his law degree at Michigan. The other was Rich Young, an outside counsel and Stanford grad who had been the primary author of the World Anti-Doping Code. USADA's legal affairs director, Onye Ikwuakor, who'd been co-president of his graduating class at Stanford Law, was the newcomer. They didn't bill at $1,000 an hour, as some of Armstrong's lawyers did, but they were resourceful, plucky and on a mission.

In early 2012, USADA's board, led by Olympic hurdling champion Edwin Moses, approved USADA's move against Armstrong. Tygart would have picked up where the federal case ended, but the feds wouldn't hand over their case files. The civil division of the Justice Department was still considering joining Landis as plaintiffs in a whistle-blower suit. They didn't want to risk the testimonies they had gathered for the criminal case becoming public and tainting a civil case that could be worth more than $100 million to the government.

At the end of April 2012—nearly three months after it reopened its Armstrong inquiry—USADA had done only two new interviews, with Betsy and Frankie Andreu. Tygart already had Landis in hand, though the Landis testimony was corrupted by both his own lies and his public hatred of Armstrong.

Tygart needed to start gathering witnesses who were more believable than Landis—not a hard task, really—but they also needed to have firsthand evidence of Armstrong's doping. It was a huge coup for Tygart, then, when Tyler Hamilton decided to cooperate with USADA's investigation.

A few weeks before the *60 Minutes* interview, in the spring of 2011, Tygart and Hamilton met secretly in Denver. For the first time since Landis, Tygart heard a rich, textured story of the Armstrong doping program from someone who'd been very close to Armstrong.

Tygart heard about the double lives built around PEDs and little red capsules of testosterone oil. Hamilton said team doctors handed white paper lunch bags to riders, filled not with sandwiches and juice boxes but with EPO, growth hormone and testosterone. When riders feared being overheard, they didn't ask for EPO, they asked about "Edgar" or "Poe," as in the poet Edgar Allan Poe.

Hamilton's lawyer, Manderson, said that throughout the

meeting, Tygart's expression seldom changed but that he grew pale. He looked like a guy who had spent years trying to track down Bigfoot, only to have the big guy show up at his front door.

Still, Tygart needed more than Landis and Hamilton. So he did what he had to do to get others to talk: He cut some deals.

Vaughters had already guaranteed the cooperation of his riders, though they were reluctant. They didn't want to be labeled dopers or be known as the riders who took down Armstrong.

Tygart threw in an incentive. Because those riders had volunteered to confess their doping to the federal investigators, USADA would go easy on them. He was even willing to bend the rules. The World Anti-Doping Code says that an athlete who provides "substantial assistance" in a doping investigation could have his sanction reduced by up to 75 percent. In this case, that would have meant a six-month ban. Instead, Tygart went one better: no ban at all.

Vaughters, Zabriskie, Danielson and Vande Velde testified. All were told they would not be penalized—on the condition that they remove their names from consideration for the 2012 Olympics. If the Armstrong case went public, their doping past could embarrass the U.S. team.

When Tygart had trouble convincing Hincapie and Leipheimer to come forward, he talked to their lawyers. He said, "Look, the system of doping in the sport is coming down, and all the riders, including Lance Armstrong, are going to be given the opportunity to get on the lifeboat. Are you on it?"

Leipheimer was looking at a minimum two-year ban. That would end his career and forever label him as a doper. By "lifeboat," Tygart meant a mitigated sanction. Leipheimer hopped on.

For Hincapie, it was a more difficult decision. He still considered himself one of Armstrong's best friends and had built his reputation on being Armstrong's loyal sidekick.

Armstrong wrote in his second book, *Every Second Counts*: "There have been times when I've practically lived out of the same suitcase with George Hincapie. In cycling, we're on the side of a mountain for weeks, in small hotel rooms, sharing every ache, and pain, and meal. You get to know everything about each other, including things you'd rather not." Hincapie did not relish having ratted on his good buddy, and he did not particularly like the idea of doing it all over again to a new pair of ears.

USADA needed Hincapie. He was credible. He had never tested positive. He had never been linked to doping, save for Landis's accusation. The public loved him and trusted him as the humble Big George who sacrificed himself for Armstrong Tour after Tour, the loyal lieutenant who would never let the general down. He was likely to know more about the behind-the-scenes activity on Armstrong's squads than any other rider. (And that may be the case. For instance, he told me that Armstrong and some of his teammates once brazenly received blood transfusions while the team bus was still parked at the finish line of one Tour.)

He would be the linchpin of USADA's case.

If Hincapie spoke out against Armstrong, people would listen. "You're talking about the most liked and respected American cyclist, maybe ever," said Bob Stapleton, who owned Hincapie's former team, HTC-Highroad. "We called him Captain America, for all the good reasons."

With Big George's testimony, USADA could convince the public that Armstrong was no hero, that he was a cheater and a liar, the biggest cheater and liar on the Postal Service team. But they needed Big George to say it.

Big George didn't want to say it. USADA called his lawyer, David Anders—whose services Hincapie had secured for virtually nothing, thanks again to the Wall Street bigwig Tiger Williams, who was also advising Landis.

USADA asked if Hincapie would provide testimony against Armstrong. Hincapie said, "Hell no."

Tygart came back with an ultimatum: Talk, or be banned for life. Tygart said USADA was prepared to charge Armstrong, Bruyneel, the trainer Pepe Martí and Drs. Pedro Celaya and Michele Ferrari with major doping violations because of their alleged involvement in the Postal Service's program. Did Hincapie want to join them?

"You need to tell us everything that happened," Tygart said.

In exchange for his testimony, Hincapie would get a six-month ban.

"They said they had enough on Lance and are going to take him down anyway," Hincapie told me. "It was, 'Either join us or be taken down also.' Those were my options. They certainly took advantage of my relationship with Lance, for sure. They knew that it was going to be the groundbreaker."

He was seething. It wasn't fair. He said he had stopped doping in 2006 and joined a "clean team" in HTC-Highroad. There, he said, he tried to convince younger riders that doping wasn't the way to go, that the dirty past needed to be forgotten. But a lifetime ban would've negated that work, in addition to ruining his reputation, his career and maybe his company, Hincapie Sports.

He was so angry that he considered coming clean publicly. He told his lawyer, "Fuck it, I doped and I will not cooperate with them. I'll come out and say, 'Look, I've made these mistakes and look what I've done since.'"

But he knew if he did that, USADA would have banned him then and there. It would have ended his career, and he didn't want that to happen. He wanted to ride again in the Tour and extend his record to seventeen Tour starts. He would talk, but just not yet. As a sign of his good intentions, Hincapie's lawyer sent Tygart his notes from Hincapie's interview with the federal prosecutors in 2010. With that information as a starting point, USADA allowed Hincapie to ride in the 2012 Tour, where he commiserated with the members of Vaughters's team who also were testifying against Armstrong.

The day of the fifth stage of the 2012 Tour, a news report from the Dutch newspaper *De Telegraaf* said Hincapie, Zabriskie, Vande Velde and Leipheimer would receive delayed six-month bans for testifying against Armstrong in USADA's case. The news was the main subject that day at the Tour as reporters rushed to confirm that the story was true.

On the miles of rolling roads in northern France, between the towns of Rouen and Saint Quentin, the riders chatted about it, too. At one point, Hincapie rode alongside Danielson and Vande Velde during their 122-mile workout on roadways that cut through green fields and hugged canals.

"Can you believe all this shit? It's not even true," Danielson told Hincapie. "We're not getting suspended."

"Really?" Hincapie said. "Um, that's fucked up. I'm getting suspended."

As soon as the stage ended, he was on the phone to his lawyer. He told Anders that it wasn't fair that he was being suspended for six months, while Vaughters and his riders were getting off without any penalty whatsoever. He complained that Vaughters was getting special treatment from USADA because he was just a kiss-up and that he obviously had been talking to USADA for years to paint himself as a good guy. After a multitude of phone calls back and forth between Hincapie's lawyer and USADA's lawyers, USADA decided to back down and dole out penalties that were equal.

After the Tour, Tygart contacted Vaughters with bad news: The immunity deal was off. His riders would be suspended for six months, at the conclusion of that season. Tygart said he and his colleagues had discussed it, and they were taking too much of a chance by granting immunity to some riders but not others. Bending the World Anti-Doping Code like that would require the blessing of the World Anti-Doping Agency, and also the UCI, an institution that seemed to be allied with Armstrong. And if the UCI appealed the riders' sanctions, every one of them could end up with two-year sanctions instead.

Zabriskie, Danielson and Vande Velde had no choice but to say yes to the six-month ban. They felt let down and duped. But there was no use in their griping about it now. USADA and Tygart were on a roll.

Armstrong's lawyer, Tim Herman, received a letter from USADA on June 4, 2012. It asked Armstrong to disclose everything he knew about doping in cycling. Or else. Armstrong didn't think much of USADA. How could it catch him when even Novitzky and the federal government hadn't been able to?

Herman didn't know much about how USADA worked and wasn't familiar with the nuances of the World Anti-Doping Agency's set of rules. He handed off the request to another lawyer on Armstrong's team.

Armstrong's response came from Robert Luskin, a Washington, D.C., white-collar defense lawyer who had represented Karl

Rove in the CIA leak case in 2006. He said USADA's request to talk to Armstrong was "a vendetta, which has nothing to do with learning the truth, and everything to do with settling a score and garnering publicity at Lance's expense."

"We will not be a party to this charade," he wrote to USADA. He said the antidoping agency was vilifying Armstrong and trying to lynch him, and warned that if the agency continued to do so, "We will not hesitate to expose your motives and your methods." He claimed that USADA had "bought and paid for" witnesses' testimony in the case against his client.

When Armstrong refused to confess, USADA said it would seek to charge him with a doping violation. The agency's three-man review board, which determines if there is enough evidence for USADA to move forward with a doping case, began compiling a report.

On June 28—after calling USADA's case against him "unconstitutional" and "a witch hunt"—Armstrong received a fifteen-page letter from the antidoping agency. He was in France preparing for a full-length Ironman triathlon—the sport that had become his new career. He had already won several half-distance Ironmans, and his goal was to qualify for the Ironman World Championship in Kona, Hawaii. NBC had bought rights to broadcast a two-hour special of that race, just because Armstrong was going to be in it.

If Armstrong's lawyers had thought they could bully USADA into backing down, they were mistaken. USADA's review board had found enough evidence to charge Armstrong with a doping violation. The agency then moved forward with a case against Armstrong, Bruyneel, Martí and Drs. Ferrari, del Moral and Celaya.

More gravely, it claimed that Armstrong was at the center of a doping ring on his teams, and that he had broken antidoping rules by using EPO, blood transfusions, testosterone, cortisone and saline infusions. The charges against him weren't focused only on his Tour-winning years, either. They spread from 1996 through 2010, meaning they included the two years of his comeback. USADA claimed that Armstrong's blood records from those seasons were "fully consistent with blood manipulation."

Armstrong only needed to read the second paragraph to know he was in big trouble: "The witnesses to the conduct described in this letter include more than ten (10) cyclists as well as cycling team employees." Tucked into the letter's second-to-last page, Armstrong saw a line even more chilling: *lifetime ban from Olympic sports.*

That meant if he lost the case, he wouldn't be allowed to compete in any sport that followed the World Anti-Doping Code— which is basically every sport he'd ever want to compete in. Cycling. Triathlons. Marathons. Swimming meets. Not even just the Olympic-level ones, either. Smaller events, like a 10-kilometer race to raise money for cancer, are usually sanctioned by the sport's national federation. And national federations of sports that are in the Olympics follow the WADA code.

Longtime friend Dan Empfield, who had met a young Armstrong during his early triathlon days, told me that a lifetime ban for Armstrong would be "very painful for him, very painful, big-time painful" because Armstrong is an "eating, breathing, sleeping athletic machine . . . It'd be like ripping an organ out of your body."

The week in June leading up to USADA's charges would have been even more painful for Armstrong if he had cared at all about his biological father, Eddie Gunderson.

The ever-stubborn Gunderson had been pulling up wet carpet from the screened-in porch of his mother's house in Tool, Texas—home to the brown recluse spider, a poisonous arachnid that happens to find wet carpet an ideal place to live. Gunderson should've been wearing long pants, and he knew it. As he'd worked, he felt a stabbing pain in his shin and saw a spider scurrying away. Damn thing had bitten him.

He waited two days before going to a hospital. He'd never liked going to the doctor. Months before, Gunderson's legs had swollen so much that they looked like overinflated balloons, a common side effect of liver failure. A doctor had told Gunderson he would treat him, but only if he could stop drinking for at least six months.

"I can't assure you that, so I don't want to take up your time," he told the doctor. His inflexibility doomed him. He should have gone to the hospital right after the spider bit him. Instead, precious time had elapsed by the time he made it to Methodist Hospital in Dallas, the same hospital in which Armstrong was born. His kidneys and liver gave out. His heart was working so hard to make up for the deficit of the other organs that it went into cardiac arrest.

On June 25, 2012, Eddie Charles Gunderson, the man whose family called him "Sonny," died. His funeral was held three days later, the day USADA officially charged Armstrong with being the kingpin of a sophisticated doping program on his Tour-winning teams. Armstrong used EPO. He received blood transfusions. He forced other teammates to dope and even gave them drugs, to give himself a better chance at winning and glory. In short, he was a lying, cheating bully. Nothing like the Lance that the Gunderson family remembered.

Micki Rawlings delivered the eulogy for her brother. Looking into the crowd gathered inside the Eubank Cedar Creek Funeral Home south of Dallas, she said her brother was loud, proud, stubborn, opinionated, obnoxious, sarcastic, bombastic.

"Sonny was his father's son," she said. "He loved fast cars, fast motorcycles, fast times. He loved family, music, sports, a good fight now and then and a cold beer. He was his mother's son. He had a huge, loving heart. He had caring and kindness to spare."

She said her brother had lived a wonderful life full of family who loved him. He had a wonderful wife and two wonderful children who adored him and "a son, Lance, who will never know how much he missed and how much he *was* missed."

Armstrong was not at the funeral.

The next month, Doug Ulman, the chief executive of the Lance Armstrong Foundation, met lawmakers on Capitol Hill. He and a lobbyist from the powerful law firm Patton Boggs were to speak about the foundation, cancer care and cancer awareness.

On the unwritten agenda: how USADA's investigation would negatively affect the foundation's mission.

Armstrong's efforts to reach lawmakers and raise concerns about Jeff Novitzky and his investigation never materialized, a lobbyist involved in the effort said. But that didn't stop Armstrong or his supporters from again trying to enlist Congress's help.

Ulman chatted with Senator Kay Bailey Hutchison, a Republican from Texas, about the consequences the foundation would face in light of USADA's inquiry. Among his next several stops was Representative Jose Serrano (D-N.Y.), the ranking Democrat on the House Appropriations Subcommittee on Financial Services and General Government, which decides how much the government will give to USADA each year. That conversation was "substantially if not all about USADA and Livestrong's concerns about the process that Lance Armstrong is being put through," said Philip Schmidt, the congressman's spokesman.

When the Livestrong representatives left Serrano's office, Serrano's staff members talked about how bold and inappropriate the meeting had been. "Livestrong was supposed to promote cancer awareness—right?—not spend its time and money trying to protect Lance Armstrong," a staffer said. "Totally inappropriate."

In July, F. James Sensenbrenner, a congressman from Wisconsin whose district includes the home base of Trek Bicycle Corporation, Armstrong's longtime sponsor, sent a letter to the White House Office of National Drug Control Policy, which gives $9 million a year to USADA—most of USADA's $13.7 million annual budget. In questioning USADA's investigation of Armstrong, the congressman relied on arguments identical to those used by Armstrong's legal team.

He said USADA was depriving Armstrong of his basic due process and that "USADA's authority over Armstrong is strained, at best." He called USADA's case "a novel conspiracy theory" and said that Armstrong had been tested "over five hundred times" without ever testing positive. (A theme Armstrong had fallen back on for years, though the number of times he had been tested was less than three hundred, according to the UCI.)

Tygart was called in to talk to Sensenbrenner and his staff several times. The gist of the conversations went like this:

> **SENSENBRENNER:** What in the hell are you doing to a national treasure?
> **TYGART:** I'm doing my job.

In the meantime, Armstrong and his team were working to discredit USADA, convince the government to cut the agency's funding and discourage the agency from continuing the case. Armstrong posted on his Twitter account that USADA review board member Clark Griffith had been charged earlier in the year with exposing himself to a young law student and telling her to fondle him.

"Wow. @usantidoping can pick em," Armstrong wrote. He marked the tweet with "#protectingcleanathletesandpervs."

Stapleton supposedly asked USOC officials for help in getting USADA to back down. His argument raised eyebrows, because Stapleton had been part of the group that drafted USADA's original rules.

Armstrong then sued USADA and Tygart in federal court, asking the court to end USADA's investigation on the grounds it was unconstitutional. The lawsuit ran to eighty pages and alleged that USADA had violated Armstrong's right to due process and was prosecuting a "big fish" to justify its existence.

In a swift smack-down rarely seen in federal court, United States District Court Judge Sam Sparks dismissed the lawsuit only hours later. He said Armstrong's unnecessarily lengthy allegations "were included solely to increase media coverage of this case, and to incite public opinion against" USADA and Tygart.

Armstrong's lawyers tried again, this time filing a shorter lawsuit and asking the court to stop USADA's prosecution of Armstrong. They argued that USADA was depriving him of his due process and didn't have jurisdiction over him anyway—that the UCI did. Though Pat McQuaid at the UCI initially said the case was USADA's to handle, he did a quick about-face—without explanation—and said that the UCI alone should deal with Armstrong.

Judge Sparks again ruled against Armstrong, allowing USA-DA's case to continue. He said USADA's arbitration rules were robust enough to deal with the matter and that the federal courts should stay out of the dispute. "To hold otherwise would be to turn federal judges into referees for a game in which they have no place, and about which they know little."

Tygart had won in federal court.

The fight was on.

It ended quickly.

Three days later, Armstrong did something he never had before: He stopped fighting.

"There comes a point in every man's life when he has to say, 'Enough is enough.' For me that time is now," he said in a statement.

Upon advice from Washington lawyer Mark Levinstein—who said never go to arbitration with USADA because athletes never win—Armstrong accepted USADA's charges and agreed to a lifetime ban from Olympic sports. His seven Tour titles would be stripped from him. Gone, too, would be the bronze medal he won at the 2000 Olympics, along with all other titles, awards and money he'd won from August 1998 forward. But Armstrong had a hard time accepting the implications.

"Regardless of what Travis Tygart says, there is zero physical evidence to support his outlandish and heinous claims," he said. "The only physical evidence here is the hundreds of controls I have passed with flying colors."

CHAPTER 24

Lance Armstrong had once known what to expect: nothing more than the usual letter from the United States Anti-Doping Agency informing an athlete why sanctions had been levied against him. Maybe a page or two of bullet points, outlining the evidence USADA had gathered in the case. But this report from the antidoping agency was different in an important, unprecedented way. This time, USADA would issue much more than a private letter of explanation to an athlete. It would be an open letter to the world. It would include every piece of evidence, every document, every bit of testimony from Armstrong's teammates who cooperated with USADA.

On October 10, 2012, in a conversation between USADA's Bill Bock and Philippe Verbiest, the main lawyer for the UCI, Verbiest asked Bock when the UCI would see the report. The cycling union had been publicly chastising USADA for taking so long to generate the document.

UCI officials were anxious to review the evidence USADA had gathered in its investigation of Armstrong, to determine if the cycling union would appeal the matter—but more so to see if they had been implicated in any wrongdoing. They expected a bit of professional, confidential decorum between the agencies.

When Verbiest asked for the report for what seemed like the hundredth time, Bock gladly revealed USADA's plans.

"Well, we can send it to you," Bock said, "or you can just get it when it goes online in an hour."

Verbiest fell silent.

"You still there?" Bock said.

Silence.

Finally, incredulous, Verbiest said, "What? You can't do that!"

Armstrong's attorneys were aghast when they heard the news from Verbiest. They thought releasing the report would be tantamount to a prosecutor's making public the government's evidence against a defendant before a trial. Herman, Armstrong's Austin lawyer, thought USADA's decision to go public would unfairly prejudice any juror—in this case, the public at large.

The Armstrong team was in disarray. *The evidence was going online? In an hour!*

Fabiani, the spokesman, blamed Herman for not anticipating USADA's move. Herman in turn thought the beginnings of the whole mess could be laid at the feet of Levinstein, who had convinced Armstrong to accept USADA's sanction in the first place. Now, USADA had risen to the challenge with a vengeance.

Armstrong had always beaten the system. He had outsmarted, outlasted, outmaneuvered and/or outspent all the critics. Even the United States government had failed in an attempt to indict him. He thought he could fight anything USADA threw at him. As always, he would use his extraordinary life story—cancer survivor, winner of seven Tour de France titles—as both shield and weapon.

"Are you fucking serious?" Armstrong said when Herman told him about USADA's plan to go public. "How the fuck did we let this happen?"

Tygart knew that if they failed to bring down Armstrong their mission would be irreparably damaged. USADA's funding could be cut, something he had inferred from his meetings on Capitol Hill about the Armstrong case. Top athletes with money would be inspired to challenge the system because Armstrong would be proof that those athletes could win. Losing the Armstrong case might become USADA's death knell.

One or two eyewitnesses to his doping and the doping on the Postal Service team weren't enough—they needed nearly a dozen. A couple documents that confirmed Armstrong had consulted with an infamous Italian doping doctor—even in the years he wasn't competing in the Tour but was running marathons and doing triathlons—wasn't enough. They wanted reams.

And reams they had—in addition to e-mails, photos, videos and even the Web diary of Armstrong's first wife, Kristin.

Rich Young, USADA's outside counsel, said it best. "It's the kind of thing where if you're hunting elephants and you're up against a great, big elephant, you damn well better kill it, or you're going to get trampled."

Tygart was aware that USADA wasn't up against just Armstrong. It was also up against his millions of fans. For the agency to bring down Armstrong, it would need to convince the public—all those jurors sitting in judgment—that Armstrong had been someone other than his packaged image all those years.

To accomplish that, the three main lawyers working on the report—Tygart at USADA, Young at his Colorado Springs law office and Bock in Indianapolis—pulled all-nighters and circulated electronic drafts every twelve hours. They wrote and rewrote the text until the report took on a character they hadn't really expected. It had begun as a report on a sports hero's misdeeds. It wound up sounding like a script for a mob-ster movie.

Tygart suggested, in a late-night joke, that the Mafia's wise guys fled Las Vegas and ended up working on Armstrong's team. Young congratulated Bock, the primary author, for turning the usual dry legal document into a suspenseful crime novel.

They wanted to make the report simple yet dramatic, so the public would read it from cover to cover and understand, once and for all, who Lance Armstrong really was: a pathological liar who had set an example of doping, not only on his team, but for the entire sport. He was the despot of cycling who had no qualms about crushing those who dared to question him. He was the boss of bosses in a corrupt organization, the undisputed champion of a sport built on lies.

Tygart no longer cared what Armstrong thought. He and his team had outmaneuvered the champion who smugly asked, "What are you on?" in the poster that had hung above Tygart's desk at USADA before the agency moved across town. Armstrong could make his threats. He could smear USADA. He could play the victim card as well as he ever had. But this time all the evidence would be on the Web, there for everyone around the world to see.

Early in USADA's investigation, Armstrong told me that he was concerned about Tygart's motivations. "I don't know his agenda, or if he's got other ambitions, but these guys are not honest and are not straight shooters. They are not out for the integrity of cycling or the integrity of the sport. He's just out to screw one guy and make an example out of him."

Armstrong believed USADA wanted to bring him down for

its own glorification. "C'mon, this is what our taxpayer dollars are funding, a witch hunt?" Armstrong asked me. "They're just out to get me because they want to get a big celebrity so they can justify their existence. Listen, it's bullshit. Total lies. Total lies."

Among his dwindling circle of friends and colleagues—he was no longer talking to his close friend and "coach" Chris Carmichael because Carmichael had turned his back on him—Armstrong was less confident. He knew that Floyd Landis and Tyler Hamilton were among the riders who had crossed him. Both had spoken publicly. They didn't worry him. He could impugn their credibility because they had lied for so long about their own doping.

Other witnesses, however, were riders with clean reputations, good guys such as fellow American riders David Zabriskie and Christian Vande Velde. Armstrong was most worried about George Hincapie—Big George, his most trusted partner on two wheels. In the weeks leading up to the morning of October 10, 2012, Armstrong and his lawyers had learned that Hincapie had talked to USADA. And while they had no idea what he had said, they wanted no one else to hear it, either.

Several months earlier, they had designed a plan to keep any confessions from going public. The key to that strategy was to accept USADA's sanctions.

By accepting them, Armstrong would forgo his right to an arbitration hearing—but that was part of the plan. At such a hearing, all of USADA's evidence—including teammates' testimonies—might be aired publicly. Without a hearing, Armstrong and his lawyers thought, USADA's evidence would remain confidential, and the bomb would stop ticking right then and there.

Armstrong and his team were banking on the UCI not appealing USADA's sanction. That would give Armstrong enough plausible deniability to persuade his legion of fans that, yes, once again he had been the victim, not the perpetrator.

But Armstrong and his lawyers had underestimated Travis Tygart's resolve to tell the world what he had learned about Lance Armstrong.

Tygart had hired a private security company after receiving three death threats, including one by someone who wanted to "put a bullet" in Tygart's head and another that said, "Hope you have a bodyguard and a bulletproof vest. Your [*sic*] a dead man motherfucker. You just don't know what you've done." Tygart had thought of putting all of his assets in his wife's name. Thousands of e-mails from Armstrong's fans streamed into USADA's office. An agency spokeswoman, Annie Skinner, received one wishing she'd get "ass cancer."

In advance of the report, Armstrong lawyers Tim Herman and Sean Breen rushed out a response.

"We have seen the press release from USADA touting the upcoming release today of its 'reasoned decision,'" Breen said, calling the report "a one-sided hatchet job—a taxpayer-funded tabloid piece rehashing old, disproved, unreliable allegations based largely on axe-grinders, serial perjurers, coerced testimony, sweetheart deals and threat-induced stories.

"USADA has continued its government-funded witch hunt of only Mr. Armstrong, a retired cyclist, in violation of its own rules and due process, in spite of USADA's lack of jurisdiction, in blatant violation of the statute of limitations."

At his computer at 10 a.m., Armstrong posted a message on Twitter, saying, "Heroes in combat and beyond, #SemperFi." He included a link to a story about a Marine in Pensacola, Florida, who had carried an eleven-year-old boy across the finish line of a triathlon. That boy had lost his right leg to bone cancer.

One of Armstrong's 3 million-plus Twitter followers posted an ominous response to that message: He referenced the scene in the movie *Jaws* in which the protagonists realize that the great white shark they are trying to capture is much bigger than they expected.

The Tweet said: "You know that line in *Jaws*, 'We're going to need a bigger boat'? Well, today, you're going to need a bigger boat."

Inside a squat, rose-colored office building in Colorado Springs, Colorado, across the street from the Pro Rodeo Hall of Fame, Tygart was at once giddy and anxious. He drove from his office to a local television station. There he would go live on ESPN's *Outside the Lines*. The plan was to appear on national television moments after USADA's report went live on the Internet. His staff had worked for days preparing the case file for publication. To finally publish the report, all they needed was a final blessing from the boss.

Just before 2 p.m. Eastern time, he called his office from his cell phone and gave the go-ahead.

"Let's do it," he said.

About 870 miles southeast, the report popped up on Armstrong's laptop. On the right side of the home page of USADA's Web site, there appeared a 2-by-2-inch sky blue box with the words "Pro Cycling Investigation Reasoned Decision and Supporting Materials." An arrow pointing to the box invited all users, "Click to view information."

Armstrong clicked.

The report portrayed Armstrong as an infamous cheat, a defiant liar and a bully who pushed others to cheat with him—join him, or be gone. USADA called the doping on Armstrong's United States Postal Service team "the most sophisticated, professionalized and successful doping program that sport has ever seen."

The evidence of Armstrong's doping was overwhelming. More than two dozen witnesses. Eleven former teammates, including the venerable Big George. Blood test results that experts said proved that during his comeback Armstrong had manipulated his blood for an edge in endurance. Banking and accounting records showing payments to EPO master doctor Michele Ferrari, including one payment that appeared to come from a bank account Armstrong shared with his mother. USADA had included proof of more than $1 million in payments to Ferrari, including at least $210,000 in payments after 2004, when Armstrong said he had severed his working relationship with the doctor.

The report ran 202 pages. With the supporting materials, there were more than 1,000 pages of information. It was all there, even George Hincapie's question to Armstrong, "Any EPO I could borrow?" and Armstrong's answer, "Yes."

Some friends and others close to Armstrong said that once he clicked on the report, he read it all and even memorized parts of it.

Yet he insisted to me that, in fact, he had not read a single word.

CHAPTER 25

One month before the USADA report was made public, Armstrong unexpectedly had learned about some evidence the antidoping agency would use against him. Those sordid details were in Tyler Hamilton's tell-all book, *The Secret Race*, which was published in September 2012.

Early in 2011, an entire year before the U.S. Attorney's Office in Los Angeles would drop its criminal investigation of him, Armstrong heard rumors that Hamilton was working on a book with author Daniel Coyle, who in 2005 had written an in-depth book about Armstrong—minus his doping, of course. One of Armstrong's lawyers called Hamilton's lawyer to find out if a Hamilton tell-all was in the works.

There was never official confirmation, but Armstrong braced himself for months and months as he waited to read what Hamilton might write. He was incensed that Hamilton, the former teammate Armstrong called "the dirtiest fucking rider," would violate the omertà—and would make money off of it.

Hamilton's *60 Minutes* interview in May 2011 gave a hint about what the book contained. He cracked open the inner workings of cycling—the doping, the lies—but focused on the Postal Service team's doping program. He told of Armstrong and the team using testosterone, "Poe" and blood transfusions. He said it had been a proud moment for him to receive from the team a white paper bag that contained performance-enhancing drugs because it symbolized his success: Finally, he was being given the chance to do what Armstrong was doing to get ahead.

Mark McKinnon, the board member and political consultant, thought Hamilton looked "weird" and "suspicious" on *60 Minutes*. "It was very halting. It came across as a guy who didn't really believe what he was saying." Because of that, McKinnon—who for years had resisted the truth about Armstrong—wasn't worried that his accusations would harm Armstrong or the foundation.

McKinnon changed his mind sixteen months later when Hamilton's book showed up on his doorstep. He lived in Austin with his longtime wife, Annie, a cancer survivor inspired by Armstrong.

He read the book in one day. With each page, his anxiety grew. He thought back to 2011 and remembered reports that Hincapie had spoken to the grand jury. (He actually volunteered to give statements to the feds.) Hincapie's testimony plus the accusations against Armstrong in Hamilton's book meant big trouble for the foundation built on Armstrong's good name.

McKinnon felt that the proof that Armstrong had cheated "was incontrovertible." His first thought: Armstrong needs to go. The next day he was on the phone with other board members at the foundation: "You've got to read Tyler's book. It's going to be a major crisis." He found an early ally in Jeff Garvey, the former Livestrong chairman of the board who was a longtime supporter of USA Cycling. Garvey also thought that Armstrong had to disassociate himself from the foundation if it was to continue thriving. It was an idea that McKinnon, Garvey and the rest of Livestrong's board of directors nursed for weeks, until they finally ran out of time.

When USADA's report came out, a majority of the board members worked to protect the foundation, without Armstrong's knowledge. They held an emergency conference call and decided that Armstrong had to step down as chairman of the board. He agreed to step down, reluctantly. At least he could remain on the board of directors, he told the foundation's president, Doug Ulman, so it wasn't a complete disaster, right? He could always take over as chairman later, once the rumblings about his doping past settle down.

So, a week after the USADA report, Armstrong announced that he'd stepped down as chairman of Livestrong's board to protect the charity from negative publicity. But it signaled much more than that. His stepping down sparked the most precipitous, unceremonious fall of any professional athlete in modern times.

Within hours, Armstrong's sponsors jumped ship. Nike was gone. Trek Bicycle Corporation. Oakley. Giro. RadioShack. Anheuser-Busch. FRS, a sports drink maker. Honey Stinger, an energy bar maker.

Nike released a statement all but accusing Armstrong of hiding information from the company: "Due to the seemingly insurmountable evidence that Lance Armstrong participated in doping and misled Nike for more than a decade, it is with great sadness that we have terminated our contract with him."

Of course, Nike had heard suggestions of Armstrong's doping along with everyone else—his cortisone positive at the 1999 Tour, the six positive EPO samples from that Tour, the testimony of teammates Stephen Swart and Frankie Andreu. All of that evidence, however, seemed to get buried under the brilliant marketing strategies that made him one of the world's most recognized athletes.

Now Nike was shocked—shocked!—that Armstrong had deceived them. It was as if one of the world's most sophisticated sports companies knew nothing of doping's history in cycling, though Tour winner after Tour winner had admitted to doping. (Most recently, in 2007, the 1996 winner Bjarne Riis confessed to doping to win the Tour.)

It was as if past cycling champions such as Belgium's Eddy Merckx, France's Jacques Anquetil and Italy's Fausto Coppi, or perhaps most winners of this hundred-plus-year-old race, had not tested positive and/or admitted that doping was engrained in the sport. (Merckx publicly claimed he was disappointed in Armstrong, though he was the person who Armstrong claimed introduced him to the doctor Michele Ferrari in the first place.)

Within two weeks of the USADA report, even Armstrong's allies bailed. The UCI, the cycling federation that had long supported him, turned on him. Pat McQuaid said USADA's report "sickened" him. "Lance Armstrong has no place in cycling. He deserves to be forgotten in cycling. Something like this must never happen again." The UCI would not appeal USADA's sanction against Armstrong.

McQuaid was hardly pure. He had been barred from the 1976 Olympics after using an assumed name to race in South Africa in violation of an international antiapartheid sporting boycott. He and his predecessor, Hein Verbruggen, had overseen cycling in its darkest days of doping. But it was Armstrong in the public eye, taking the hit for all the sport's sins.

Several weeks later, on November 10, 2012, Armstrong posted a photo on his Twitter page, trying to show that he could not be defeated. It showed him at home lounging on a couch beneath his seven framed yellow Tour jerseys. It came with the comment, "Back in Austin and just layin' around." No matter what USADA could do to him, he would not let himself be humbled. Not that other people didn't try to do it for him.

In early November 2012, foundation board members who had formed a cabal against Armstrong talked to Ulman about a way to completely extricate Armstrong from his own organization. Outing Armstrong as board chairman hadn't been enough. The board realized that Armstrong needed to cut all ties.

The decision wasn't simple to make. Armstrong had accomplished a lot with the Livestrong Foundation. He made it cool to survive cancer, and removed a stigma from those who had gone through months and years of pain and hospitalization. He personally donated $7 million, and the foundation raised a total of $500 million to help families touched by cancer. Without him, Nike would never have cobranded all those yellow bracelets or the entire Livestrong sportswear collection, which included things like sneakers, shirts, hats, etc.

Now, though, the foundation had evolved out of his hands. Actually, it was taken out of his hands.

Those board members gave Ulman an ultimatum: "If Lance doesn't leave, then we're leaving."

About a month after the USADA report was published, Ulman told Armstrong that most of the board members wanted him to step down as chairman. Armstrong blew up. First he blamed Ulman for betraying his loyalty. Then the man with a quick temper and no impulse control went to his laptop. He wrote a scathing e-mail to board members. He reminded them he had built the foundation from scratch and that the charity would be nowhere without him. He called them "cowards" for not sticking by his side. McKinnon said Armstrong's e-mail showed "a lack of remorse or any notion that he has to serve a cause greater than himself."

Though he apologized the next day for his language in the e-mail, the board members weren't about to change their minds. So Armstrong abandoned the organization.

Two days later, the Lance Armstrong Foundation officially was renamed "Livestrong," as the organization began to scrub itself of its founder. The charity no longer displayed a duplicate set of Armstrong's seven yellow jerseys in its lobby.

Armstrong stopped talking to the board members, including some, like Garvey, who had been personally close to him. He removed more than a dozen pieces of his art collection from the foundation's headquarters, leaving large rectangles of blank space on the walls.

He felt hurt that his own charity had forsaken him. But if Livestrong didn't want him, he didn't want Livestrong, either.

Betsy Andreu was at home in Michigan waiting for the USADA report. When it went live, she took her laptop and clicked to the page listing which riders and other witnesses had submitted affidavits for the prosecution.

As she saw the names on sworn affidavits from eleven of Armstrong's former teammates, she said, "Oh, my God. Oh, my God." She called across the room to Frankie and said, "All of our work paid off!"

For more than a decade, Betsy had called reporters, antidoping officials like Tygart and federal investigators like Novitzky with tips. Check out these documents, she'd say. Call this cyclist, call that lawyer. During that time, I estimate, we easily spoke more than two hundred times, mostly after she sent me a link to a story about Armstrong or doping, or both. She always told me, "Don't tell anyone I told you this," and wanted me to chase every one of her leads in the hopes it would prove Armstrong had doped. It was clear that on some days she spoke to reporters nearly nonstop because while we were speaking on her home phone, her cell phone would ring and ring, as if she were a switchboard operator.

All good, Frankie agreed. But he was less than happy. So what, he asked his wife, if ten other riders had admitted to doping and had testified against Armstrong? While he'd been shunted aside, other guys still rode. "Yeah, yeah, but every one of those guys still has their money, and where does that leave us?" he said.

The Andreus weren't millionaires, like some of the riders. They didn't have a a $105,000-plus Maserati parked in their driveway or own a boutique hotel, like Hincapie did. Nor did Frankie Andreu ever own a Corvette and eight acres of land outside of Chicago, like Vande Velde did. He never made upward of a half-million dollars a year, like most top Postal Service riders eventually did.

But after the USADA report, Betsy Andreu was rewarded with intangibles. She had regained her dignity. She was no longer the "crazy bitch," as Armstrong had told so many reporters. In tears, she told her children, "Mom stood up to the bully. Always stand up to the bully."

In the weeks after his fall, Armstrong went into seclusion on the Big Island of Hawaii. He let his closely shorn hair grow into a wild mess. He stopped shaving. He looked lonely and, truth be told, like a man who didn't care about anything anymore.

As the federal whistle-blower case creeped ever forward, Armstrong worried what it could cost him. If he was found guilty, it could mean that he'd have to pay the Postal Service $120 million out of his pocket.

Bad enough, the money. Worse, the lifetime ban from sports. He had expected to start a second career in triathlons, but USADA's order made that impossible. He wanted to get the ban lifted or at least mitigated. His complaint to anyone who would listen: *Why should teammates like Vande Velde and Hincapie get six months while I get the death sentence?*

Tygart said USADA might reduce the ban in exchange for information about people in cycling who facilitated or condoned his doping. From USADA's perspective, Armstrong would have to give up big names that the antidoping agency suspected were involved in his doping scheme. As Armstrong hesitated, at least one advisor told him to come clean for the simplest of reasons: Americans were a forgiving bunch.

That man was Steven Ungerleider, a visiting scholar at the University of Texas, a sports psychologist and an antidoping expert who had written a book on the East German doping machine, *Faust's Gold*. Ungerleider had met Armstrong through a friend, Armstrong's lawyer Tim Herman.

Herman had enlisted Ungerleider, who had extensive experience working with Olympic athletes, to be a volunteer consultant in the matter and help talk to Armstrong about coming clean. Ungerleider spoke with Armstrong about how his confession would unburden him and how it would be beneficial for his children in the long run. He suggested that he look the public straight in the eye and say, "Look, I really fucked up. Please don't hurt my foundation."

Armstrong wanted to know two things—how he could rebuild his reputation and how he could mitigate his lifetime ban from Olympic sports. Ungerleider told him that he could turn around his reputation in a second if he came clean. Telling US-ADA everything should be a part of that deal, he said.

If Armstrong confessed to the antidoping agency, it could help the sport of cycling and USADA might reduce Armstrong's suspension. It would be good for both parties, Ungerleider said. Armstrong could set an example for other riders to come forward with their own doping tales. The entire sport would come clean and start anew.

They went back and forth for days. Armstrong: "Oh no, these motherfuckers are out to destroy me. They are sleazebags out to destroy me, my home and my children."

> **UNGERLEIDER:** "You need to trust the system."
>
> **ARMSTRONG:** "Why did they break out that report on me? It just ruined me."
>
> **UNGERLEIDER:** "You left them no choice. If you had come forward in June, it would have been another story."
>
> **ARMSTRONG:** "Screw them."
>
> **UNGERLEIDER:** "You should give back your Olympic bronze medal. It would be a gesture of good faith."
>
> **ARMSTRONG:** "Fuck you, I'm keeping it."

In the end, Ungerleider helped broker a meeting between Armstrong and Tygart. They met on Friday, December 14, 2012, at noon, at the former Colorado governor Bill Ritter's office in downtown Denver. Ritter agreed to host the gathering because he was a cycling fan who years before had befriended Armstrong.

They gathered in a conference room on a quiet floor of

the building. Armstrong was late, worrying everyone that he wouldn't show. When he finally walked through the door, he looked unkempt and unshowered. He looked like "Robinson Crusoe," one person said. No wonder his close friends had been worried about how he was handling the aftermath of the US-ADA report. Those friends saw that Armstrong was depressed and that he had turned to alcohol for solace. Even USADA was nervous that he'd do something to hurt himself, based on how quickly his kingdom had collapsed and how quickly the public had turned on him.

Herman, Armstrong's lawyer, was there to help Armstrong navigate the situation. Tygart was there with his colleague, Bill Bock. Ungerleider was there as someone who had been authorized to speak on Armstrong's behalf. Ritter were there acting as a neutral party, though everyone knew he was buddies with Armstrong.

For a few minutes, everyone exchanged pleasantries. *How was your flight? Did you find the building OK? Anyone want coffee?* But Armstrong couldn't remain civil. He was face-to-face with Tygart, his nemesis, for the first time.

"Travis, you're a motherfucker," he said. "I can't believe that shit you put in that report. You know that's all garbage. You called me the Bernie Madoff of sports? [Which he hadn't, actually.] You're putting me in the same category as that motherfucker! He ruined and destroyed lives! He's like Adolf Hilter!"

He began to cite certain points in the USADA report with which he disagreed, speaking as if he had committed them to memory. He mentioned that the report had called his doping program "the most sophisticated and professionalized" in sports history. "It's the most sophisticated doping program ever? C'mon, how about the East Germans?" He pointed to Ungerleider's book on the East German doping machine, which Ungerleider had placed in front of him. "Fuck, they were doping *children*! They were *real* criminals doing real harmful things to people! That's not at all what we were doing!"

To Herman, who had grown close to the troubled star, Armstrong was both a client and a de facto son. He grabbed Armstrong's arm and said, as if talking to a toddler, "Lance, remember we talked? You have to be nice." Herman smiled. "All right, Lance, you feel better now? Are you OK, buddy?"

Bock interrupted. "Lance, we just want to tell you how much we appreciate your coming here. It took a lot of courage for you to come. We're here to help you and help you restore yourself in the community. We don't know what we're capable of doing about your lifetime ban, but we're here to start the conversation."

"What kind of promises can you make?" Armstrong asked.

Tygart answered, "None, right now, but we need to take baby steps."

Armstrong was set off again, "Why the fuck am I here? This is fucking bullshit! I knew Travis would do this!"

Herman put a hand on his shoulder, telling him he should just let it all out, if he wanted to. Embarrassed, Armstrong fell quiet.

In the next several hours of the meeting, they discussed how Armstrong could rid himself of his lifetime ban. He wanted to, he needed to, get back into triathlons and bike races, and to race in running events like the Chicago Marathon. (Three months before, he had been denied entry into that marathon because of his suspension.)

Tygart said he could possibly lower Armstrong's suspension to eight years, if Armstrong gave USADA enough information about the people who'd helped him dope and helped him avoid detection. Tygart said the ban could be even less, maybe four years, if he got the cooperation of the UCI and the World Anti-Doping Agency in determining his ban. He encouraged Armstrong to point fingers at those people who facilitated his doping. It was the perfect opportunity for him to give back to the sport he loved, to leave a positive legacy and start changing the public's perception of him, Tygart said.

Tygart said USADA worked closely with the Justice Department and could put in a good word for him in the whistle-blower case. Former governor Ritter mentioned the power in the room, including himself, and said they could help Armstrong, but only if he cooperated.

Armstrong grew introspective. He said he was unfairly blamed for a whole era of cheating in cycling. But he allowed that he was part of a toxic system and admitted that the culture needed to be dismantled. "At the end of the day," he said, "I can get you skeletons and dead bodies. I know where all the bodies are buried."

But if Armstrong was going to talk, he wanted a guarantee that he would receive a ban that was exactly the same ban his teammates had received for talking: six months. Worst-case scenario: two years.

When Tygart said that wasn't really a possibility—that any sanctions which would vary from the World Anti-Doping Code needed to be approved by WADA and the UCI—Armstrong's voice rose: "You don't hold the key to my redemption. *There's only one person who holds the key to my redemption, and that's me!*"

"I don't need to work with you, I think I can do this on my own," he said. "I'll just go out and tell the public what I know, and that will pressure you guys to give me a lesser ban. I'm the only one who can clean up the sport!"

He mentioned that the UCI was going to form what was being called the "Truth and Reconciliation Commission," a program that would allow riders to talk about all the doping they'd done and who'd helped them do it, in exchange for immunity from prosecution by antidoping authorities. *He would give his information to* them *and his ban would be lifted, right?* (Wrong: The UCI backed out of a commission, though in late 2013 there was talk to establish another one.) He didn't need USADA—he was Lance Armstrong, for God's sake, and he could fix things himself.

As the meeting went into its fifth hour, Armstrong seemed to realize that his aggressive posture was getting him nowhere. He softened and said that the ban would kill him. He wasn't allowed to even run with his kids in USA Track & Field–sanctioned races in Austin. He was a man who thrived on testing himself against others in an athletic arena. Basically, he told USADA, the ban meant that he couldn't be Lance Armstrong.

"I can't get up in the morning without knowing that I have something to live for," he said. "For me, that's training and competition. I'm not training because I enjoy it—I'm training because I have to. I need to train more than just to stay in shape—I need to know that I'm going to compete. This has been my whole life. I've been a competitive athlete my whole life. I need to know that you will help me back into competition."

For a moment, nobody said a word. Armstrong had just laid it out for them. He wasn't just asking for a mitigated ban. He was begging for his self-esteem, his identity, his life.

Ungerleider, the psychologist, later told Tygart: "I hope you guys got that memo. What he's trying to say is that you are taking away his coping mechanisms. This is who he is as a human being. Any way he can get back into it, with a 10k or a swimming race, that might be healthy and give him the skills to cope better in life. I'm not asking you to do anything, I just want you to be aware of that."

With Armstrong seeming to lean toward confessing to US-ADA, the parties arranged another meeting in Austin for a week later. Armstrong went back to Texas to bide his time until then. When he did not receive a written guarantee that his ban would be reduced, he refused to meet again.

A little less than three months after the USADA report came out, Armstrong called his longtime friend Oprah Winfrey. Both were in Hawaii. Armstrong was there with his family during a self-imposed exile from the United States mainland. *Could he come over to her estate in Maui and have lunch?* He had a business proposal for her. She jumped at the chance.

Armstrong trusted Winfrey. She had been an admirer and had worn a Livestrong yellow band, had even sold the bands on her Web site. She had hosted the Armstrongs, including his mother, at her house for dinner. (Armstrong had grown closer to his mother since his divorce from Kristin in 2003, but their relationship, at times, was still strained.)

He and Sheryl Crow had gone on her talk show when they were still a couple in February 2005, and it had been nothing but positive. Winfrey asked Crow, "Is he a big romantic?" Oh, yes, she answered. Armstrong's mother, Linda, appeared also, and Winfrey cooed, "The thing that I love about Linda is that she was a single mom."

Weeks before their meeting on Maui, Winfrey had reached out to Armstrong to ask if she could interview him on her struggling Oprah Winfrey Network (OWN), and he declined.

But it got him thinking.

He was sick of listening to lawyers who told him to keep quiet about his past, sick of waiting to hear back from spin doctors trying to gauge what the public thought he should do next. Most of all, though, Armstrong couldn't stand Tygart's wielding so much power over him: There would be no mitigated lifetime ban unless Armstrong came clean to USADA.

He knew he'd eventually have to tell the federal prosecutors in the whistle-blower case about his doping. But he hated the fact that some no-name prosecutor desperate for fame would get the glory for outing him. He wasn't ready to give up that control. He wanted to confess on his own terms.

Besides, that fall Armstrong had had an upsetting experience with his teenage son, Luke. The boy had been teased at school for having a cheating, doping father, and then got into a fight at the bus stop defending him. Armstrong was shaken when Luke said, "So-and-so said this about you. Is it true?" The father wanted to set the story straight in the eyes of the public.

So, he told his old friend Oprah: *I want to come clean and I want to do it on your show, with you asking the questions and the whole world watching.*

Armstrong's handlers were in disbelief that he'd gone ahead and set up an interview with Winfrey without consulting them. But he was adamant that there was no turning back. So his PR and legal team, plus a psychiatrist, streamed into Austin to prepare him for the show.

The day of the taping, he made a special trip to Livestrong's headquarters to apologize to the staff for what he had done and what he was about to do. "I'm sorry for everything that you've been through because of me." He texted the *soigneur* Emma O'Reilly, hoping she would call him back so he could apologize for publicly vilifying her and calling her a whore. She didn't.

He called Betsy and Frankie Andreu and said, "Look, I know I called you guys ugly liars forever, and I'm sorry about that."

"How could you do this to us? We were friends. You ruined our lives!" Betsy Andreu said.

"I know, I'm sorry."

Armstrong talked to Frankie for ten minutes. For another forty, he spoke to Betsy, only because she made him listen to her tirade against him. She cried. Then she laughed, then she cried— and then they promised to stay in touch by e-mail. After years of not speaking, years during which he wanted her dead if not worse—and vice versa—Armstrong had done the equivalent of climbing Mont Ventoux in eight turns of the pedals.

He had charmed Betsy Andreu.

"Yes or no, did you ever take banned substances to enhance your cycling performance?"

Sitting just feet away from Oprah Winfrey for a two-part blockbuster that had been billed as a "no holds barred" television interview, Armstrong took a breath in front of 4.3 million people.

"Yes."

"Was one of those banned substances EPO?"

"Yes."

"Did you ever blood-dope or use blood transfusions to enhance your cycling performance?"

"Yes."

"Did you ever use any other banned substance such as testosterone, cortisone or human growth hormone?"

"Yes."

"In all seven of your Tour de France victories, did you ever take banned substances or blood dope?"

"Yes."

"Was it humanly possible to win the Tour de France without doping, seven times?"

"Not in my opinion."

Armstrong met Oprah Winfrey halfway. He told his version of the truth. He neither shed the obligatory Winfrey tear nor offered the anticipated apology. He didn't feel bad for cheating and, to prepare for the interview, had even looked up the word in the dictionary to make sure he understood it. "Cheating" meant gaining an unfair advantage over your competitors, and he didn't think he ever did that. The doping program was "very conservative, very risk-averse" on his teams, he insisted. And, he said, it was so necessary that it was like "putting air in your tires."

He confirmed Emma O'Reilly's stories about the cover-up of his positive cortisone at the 1999 Tour. He apologized to her for what he'd put her through. He said he never tested positive for EPO at the 2001 Tour of Switzerland, as Landis and Hamilton suggested. No, he did not pay off the UCI to bury that supposed positive test. No, he never offered a bribe to USADA, either. He also said he was clean during his comeback in 2009 and 2010, which Tygart and prosecutors later said was just his way of protecting himself from criminal charges. He defended his former doctor Michele Ferrari. He admitted that he didn't like the man he had become—a liar and a bully—and that he was the type of person who needed therapy.

When asked if he ever confessed to doctors in an Indianapolis hospital room that he doped—as Betsy and Frankie Andreu had asserted he did—he said he couldn't answer that question. Then, in another awkward moment amid 180 minutes of discomfiting half-truths, he addressed Betsy directly, saying, with a smirk, "I called you crazy, I called you a bitch, I called you all those things, but I never called you fat." He was trying to be funny—because Betsy is actually rail thin—but the sound of the joke falling flat echoed throughout the country, maybe even the world.

Only once did Armstrong show emotion or contrition: when he relayed how he had sat down his three eldest children— thirteen-year-old Luke and the eleven-year-old twins, Grace and Isabelle—to tell them why there had always been so much controversy following him. The conversation happened just before the Christmas holidays, a few weeks after Luke had gotten into that fight at the bus stop.

"I said, listen, there's been a lot of questions about your dad, my career and whether I doped or did not dope, and I've always denied, I've always been ruthless and defiant about that, which is probably why you trusted me, which makes it even sicker. I want you to know that it is true."

He then told Luke, who had been in other fights over his father's reputation, "Don't defend me anymore." Glimmers of tears appeared in his eyes.

There were no tears, though, when he spoke of the impact his lies might make on his foundation or on the millions of people who considered him a hero. His summary for Winfrey: "The ultimate crime is the betrayal of these people that supported me and believed in me."

He walked off the set a little lighter, but his friends saw him as a shadow of the man from even a few months before. McKinnon called Armstrong's performance "hall-of-fame horrible . . . I'm sure that will become an exhibit for people who do crisis management on what not to do."

Betsy Andreu watched the first night of the Oprah interview from the CNN studios in New York City and went live on *Anderson Cooper 360°* afterward. "If he can't say the hospital room happened," she said, again brought to tears, "how are we supposed to believe everything else he said?"

Armstrong had thrown himself, yet again, between his dwindling supporters and the story being told by reporters, lawyers, prosecutors and USADA. And it may have broken him once and for all.

After the Winfrey confession, SCA Promotions filed a lawsuit in Dallas to recoup the $12.1 million that Armstrong had received from the company, legal fees and interest. He offered them $1 million to settle it, but SCA's bridge master, Bob Hamman, would no longer be satisfied by moral victories. Several other insurance companies filed lawsuits to get their money—more than a million, in each case—back from him, too. A group of readers sued him for more than $5 million, claiming that his autobiographies, *It's Not About the Bike* and *Every Second Counts*, were based on lies. They wanted refunds. A judge ruled that Armstrong's books, filled with lies or not, were protected by free speech.

A group of Livestrong supporters prepared to sue for a return of their donations because, they said, the foundation was based on lies. "We're all suckers," said Michael Birdsong, a donor who gave at least $50,000 to Livestrong and came up with the idea for the lawsuit.

David Walsh, the *Sunday Times* of London and its then–sports editor Alan English, sued Armstrong to get back the more than

$450,000 they gave Armstrong in 2006 in his libel case against them. This time, they won and received about $1.56 million.

In February 2013, the government decided to join Floyd Landis as a plaintiff in the federal whistle-blower lawsuit against defendants that include Armstrong, team manager Johan Bruyneel and Tailwind Sports, the company that managed the Postal Service team. The plaintiffs claimed that Armstrong, Bruyneel and Tailwind had defrauded the government by engaging in systematic doping in violation of the team's contract with the Postal Service. To Armstrong's dismay, the chances of Landis winning the case rose steeply with the government on his side.

The year before, Armstrong had told former Postal Service rider Mike Creed that he wasn't sweating the federal criminal investigation of him because he had "$100 milski" in the bank. But with the payout in the federal whistle-blower case possibly $120 milski, $100 milski doesn't seem all that much.

He tried to limit his losses. First, he offered the government $5 million to settle the case, but it refused the offer—too low. Next, he offered $13.5 million. That didn't work, either. For the government to walk away from the case, it wanted $18.5 million and his cooperation against the other defendants, which included Bruyneel, his trusty team manager.

Though it could have saved him a multitude of grief and legal fees, Armstrong turned down that deal. The case might end up bankrupting him, but, he told me, he'd rather be poor than a rat.

Closer to home, friends of Armstrong's mother, Linda, said she took news of her son's confession badly. She took down her Web site, called "Force of Nurture," which promoted her motivational speaking. She stopped posting on Twitter—her account was @LindaASpeaker, with a photo of her in a Tour de France–yellow shift dress.

Terry Armstrong watched the *Oprah* confession and wept. "Lance is asking the country to forgive him," he said. "It might be a good idea if he forgives his dad." As his adopted son explained how he became involved in cycling's most successful doping program, Terry thought, "Oh my God, this is me, I instilled that."

He said, "I could see him showing up going, 'You know, everybody is cheating, well, I'll do it better. I'll find whoever I got to find that's the best.' Then the money just rolled. I taught him to win. I gave him that drive, but I never taught him to be a bully. I never taught him to cheat."

Armstrong himself didn't watch his confession. He retreated to a bedroom to sleep while the show aired in front of his girlfriend, Anna, and his good buddy John Korioth.

The next day on the golf course, Armstrong asked Korioth, "What did you think?"

"Man, Lance, I got to tell you, watching that interview, you are a really good liar."

"Huh?"

"Yep, you are a really good liar, but you're horrible at telling the truth."

EPILOGUE

I n my four hours of conversation with Lance Armstrong on his
final day inside his Austin mansion, he gave profanity a bad
name.

Here, compressed into a sentence, is an abbreviated compila-
tion of what he had to say about old friends, family members,
teammates, journalists and cycling officials.

The spineless pussies included a blowhard, prick, fool,
fuckin' weasel, piece of shit and weak, ass-covering motherfuckers who are crazy, batshit crazy, certifiably crazy,
loopy, toxic, psycho and, anyway, calling her a whore was
just shorthand for saying she likes sex, and no, he didn't
sleep with his idiot teammate's wife but the thought crossed
his mind.

Only when I reviewed my notes did I realize how often Armstrong had dehumanized the people close to him. They were
transformed into aural manifestations of his anger. But to feel the
heat of his rage was to understand another thing as well: Here was
a man who didn't glide into cycling history. He beat the living
crap out of it.

I came away from my visit with him in June 2013 suspecting

that Armstrong, in his heart of hearts, believed absolutely, and will believe forever, that he won those Tours de France because he was the best.

Hear him now: "The most successful people in the world, the true killers in the world, they weren't handed anything, they didn't grow up with anything, they had to fuckin' scrape and fight for it."

In Armstrong's view, you can pour EPO by the gallons into a man without Armstrong's obsessions and that man might still lag way behind the leaders, might still be at the bottom of the mountain. But give it to an extraordinary athlete willing to scrape and work beyond human comprehension and that man becomes an unstoppable force.

Armstrong did whatever it took, no matter the rules. And he lied about it so often and with such vehemence that the only explanation people had for his aggressiveness was that he had left the oncology ward reborn, like a phoenix, with a supernatural motivating drive that pushed him to crush anyone in his way. "If that's a sociopath, then fuck it, I'm a sociopath," he told me. "I definitely wanted to win at all costs. But so did Michael Jordan, so did Muhammad Ali, so did Wayne Gretzky."

Even as he said that, I didn't believe he was convinced. Had he been more forthcoming, and less hateful, had he not savaged anyone who dared suggest he had a long and intimate relationship with winning by any means available, maybe he would have built enough goodwill to survive the USADA investigation. Maybe he would still possess a legacy commensurate with those of our nation's greatest athletes.

But he hadn't, and he didn't.

"I hated those motherfuckers—the Betsys, the LeMonds. Walsh, I hate him. Bad guy. Cheater. Got some stuff right, lied about a lot . . . Yes, I doped. Yes, I was doping. These people, the lengths that they went to . . . it's the reason I picked on these people. I really hated them. These people sucked. This is just so dirty, so dirty you just feel like you need a shower. Honestly, I hated these people and I still hate them. I couldn't let them get away with it because they are so awful."

Get away with what? They'd only accused him of truths he spent decades obscuring. They "got away" with exposing a game built on a century of lies. And in their revelations—here, I think, is the crux of the matter—they hadn't placated his ego by marking his place in history.

June 6, 2013: on a couch in the media room of Lance Armstrong's expansive Austin estate. Soon, the place will be empty, the moving trucks having packed up Armstrong's belongings. By the fall, his things will be moved into a lesser place, one in Old West Austin, a historic district filled with many grand old homes and within walking distance to downtown. The new place is nice, for sure—especially at more than $2 million—but it has no gate or fence, no circular or even paved driveway, no lawn, certainly no sprawling oak tree that has been transplanted from one side of the property to the other. While we talk, Armstrong is, as ever, ferocious and charming, spectacular in his ability to spin brutal lies from a thin strand of truth.

Armstrong shrugs off the notion that USADA's long-running war has ruined him. Under the seven framed yellow jerseys that in a day's time will be stripped from the walls, he insists that he is OK. Look at this house, he says. Look at his kids. Look at the life he's built for his family. What's not OK? He says he's OK so often that it seems clear that he's not OK.

He stares at me, giving me the infamous and cold expression that has been dubbed "The Look." People may have forgotten all the good he did at Livestrong, he says, but that won't last. People will remember. People still love him, he says, almost hypnotically. Look, he tells me, here's a letter from one former Livestrong donor who still supports him. Below the strange return address, the sender wrote, "Yep, it's prison."

Armstrong says, "There's millions of people who might not be empowered right now to say it, but there's still people that believe." He jams a finger against his chest. "This is the fucking guy who overcame his disease. He came back to his sport and did what he had to do. Are we all better off that I was here, or are we worse off?"

He waits, then says, "It has to be better."

I ask him how secretive he had been while he doped. Who else knew?

"Everybody," he says.

Everybody?

"They knew enough not to ask."

Bill Stapleton, his agent?

Silence.

Nike, his primary sponsor?

Nothing.

The board of directors of Livestrong?

Not a word.

"I ain't no fucking rat," he says, "like these other pussies."

Maybe not at the moment. But in exchange for the right to resume his athletic career—held hostage, as he sees it, by US-ADA—he says he would barter the necessary information to reduce his lifetime ban to four years, maybe two, maybe even less.

Only thing is, Armstrong doesn't want to talk to Travis Tygart. "Just a blowhard," Armstrong says. "He got what he wanted. He got me. I know where all the bodies are buried. I'm not saying anything. Fuck them until they treat me like everybody else."

I'm told by Armstrong that our meeting this week has been a highlight of "Act III" of our professional relationship. Act I was comprised of the years I wrote about the accusations that he had doped to win, a time when he still thought he could win me over. That was before I ever met him or covered the Tour de France. The defining moment of Act I was in 2006 when I reported Frankie Andreu's admission that he had used EPO to help Armstrong win the 1999 Tour de France.

Several days after that story ran—that's several days after his lawyer threatened to sue me—I was walking my dog at 7 a.m. when my cell phone rang. I didn't recognize the number.

"Good morning!" someone said.

"Uh, good morning," I said. "Who's this?"

"It's Lance!"

For the next several weeks, we talked about both cycling and his plan to run the New York City Marathon. I'd ask him how he could be a clean rider when so many of his top competitors at the Tour had been caught for doping. His reply: "Some of us are born with four cylinders and some of us are born with twelve, honey." He'd shoot me an e-mail asking me to guess his latest workout time for a mile. I guessed 10 minutes, 30 seconds, then 5:13, and added that he'd need to down a bunch of Advil afterward because he was so old.

He wrote back, "4:51 . . . no advil. Ha! Nope, no drugs. How many times do I have to tell you that?!?!?"

That was the beginning of Act II: The years writing about him basically became my entire beat, covering his comeback to the sport after his short retirement and breaking news about the various formal investigations into his doping.

Over the course of our encounters, he was sometimes irritated that I didn't buy into the fairy tale he spun about his life and career. At the 2009 Tour of California, his first race in the United States after returning to the sport, he singled me out in front of hundreds of reporters, criticizing "my friend Juliet" for a story I'd written about his personal antidoping program, which he touted as a key to his comeback, and which I reported had never gotten off the ground.

We sparred a few minutes and he later left me an apology by voice mail: "I didn't mean to call you out in front of all those people, but I was just bustin' on you," he said. "I hope you know I was only kidding. Talk to you later!"

That was vintage Armstrong. He tested reporters, befriended them, and vilified them—sometimes doing all three at once, depending on what he wanted.

The first two acts were cat-and-mouse games, which ended with me writing about his unceremonious and brutally fast downfall. But Act III, he promised, would be different. No more lies. He didn't have anything to lose anymore.

It was not lost on me that the setting for Act III would be his emptying manse. It was as if I was there to see his superhero emblem being stripped from his chest. In the previous acts, he never would have let me witness these humbling moments.

"I didn't cheat," he tells me. "Who got cheated?"

He proclaims Jan Ullrich, the German, as cycling's strongest rider. (Several weeks later, Ullrich will admit to doping during his career and say that Armstrong should have his Tour titles reinstated because doping was so prevalent.) Yet Armstrong perennially left Ullrich in his slipstream. No, not by cheating, he says, but rather by organizing his team better—training harder and more ruthlessly, and with meticulous attention to detail. Armstrong said it all so casually he might have been saying the sky was blue. He ran his team like a high-powered corporation. That's how he won. It wasn't the drugs, he says. Ullrich had the drugs, too.

"If people think I cheated to win the Tour de France," Armstrong says, "they're fucking dumb. I didn't cheat."

You broke the rules.

"I did, but we all did," he says. "All two hundred guys that started the race broke the rules."

Isn't that cheating?

Again he fixed that stare on me. It pretty much said I was fucking dumb.

I ask if he was sorry.

No answer.

I ask if he had ever felt apologetic about anything in his life, ever.

He laughs. "I'm sure there have been plenty of moments."

He is sorry he came out of retirement to push his luck and ride the Tour in 2009 and 2010. If he hadn't come back, he believes, he never would have been caught.

He is sorry he hadn't been nicer to Floyd Landis and was sorry that he didn't remain silent after Tyler Hamilton appeared on *60 Minutes* to talk about the doping on the Postal Service team. Instead, he and his public relations team attacked Hamilton as an idiot and liar. "That was over the top," Armstrong says. He was also sorry that he called Emma O'Reilly a whore when he testified under oath in the SCA Promotions case. "I didn't know it was going to be broadcast all over the world," he says.

He isn't sorry for lying. Not for the original lie or any other in the cycle of lies that followed. "We all would have lied," he says. "You would have lied."

In 1999, he sat in front of reporters at the Tour and made his first denial of doping. After that, he says, he could never turn back—he had to keep denying. But, really, he says, everybody would have done what he did. You, me, the guy down the street—if it meant you could win the Tour de France, anybody and everybody would have denied doping. In Lance Armstrong's moral universe, anyone will sell his or her soul to win.

"Nobody would have said, 'Well, you know, since you asked me that question, I might as well tell you the truth,'" he tells me. "I should have just had a quiet denial."

Instead, he has spent years shouting denials and confronting critics and filing lawsuits to quiet anyone who dared question him. It was not in his nature as a rider to dismount and walk his bike down the road past Joseba Beloki in the 2003 Tour de France, nor in his personality to accept accusations in silence. So he attacked anyone who went public with reports of his doping, and still hasn't spoken with Tygart since their meeting in Denver. Was there anyone, I ask, who could have and should have censored him? Anyone who could've saved him from himself?

"It probably should've been Bill," he says, naming his agent. "I think Bill could've said we need to not be picking any fights here because that's Pandora's box. I think we all felt invincible. 'Yeah, fuck, just call them fucking liars, yeah!' "

Most of the people who testified against him in the USADA case, including his former teammates, have received especially cruel treatment from Armstrong.

He calls Hamilton "an ungrateful, selfish prick" who hid his recklessness behind his preppy New England upbringing. While the Postal Service team doped during the season, Hamilton's doping calendars revealed that he doped even in the winter, even on Christmas Eve. "He's the exact opposite of the image he portrays," Armstrong says.

He calls Zabriskie a classic follower who trailed Landis around "like a little puppy" and did whatever Landis did. He scoffs at Frankie Andreu, a former doper who came to be considered one of the good guys. (Andreu now works as a cycling team director.) How antidoping can Andreu be, Armstrong asks, if the lead rider on his team, Francisco "Paco" Mancebo, is one of the riders implicated in a Spanish doping ring, an athlete who maintains his innocence but is thought to have stored more blood bags than anyone else implicated in that scandal?

"No good guys and bad guys," Armstrong says. "We've all done something wrong. I handled myself in the wrong way and I'm paying for it."

He still has friends, even some, like George Hincapie, whose damning testimony can be found in USADA's report. The day after the report was published, Armstrong sent Hincapie a text: "How are you doing?" The two had won seven Tours together, and are sticking together.

Hincapie is saddened that the killer in Lance Armstrong has

been silenced, and that he was one of the main reasons for it. He didn't think it was fair, the way USADA used him to take down Armstrong. The two talk often and commiserate over how ridiculous it is that they have been singled out in a sport with such a rich doping past. It's even more ridiculous, they say, to see Landis considered a proponent of antidoping.

"That," Hincapie says, is "like Osama bin Laden hosting an antiterrorism conference."

When I ask about Armstrong's family, he tells me he hasn't seen his father in nearly forty years. He insists that he never, not even once, asked his mother about his father or that side of the family. Why would he have gone to the funeral?

"Ninety percent of what I know about that family I've read from her book," he says.

I ask the question a dozen different ways. I wonder if his turning his back on his father, and basically saying he had never been a Gunderson, was the denial that began the pattern of lies that would come to symbolize his life.

You never were curious about your dad? You never thought about him or his family? You never wondered about your roots?

He stops me midsentence. "You're asking me a question," he says. "'Did it ever cross my mind to look up those people?' I'm going to answer the question, then I'm going to follow up. The answer is no. You are asking me, so I'm thinking about it now: No. I mean, I go on long bike rides and think and never in my life have I said, I got to go home and find these people. Never. The follow-up is maybe that means I'm just extremely fucked up. I don't know."

I ask about his adoptive father, Terry Armstrong, and he stops me again. "Terry Armstrong was batshit crazy, certifiable, eew! So weird, such a weirdo. I'll never talk to him again."

Does he remember anything about Terry coaching him or pushing him as an athlete?

No, Armstrong says. He doesn't remember ever playing youth football or Terry being involved with his sports. "I do remember him showing up here at the ride in Austin and we had to call the police to have him escorted out," he says, though there is no record of police ever being involved. "Oh, yeah, he was making a lot of people very uncomfortable."

By the time I arrived in Austin, Armstrong had lost his status as the city's superstar. The mayor had removed Armstrong's autographed yellow Tour de France jersey from a trophy case in city hall. There is talk of renaming the city's main bike route, which is now called the Lance Armstrong Bikeway. Once, people were proud of him. Now, when he tried and failed to enter a U.S. Masters swimming race here in the spring of 2013, the registrar saw his application and said, "This poor guy has the same name as Lance Armstrong, the cyclist. Oh, how unfortunate."

All that, Armstrong can take. He can rebuild his life. But it's going to be tough without the blood rush of competition. As it stands, his lifetime ban from Olympic sporting events means he is disqualified from most running events, triathlons and swimming meets.

But Armstrong is convinced that a lifetime ban in cycling doesn't mean his athletic career is over. The way he and his lawyers see it, it's only a few years before he'll be free to compete in another sport, before he'll return to triathlons and win the Ironman World Championship. "It's fucking rock and roll, baby," he says.

The thought stirs in him the old urge to bend the future his way. As he sits on his couch, under those yellow jerseys, reminders of who he had once been and what he had once accomplished, I see Armstrong's hands curling into fists.

ACKNOWLEDGMENTS

This book exists because my former editors at the *New York Times*, Tom Jolly and Kristin Huckshorn, assigned me to write about Tyler Hamilton, who tested positive for blood doping in 2004. That story kicked off years of reporting about cycling, doping and Lance Armstrong. Tom and Kristin, I am grateful for your guidance. Thanks to you and Jill Abramson for bringing me to the paper, an exhilarating place to work. I am also indebted to those editors who approved my leave for this project: Joe Sexton and Phil Corbett for their initial go-ahead, and Jason Stallman and Janet Elder for their blessing. Jason, I appreciate your ongoing support, encouragement and sense of humor. Janet, you are a lifesaver.

I am so lucky to have such exceptional colleagues, including Harvey Araton, Filip Bondy, John Branch, Joe Drape, Sandy Keenan, Jeré Longman, Bill Rhoden and George Vecsey. They told me to write this book because "It's so easy!" They lied, but I forgive them. Special thanks to Fern Turkowitz and Terri Ann Glynn, who always have my back, and to Patty LaDuca, backfield editor extraordinaire and fellow Jersey girl, who stood by my side throughout the Armstrong coverage. Sandy Padwe, my former professor at Columbia Journalism School, provided invaluable advice. He has guided me through every big career decision, and

I've relied on him so many times that it's not even funny. Thank you, Sandy, for always being right.

When assigned to cover the Tour de France and Giro d'Italia, I would have been lost if not for the help of generous people. The talented Bonnie Ford has been a wonderful friend. Ian Austin, Rolf Aldag, Connie Carpenter, Davis Phinney, Bob Stapleton, and Matt White were great resources. The wonderful band of brothers and sisters who cover cycling were kind in sharing their knowledge and offering friendship.

I appreciate the people with ties to Lance Armstrong who let me bombard them with questions. Some didn't want their names used, but their insights guided me. Some allowed me to quote them at length and spend days following them. They include Jonathan Vaughters, David Zabriskie, Allen Lim, Betsy Andreu, Micki Rawlings and J.T. Neal and his family, Frances, Scott and Caroline. Thank you for trusting me with your stories.

All that reporting would never have become a book if not for my plucky agent, PJ Mark at Janklow & Nesbit, who is an unparalleled advocate. PJ, you were a delight to work with, as were all of Janklow's phenomenal people, especially Dorothy Vincent, Bennett Ashley, Stefanie Lieberman and Marya Spence.

My eternal gratitude to Jonathan Burnham and David Hirshey at HarperCollins for bringing this book to life. Thank you, David, for putting your confidence in me early on. You and Barry Harbaugh helped distill this book into the best narrative it could be, and I'm grateful to you both. Thanks also to others at HarperCollins: Martin Redfern, who made the British publication of the book possible; Fabio Bertoni, Elissa Cohen, Arthur Heard and Chloe Strong for their valuable counsel; Tom Cherwin for his meticulous copyediting; Tina Andreadis, a Barnard sister; Katie O'Callaghan and Kate Blum for their energetic marketing and publicity efforts; and the incomparable Sydney Pierce for cracking the whip.

How can I ever thank my friends and relatives who for years have heard me drone on about cycling? Wendy Dalchau, Rose Greco, Cynthia Grilli, Catherine Ivey, Sylvia Curiel and Jade-Snow and David Joachim deserve awards. Medals for exemplary moral support should go to Christine Macur; Rich, Debbie, David, Daniel, Meghan and Caleb Macur; Christina and Carmine Fiore; Dianna Radoslovich; Lili Lewandowski; Fran Angiola; my father-in-law, David Michaels; and Teresa Mendoza. My mom, Leokadia, and my mother-in-law, Angela Michaels, were super nannies while I was out reporting. Big hugs to Wendy and Cynthia for opening their homes to me. Another big hug to Rose, who, as she often reminds me, was responsible for my becoming a writer instead of a lawyer.

I was fortunate enough that two of my best friends, Roxanna and Andy Scott, helped with this project. Andy, you are a phenomenal photographer and the best photo editor anyone could want. Roxanna, you are an amazing person, a better friend than I deserve, and the most exacting fact-checker ever. I love you both.

There's no way I could ever give enough thanks to Dave Kindred for his help as the first reader on this book, the man who talked me through bouts of writer's block and an ever-patient friend. It seems like yesterday that he told me, "You won't have to write about NASCAR forever." I cried with happiness. More than fifteen years later, Dave is still making me cry, but only with gratitude that he has remained my mentor. I feel that I won the jackpot. Without him as a guide, I never could have finished this book, especially on such a tight schedule. Next up, climbing our second fourteener!

I have been blessed to have truly amazing parents, Poles who survived the Nazi forced labor camps in Germany and came to the United States with nothing but their faith in God, determined to build a new life.

My father, Zbigniew, has told me for years that I should write a book. One about Armstrong, a serial liar with a mouth of a sailor, probably isn't what he had in mind. Still, I will never feel more accomplished than the moment I hand him and my mother inscribed copies.

Thank you, Tata—the world's greatest soccer player—for sitting with me all those Saturdays while we watched Olympic sports on television. Thank you more for supporting me as an athlete. Your job as a diesel mechanic was not easy and not what you wanted to do with your life, but it gave you the chance to come to my afternoon games and meets. Having you watch over me made me feel so special.

I'll always remember our time together playing sports that mattered, and even some that didn't: All those trips to the track to practice hurdling and long jumping. The laid-back sessions of catch during which you taught me to throw a baseball like a rocket. The countless hours we spent shooting hoops. You are an incredible coach and father because you were always upbeat and treated me the same, whether I won or lost, and whether I performed well or not. I fell in love with sports because you made them fun.

Thank you also to my warmhearted and beautiful mother for being my biggest fan. Even when I'd lose a basketball game or a rowing race, she'd applaud with such vigor, it was as if I'd just won an Olympic gold medal. I couldn't ask for a better cheerleader. Everyone should have a mother like her, someone who believes that everything you write—even the 100-word briefs— should win a Pulitzer. Mama, I love you and Tata so very much. You are the world's best role models and will forever be my heroes.

The greatest blessings in this good life that my parents made possible are my husband, Dave Michaels, who I love more each day, and our daughter, Allegra, who makes my heart burst with joy. Our Labrador retriever, Chopper, is the best writing partner and foot warmer I could ask for.

Thank you, Dave, for performing daily superhero miracles while I wrote this book. You worked ten-plus hours a day as a brilliant journalist, then kept our household going. What would Allegra, Chopper and I have done without you? Lesser men would have cracked when I took my thousandth phone call about Armstrong, but you remained understanding. You are our guardian angel, the best husband, the best papa and the ballast of our family.

Allegra, someday you'll read this, and I hope you understand that the most valuable hours of this project were the hours I spent with you. In those happy times, you inspired Mama. I love you more than words can say.

NOTES

This book was compiled from information gathered over nearly ten years, from 2004 through 2013, with the bulk of it reported from January to October 2013. The interviews of Armstrong and more than 130 people connected to him took place at cycling races, at people's homes, in hotel lobbies and in restaurants—and once atop a frozen lake, ice-fishing in Colorado. Some sessions were done on the phone, but most were conducted in person, and many occurred over many hours, over multiple days. Some of the people I interviewed did not want to have their names used for fear of retribution from Armstrong, who they believe continues to wield power in the sport of cycling, and/or in the community because of the work he has done for cancer awareness. Where there are attributed quotes in the text that are not cited in these notes, they derive from personal interviews.

PROLOGUE

A majority of the information used in this section was derived from my one-on-one interview with Lance Armstrong on June 6, 2013, and from subsequent interviews in 2013 with his friends and former colleagues in Austin, Texas.

1   The $10 million estate: Suzanne Halliburton and Shonda No-
     vak, "Austin Home Sold to Oil Businessman," *Austin American-
     Statesman*, April 11, 2003.

3   His sponsors have abandoned him: Juliet Macur and Ian Austen,
     "After the Tears, Some Questions Remain," *New York Times*, Jan-
     uary 19, 2013; Lance Armstrong interview with Oprah Winfrey,
     January 17 and 18, 2013.

3   He would owe more than $135 million: Armstrong is facing a $120
     million payout if he loses a federal whistle-blower lawsuit. He faces
     at least two other possible major payouts—$12.5 million or more in
     a case against SCA Promotions, a company that paid him bonuses
     for several of his Tour wins, and $3 million in a case against Accep-
     tance Insurance, another insurance company that paid him a bonus.

4   Trek's revenue: Two people at the company said the revenue was about
     $300 million in the 1990s and was close to $950 million in 2012.

4   On an income of $12,000: John Thomas "J.T." Neal, audiotapes
     recorded April 2000 to fall of 2002; photos of Lance Armstrong's
     first apartment in Austin.

5   "*negative-edge* pool:" Interview with Adam Wilk, one of Armstrong's
     oldest friends, who said Armstrong scolded him for calling the pool
     an "infinity pool," April 2013.

5   "nobody's going to mess with me": Nancy Collins, "Lance Arm-
     strong's Home in Austin," *Architectural Digest*, July 2008.

5   Armstrong had sold the plane: Paul Tharp, "Third World Moguls
     Driving Jet Demand," *New York Post*, February 7, 2013.

6   In 2009, when he decorated: Mark Prigg, "In a Flap: Animal Rights
     Groups Erupt Over Bike Built for Armstrong," *Evening Standard*
     (London), July 24, 2009.

8   they would graduate: Nancy Collins, "Lance Armstrong's Home in
     Austin," *Architectural Digest*, July 2008.

9   At 4:15 a.m.: Interview with Dave Bolch, Lance Armstrong's per-
     sonal assistant, 2013.

10   carries a price tag of $70,000: Ibid.

13   As she tells it, the two of them: Linda Armstrong Kelly, promotional videos for her motivational speaking. http://apbspeakers.com/speaker/linda-armstrong-kelly.

13   The boy never met his father: Kevin Sherrington, "Mom's Support, Cancer Fight Energized Armstrong," *Dallas Morning News*, July 26, 1999.

13   She said she taught him: Linda Armstrong Kelly with Joni Rodgers, *No Mountain High Enough: Raising Lance, Raising Me* (New York: Broadway Books, 2005).

13   "How did a single teenage mom": Ibid., 7.

13   "totally biased, subjective": Ibid., Acknowledgments.

13   "Someone else might have": Ibid.

14   Both of Armstrong's grandfathers: Ibid., 72; interviews with Willine Gunderson Harroff, Lance Armstrong's paternal grandmother, and Micki Rawlings, Lance Armstrong's paternal aunt, April 2013.

14   His paternal grandfather was so mean: Betty Ann Gunderson Vowell Freeman Trednick, Gunderson Family Genealogy, January 1, 2006.

14   Armstrong's father was an alcoholic: Interviews with Willine Gunderson, Micki Rawlings and friends and other family members of Eddie Gunderson who did not want to be identified, April 2013.

14   By the age of twenty, Armstrong had had three different fathers: Dallas County (Texas) court records; Collin County (Texas) court records.

14   "stupid, self-undermining": Armstrong Kelly, with Rodgers, *No Mountain High Enough*, 223.

14   "from poverty with no money": Linda Armstrong Kelly, Web site for Harry Walker Agency promoting her public speaking engagements. http://www.harrywalker.com/speaker-bureau/video/Linda-Armstrong-Kelly/Armstrong-Linda.cfm.

14   The first step in that process: Armstrong Kelly, with Rodgers, *No Mountain High Enough*, 85; interviews with Willine Gunderson Harroff and Micki Rawlings, April 2013.

15   Linda Armstrong has said she was alone: Brad Townsend, "Finishing a Hard Ride, Armstrong Reflects on Road from Cancer to Near-Certain Race Win," *Dallas Morning News*, July 25, 1999; Sherrington, "Mom's Support, Cancer Fight Energized Armstrong."

15   only without a husband for a year: Dallas County (Texas) court records; Collin County (Texas) court records.

15   her first husband's family said they helped: Interviews with Willine Gunderson Harroff and Micki Rawlings, 2013.

15   The Gundersons had their own version: The story was compiled through interviews with Willine Gunderson Harroff, Micki Rawlings and several family and friends of Eddie Gunderson and the former Linda Mooneyham, 2013.

15   willingness to help friends steal tape decks: Interview with Micki Rawlings, April 2013; Dallas County court records.

15   nothing like: Documents from the city of Dallas show that the apartment complex that was home to the Gundersons and Mooneyhams was never government-owned housing.

16   "Make love, not war": Armstrong Kelly, with Rodgers, *No Mountain High Enough*, 51.

16   He was named after Lance Rentzel: Ibid., 72; J. R. Eggert, "Lance Rentzel: The Laughter Hasn't Died," review of *When All the Laughter Died in Sorrow*, by Lance Rentzel, *Harvard Crimson*, February 8, 1973.

16   9 pounds, 12 ounces: Lance Armstrong, with Sally Jenkins, *It's Not About the Bike: My Journey Back to Life* (New York: Berkley Books, 2003).

16   "What's wrong with his head?": Interview with Micki Rawlings, 2013.

17   As a minor, he had made frequent appearances: Ibid.

17   his first night in jail: Dallas County court records.

17   Years later, the ex-husband: Article in *Algemeen Dagblad*, the Netherlands, 2005, quoted in Françoise Inizan, "Lance's Two Fathers," *L'Equipe*, 2005.

18   "I'm the one that": Interview with Willine Gunderson Harroff, 2013.

CHAPTER 2

21   as much as $20,000 a pop: Web site for Keynote resource, http://www.keynoteresources.com/LindaArmstrong-Kelly.html.

21   Some newspapers have quoted her: David Tarrant, "Rookie Cyclist on the Fast Track to Becoming a Sports Icon," *Dallas Morning News*, July 4, 1993.

21   "Sales coached Lance's": Armstrong Kelly, with Rodgers, *No Mountain High Enough*, 108.

23   He drove himself: Interview with Adam Wilk, 2013.

23   He armed himself with: Interview with Terry Armstrong, 2013.

24   Classmates from middle school: Interviews with several people who went to school with Armstrong. They did not want to be identified for fear of retribution.

25   Although Lance did poorly: Interview with Lance Armstrong, 2013; interview with Terry Armstrong, 2013.

25   Lance Armstrong was fourteen when he learned: Armstrong, with Jenkins, *It's Not About the Bike*, 23; interview with Terry Armstrong, 2013.

27   "Screw off": Interview with Rick Crawford, 2013.

28   Crawford later was fired: Interviews with officials at Colorado Mesa University and Scott Mercier, a consultant to the cycling team there, 2013.

28   "No," he said: Interview with Rick Crawford, 2013.

28   "Can you watch over": Interview with Scott Eder, Armstong's manager, 2013.

28   "a coach meets agent": Interview with Lance Armstrong, 2013.

28   He was only thirteen: Armstrong, with Jenkins, *It's Not About the Bike*, 22.

29   with Terry Armstrong changing: Interview with Jim Woodman, former triathlon race director, 2013.

29   "Are you Mark Allen?": Interview with Scott Eder, 2013.

29   Armstrong finished sixth: Robert Vernon, "Triple Threat," *Dallas Morning News*, July 29, 1989.

29   The next year, Armstrong: Robert Vernon, "Triathlon Winners Keep on the Run," *Dallas Morning News*, June 13, 1988.

29   *Triathlete* magazine claimed: David Tarrant, "Rookie Cyclist on the Fast Track to Becoming a Sports Icon," *Dallas Morning News*, July 4, 1993.

29   making $20,000 a year: Ibid., 29.

30   Kestrel dropped its sponsorship: Interview with Scott Eder, 2013.

31   Linda Armstrong had tracked: Interview with Terry Armstrong, 2013.

32   His senior year, he: Interview with Adam Wilk, 2013; interviews with Lance Armstrong's classmates at Plano East High School, 2013. They didn't want their names used because they didn't want to be seen as kicking him when he is down.

32   he amazed everyone: Interviews with Connie Carpenter-Phinney, Olympic gold medalist and coach at those junior worlds, and Davis Phinney, Tour de France stage winner, 2013; John Wilcockson, *Lance: The Making of the World's Greatest Champion* (New York: Da Capo Press, 2009), 68–70.

32   He and his mother didn't: Interviews with school officials at Plano East High School, 2013. Those officials didn't want their names used because they weren't authorized to speak about the subject.

32   His mother argued: Ibid.

33   including CNN: Paula Zahn, Kyra Phillips, Sharon Collins, "Profiles of Lance Armstrong, Will Smith," July 19, 2003.

34   Linda said, well, you: Interview with Tami Armstrong, 2013.

34   "Really?" Interview with Terry Armstrong, 2013; interview with Tami Armstrong, 2013.

CHAPTER 3

35   Part of the information used in this chapter was gleaned from au-
      diotapes made by J.T. Neal from 2000 to 2002 about his life with
      Lance Armstrong. Much of that information was confirmed by more
      than twenty interviews of Neal family friends, people in the sport
      of cycling and Armstrong's former friends, teammates and workers
      on his cycling teams. Other details in the chapter were compiled
      through news reports, or documents, photos and memorabilia in the
      possession of J.T. Neal's family.

35   he married into money: His wife, Frances, came from a family that
      earned its wealth in the east Texas timber industry. Her grand-
      mother, Frankie Carter Randolph, was the first publisher of the
      Texas Observer, a left-leaning newspaper established in 1954.

37   "killer . . . s-o-o-o nice": David Tarrant, "Rookie Cyclist on the Fast
      Track to Becoming a Sports Icon," *Dallas Morning News*, July 4,
      1993.

37   Linda Armstrong was pleased: Armstrong Kelly, with Rodgers, *No
      Mountain High Enough*, 171–72.

39   Pulled over: Arrest report, San Marcos, Texas, August 1991.

40   In Hincapie's case: J.T. Neal audiotapes. In his 2012 affidavit in the
      United States Anti-Doping Agency case against Armstrong, George
      Hincapie recounts being stopped at customs while returning to the
      United States from Europe in 1996.

40   A coed named Nancy Geisler: Interview with Nancy Geisler, June
      2013.

41   "Had I been a part of something illegal?": Ibid.

41   fellow Olympian Timm Peddie: Interview with Timm Peddie, 2013,
      and another member of the national team who did not want to be
      identified for fear of retribution from Armstrong.

42   He insisted that Steve Penny: Interview with Steve Penny, 2013.

42   Rule #4: As it turned out, the four cyclists in the poster did use a
      back door. All four eventually admitted doping, or were suspended

for doping or, in Evanshine's case, for missing a mandatory doping test. Evanshine missed the Olympics because of it. Elliott Teaford, "He Refuses to Be Left Spinning His Wheels," *Los Angeles Times*, July 15, 1992.

43   several riders on the Motorola team: Interview with two Motorola riders who didn't want to be identified because they didn't want to "rat" on Ochowicz, who is still involved in pro cycling and wields power in the sport.

43   They allegedly offered to pay: Interview with Stephen Swart, former Motorola rider and Armstrong teammate, 2006 and 2013. *Stephen Swart affidavit, Lance Armstrong v. SCA Promotions, Inc.*, January 11, 2006.

43   Later that night: Ibid.

43   Armstrong would receive the prize money: J.T. Neal audiotapes, 2000–2002.

43    $3,000 to $5,000: Interviews with Stephen Swart, former Motorola rider and Armstrong teammate, 2006 and 2013. *Stephen Swart affidavit, Lance Armstrong v. SCA Promotions, Inc.*, January 11, 2006.

44   selling victories was a common: Joe Parkin, *A Dog in a Hat*, Velo-Press, 2008.

44   He offered Gaggioli: Marco Bonarrigo, "Armstrong, prima combine a 22 anni," *Corriere della Sera*, December 13, 2013.

45   "For God's sake": J.T. Neal audiotapes, 2000–2002.

45   Armstrong, according to a person: Interview with a person with direct knowledge of the situation who didn't want his or her name used, 2013.

46   "boy wonder" and playing up: Armen Keteyian, ABC News, interview with Lance Armstrong and Linda Armstrong, June 13, 1993.

46   "Well, being young": Ibid.

46   "We had to overcome": Ibid.

46   "Lance is just what our country needs": John Rezell, "Pedaling Toward Greatness," *Orange County Register*, June 6, 1993.

51   many team doctors write: Interviews with cyclists and antidoping experts, 2013.

52   Through the early 1900s: Christopher S. Thompson, *The Tour de France: A Cultural History* (Berkeley and Los Angeles: University of California Press, 2006), 225–26; Roger Bastide, *Doping: Les surhommes du velo* (Paris: Raoul Solar, 1970), 37, 39, 63–64, 99; Patrick Laure, *Le dopage* (Paris: Presses Universitaires de France, 1995), 26, 49, 59–60, 63–65, 69, 71, 75.

52   The abuse of those drugs: Thompson, *The Tour de France*, 190–91; Albert Londres, "Les Forçats de la Route," *Le Petit Parisien*, June 27, 1924.

52   Amphetamines became popular: Thompson, *The Tour de France*, 229; Bastide, *Doping*, 86–87; Russell Mockridge, completed by John Burrowes, My *World on Wheels: The Posthumous Autobiography of Russell Mockridge* (London: Stanley Paul, 1960), 96, 131; Mondenard, *Dopage* (Paris: Editions Chiron, 2006), 23, 105–7, 169–70; Noret, *Le dopage* (Paris: Editions Vigot, 1990), 32–33.

52   French rider Jean Malléjac collapsed: Bill and Carol McGann, *The Story of the Tour de France*, Volume 1: 1903–1964 (Indianapolis: Dog Ear Publishing, 2006), 211.

53   amphetamine-fueled breakdown: Thompson, *The Tour de France*, 228.

53   Roger Rivière, landed in a tangle: McGann, *The Story of the Tour de France*, 247–48.

53   Five-time Tour winner: *Sports Illustrated*, "Something Extra on the Ball," June 30, 1969.

53   a group of cyclists, doctors, lawyers: Thompson, *The Tour de France*, 231–32; Guillet, *Le doping de l'homme et du cheval* (Paris: Masson & Cie., 1965) 3-4, 83-85; Rapp, *Le doping des sportifs* (Paris: Editions Médicales et Universitaires, 1977), 105, 167.

53   Led by Anquetil: Thompson, *The Tour de France*, 233–34;

L'Humanité, June 30, 1966; *Le Monde*, July 1, 1966; *Le Parisien Libéré*, June 30, 1966.

54 "Get me up": McGann, *The Story of the Tour de France*, Volume 1.

54 An autopsy report: Thompson, *The Tour de France*, 237.

54 one unpublished Swedish study: Randy Starkman, "New Wonder Drug May Speed Athletes to the Killing Fields," *Toronto Star*, April 27, 1991; Lawrence M. Fisher, "Stamina-Building Drugs Linked to Athletes' Deaths," *New York Times*, May 19, 1991.

55 "Mister 60 Percent": Jeremy Whittle, "Bjarne Riis's Year Without Lying," *New York Times*, May 2, 2008.

55 five Dutch riders: William Leith, *Independent*, July 1, 1991.

55 at least eighteen professional European: Starkman, "New Wonder Drug May Speed Athletes to the Killing Fields."

55 "Stamina-Building Drug Linked": Fisher, "Stamina-Building Drugs Linked to Athletes' Deaths."

56 Riders said they'd never heard of it: Interview with Don Catlin, 2013.

56 Seven years later: Interview with Lance Armstrong, 2013.

57 Borysewicz and other team officials: Robert McG. Thomas Jr., "USOC Checking Use of Transfusions," *New York Times*, January 10, 1985; Bjarne Rostaing and Robert Sullivan, "Triumphs Tainted with Blood," *Sports Illustrated*, January 21, 1985.

57 Four went on to win medals: Rostaing and Sullivan, "Triumphs Tainted with Blood."

57 Each of them would eventually: Charles Pelkey, "Wenzel Denies Charges," *VeloNews*, April 3, 2001. Charles Pelkey, "Six Years Later, Strock Case Comes to Court," *VeloNews*, April 18, 2006; interviews with two of the cyclists on the national team at the time the alleged doping occurred. They did not want their names published.

58 Strock and Kaiter settling: Jon Sarche, "Former cyclists settling doping lawsuit," *Associated Press*, September 15, 2006.

58 Carmichael allegedly paid: Dave Philipps, "Question remains around doping ties to Armstrong's coach," *The Gazette* (Colorado Springs, Colo.), January 20, 2013.

59   There he mixed, matched: Interview with John Hendershot, 2013.

60   If Hendershot was his own lab rat: Ibid.

60   Both *soigneur* and rider were willing: Ibid.

63   the process was overseen: Ibid.; J.T. Neal audiotapes.

63   Hendershot trusted Testa: Interview with John Hendershot, 2013.

63   All became patients: J.T. Neal audiotapes; interview with George Hincapie, 2013.

63   Armstrong believed: Interviews with Lance Armstrong, 2013; Oprah Winfrey interview with Lance Armstrong, 2013.

63   As Hendershot had done: Interview with John Hendershot, 2013.

65   "I don't prescribe": Jean-Michel Rouet, interview with Michele Ferrari, *L'Equipe*, April 1994.

65   Armstrong, Andreu, Hincapie and: Interview with Max Testa, 2006.

65   "People are trying to": Ibid.

65   One day, he handed: Ibid.

65   "If you want to use a gun": Ibid.

65   "This is bullshit": Interview with George Hincapie, 2013; Hincapie's affidavit in USADA case.

66   "I'm getting my ass kicked": Interview with Frankie Andreu, 2013; affidavit of Frankie Andreu in USADA case.

66   They agreed it was time for EPO: Interviews with Stephen Swart, 2006 and 2013; interview with Frankie Andreu, 2013; affidavit of Frankie Andreu in USADA case.

66   Riders carried thermos jugs: Interviews with various riders, including Christian Vande Velde, Jonathan Vaughters and George Hincapie, 2013.

67   an ultimatum: Interviews with Stephen Swart, 2006 and 2013.

68   Armstrong himself claims: Interview with Lance Armstrong, 2013.

68   Testa gave him: Ibid.

68   The drug was available: Interview with Lance Armstrong, 2013; interview with Stephen Swart, 2013; interview with George Hincapie, 2013.

68 Testa was constantly giving: J.T. Neal audiotapes.

69 He would smile nervously: Interviews with Jim Ochowicz, 2005, 2009 and 2010.

69 Armstrong said Motorola's EPO use: Interview with Lance Armstrong, 2013.

70 team employees showed up: Interviews with Stephen Swart, 2006 and 2013.

70 Swart saw that most: Stephen Swart affidavit in USADA case; interview with Stephen Swart, 2013.

71 Andreu's was at about 50: Ibid.

71 The telephone call came: Interview with Kathy and Greg LeMond, 2006.

71 "He died for what?" Interview with Greg LeMond, 2013.

CHAPTER 5

72 In the fall of 1995: J.T. Neal audiotapes.

72 "Lance, don't get greedy": Ibid.

72 Armstrong had nearly $750,000: J.T. Neal audiotapes and documents.

73 He had asked Eddy: Interview with Lance Armstrong, 2013.

73 come from Texas: Interview with the former Monica Buck, 2013.

73 "too opinionated": J.T. Neal audiotapes.

73 some of Ferrari's clients: Ibid.

73 Merckx's son, Axel: E-mail from Axel Merckx, December 1, 2013.

73 The IOC had paid him: Paul Howard, "Past That Haunts Roche," *Sunday Tribune*, April 4, 2004; David Walsh, "Sports Chief Hails Drug Code," *Sunday Times*, March 9, 2003.

74 "amazing, amazing," J.T. Neal audiotapes.

74 $10,000 for the consultation: Ibid.

74 under investigation by Italian: Interview with an Italian investigator involved in the inquiry, who didn't want his name published because he isn't authorized to speak about the case.

74 he talked nonstop: J.T. Neal audiotapes.

74 who allegedly had been overseeing: Interview with Lance Armstrong, 2013; interview with John Hendershot, 2013; Ibid.

74 allegedly persuaded the forensic doctor: Richard Weekes, "The Hard Truth Behind a Waste of Life," *Sunday Times*, July 23, 1995.

75 "It's not about the bike": Armstrong, with Jenkins, *It's Not About the Bike*, 71.

75 the fax machine: J.T. Neal audiotapes.

75 that relationship was just a cover: Ibid.; interviews with several Motorola, Postal Service and Astana riders who never saw Carmichael working with Armstrong; interview with a former RadioShack team employee who was told by Armstrong that Carmichael hadn't coached him since Ferrari took over.

76 He offered a low commission: J.T. Neal audiotapes; interview with a person with knowledge of the situation.

76 third marriage was crumbling: Armstrong Kelly, with Rodgers, *No Mountain High Enough*, 214.

76 Neal thought Armstrong: J.T. Neal audiotapes.

76 Armstrong grew increasingly: Ibid.

77 But he didn't: Ibid.

77 Linda Armstrong and Neal had flown: Ibid.; interview with Greg and Kathy LeMond, 2006.

77 "How do I get Lance": Interview with Greg and Kathy LeMond, 2006.

78 "I couldn't breathe": Samuel Abt, "Armstrong Without Power, Withdraws from the Tour de France," *New York Times*, July 6, 1996.

78 Doctors gave Neal: Interviews with Scott and Caroline Neal, two of J.T. Neal's three children, 2013.

78 "He needed it for privacy": J.T. Neal audiotapes.

78 Neal watched as Hendershot: Ibid.

78 Armstrong was already: Interview with Lance Armstrong, 2013; Betsy Andreu deposition in *Lance Armstrong v. SCA Promotions, Inc.*, January 17, 2006.

79 He had even negotiated: J.T. Neal audiotapes.

80   On October 2, 1996: Ibid.

80   "Well, this is a serious situation": Armstrong, with Jenkins, *It's Not
      About the Bike*.

80   Between 5:30 and 5:45 p.m.: J.T. Neal audiotapes.

80   Ferrari was worried: Selena Roberts and David Epstein, "The Case
      Against Lance Armstrong," *Sports Illustrated*, January 24, 2011.

81   "It's bad": Interview with John Korioth, 2013.

81   must have had something: Interview with John Hendershot, 2013.

81   The riders. The team managers: Ibid.

81   Hendershot never called: J.T. Neal audiotapes; interviews with John
      Hendershot and Lance Armstrong, 2013.

CHAPTER 6

84   "You can't control": Interview with Betsy Andreu, 2006.

86   He said, "Growth hormone": Ibid.; Betsy Andreu deposition in
      Lance Armstrong v. SCA Promotions, Inc., January 17, 2006.

87   "Betsy, please, I've never taken": Interview with Betsy Andreu,
      2006.

87   Several of his former teammates: Interviews with Stephen Swart,
      Lance Armstrong and two other Motorola riders who wanted to re-
      main anonymous because they didn't want to be seen tattling on a
      former teammate, 2013.

88   Men have a 1-in-270: American Cancer Society, Web site primer on
      testicular cancer.

88   Growth hormone stimulates: Interview with Dr. Arjun Vasant Balar,
      2013.

88   a research paper: Lucio Tentori and Grazia Graziani, Department
      of Neuroscience, University of Rome Tor Vergata, "Doping with
      Growth Hormone/IGF-1, Anabolic Steroids or Erythropoietin: Is
      There a Cancer Risk?" January 26, 2007.

CHAPTER 7

89   Stapleton suggested: J.T. Neal audiotapes; interview with a person
      with knowledge of the situation, but who wants to remain anony-
      mous because of ongoing business dealings with Stapleton's firm and
      wanting to remain in Stapleton's good graces.

90   Knaggs encouraged: Interview with John Korioth, 2013.

90   he offered $200: J.T. Neal audiotapes and several interviews with
      people who were friends with both Neal and Armstrong, 2013.

92   Neal's oldest daughter: Interviews with the Neal family, 2013.

93   Kevin Kuehler, a competitive: Bonnie DeSimone, "From 'Big C'
      Back to Big-Time Cycling," *Chicago Tribune*, February 7, 1998.

93   "Did you call for my advice": Ibid.

94   "I think it's phenomenal": Ibid.

94   On his blog: runfordori.blogspot.com/2007/08/lance-issues-wake-
      up-call.html.

94   "I don't like that big frenzy": Interview with Lance Armstrong, 2013.

95   "Where are you?": J.T. Neal audiotapes; interviews with Neal's fam-
      ily, 2013.

95   "Um, I can't make it": J.T. Neal audiotapes.

95   He had backstage passes: Ibid.

95   to help figure out: J.T. Neal audiotapes.

96   who had been replaced: Ibid.

96   He doubted his drug: Interview with John Korioth, 2013.

97   Weisel accepted: Armstrong, with Jenkins, *It's Not About the Bike*,
      184.

97   "Lance isn't just a cyclist": Suzanne Halliburton, "Austin Cyclist
      Back on Track After Cancer," *Austin American-Statesman*, October
      27, 1997.

98   "Look how he got it": J.T. Neal audiotapes.

98   he was looking for a way: Ibid.

99   Garvey offered: Ibid.

100   Steffen had been in: Interview with Prentice Steffen, 2013; David Walsh, "Saddled with Suspicion," *Sunday Times*, July 8, 2001.

100   Steffen considered this: Interview with Prentice Steffen, 2013.

101   which was known as: Interview with Jonathan Vaughters, 2013; interview with Christian Vande Velde, 2013.

102   Darren Baker and Scott Mercier went: Interviews with Darren Baker and Scott Mercier, 2013.

103   At the 1992 Olympics, he received: Affidavit of George Hincapie in USADA case.

103   he saw a teammate: Interview with George Hincapie, 2013.

103   Another teammate: Ibid.

105   so fierce that: Matt Smith and Lance Williams, Center for Investigative Reporting, "Will Thomas Weisel, Who Owns Lance Armstrong's U.S. Postal Team, Get Charged With Fraud?" *Bloomberg Businessweek*, January 15, 2013.

105   Baker said: Interview with Darren Baker, 2013.

105   Armstrong feared that: Matt Lawton, "She Was the Whistleblower Who Hauled Him Down, Lance Armstrong Was the Drug Cheat, So What Happened When They Were Brought Together Again by MailOnline?" *Daily Mail*, November 18, 2013.

107   Celaya handed: Interview with Scott Mercier and his wife, Mandie, 2013.

109   "I was strong most of": Samuel Abt, "Tour of Spain Is 'Last Chance': U.S. Rider Hopes for a Happy Finale," *New York Times*, September 4, 1997.

111   She supposedly helped the entire: Interviews with Jonathan Vaughters and Christian Vande Velde, 2013.

111   "Lance's wife is rolling": Affidavit of Jonathan Vaughters in the USADA case; interview with Christian Vande Velde, 2013.

112   He carried: Willy Voet and William Fotheringham, "Observer Sports Monthly: Drugs in Sport," *Observer*, May 6, 2001.

113   "Maybe the reason": Interview with Jonathan Vaughters, 2013.

113   Celaya, a mild-mannered: Interview with a rider who was in the camper with Celaya, but who didn't want his name published because he wanted to stay out of the doping controversy.

114   was dead set on flushing: Affidavits of Emma O'Reilly and George Hincapie.

114   "one last huge dose": Interview with a rider who was in the camper with Celaya, but who didn't want his name published because he wanted to stay out of the doping controversy.

114   Viatcheslav Ekimov, a Russian: Ibid.

114   "My God, I thought he'd": Ibid.

115   "He wants to take your": Affidavit of Jonathan Vaughters in US-ADA case.

115   They also shared: Interview with Jonathan Vaughters, 2013.

115   feigned laughter: Interviews with Jonathan Vaughters and Christian Vande Velde, 2013.

116   "Hey, do you want": Affidavit of Christian Vande Velde in USADA case.

116   Vaughters's bottle read: Affidavit of Jonathan Vaughters in USADA case. Interview with Christian Vande Velde, 2013.

116   "You're going to need": Interview with Christian Vande Velde, 2013.

117   Armstrong just said: Affidavit of Christian Vande Velde in USADA case.

117   Now he understood why: Interview with Christian Vande Velde, 2013.

117   "What the hell": Ibid.

118   Nuñes allegedly gave in: Interview with Jonathan Vaughters, 2013.

118   "We're going to use EPO": Ibid.

119   Like Armstrong, Vaughters: Ibid.

120   a Postal rider left: Affidavit of Emma O'Reilly in USADA case.

121   "Ten years down": Samuel Abt, "Tour de France Ends for Riders on the Storm," *New York Times*, August 3, 1998.

121   "Hey, 49, JV?": Interview with Jonathan Vaughters, 2013.

121   to fetch him a cortisone pill: Ibid.; affidavits of Jonathan Vaughters and Christian Vande Velde in USADA case.

CHAPTER 10

125   In the weeks before: David Walsh, *Seven Deadly Sins: My Pursuit of Lance Armstrong* (London: Simon & Schuster, 2012), 41.

125   It has ten wooden: Photos of the chapel on the Web site of *Le Figaro*, lefigaro.fr.

125   "the Tour de Farce": David Walsh, "Inspired Armstrong Brings Hope to Beleaguered Tour Organizers," *Sunday Times*, July 4, 1999.

126   "It's been a long year": Ibid.

127   "Riders take them when": David Walsh, "Racing Clean, Riding High," *Sunday Times*, July 11, 1999.

127   the aggressive new doping: USADA reasoned decision, 115.

128   which had a reputation: Interviews with Jonathan Vaughters and Christian Vande Velde, 2013.

128   Armstrong and his teammates: Interview with Jonathan Vaughters, 2013.

128   "Um, I'm peeing": Ibid.; affidavit of Jonathan Vaughters in USADA case.

129   "no-holds-barred": Interview with Jonathan Vaughters, 2013.

129   While Celaya may have: Interview with Jonathan Vaughters, 2013.

130   "It's a professional": Ibid.; interviews with Jonathan Vaughters, Christian Vande Velde and David Zabriskie, 2013.

130   "was like looking in": Johan Bruyneel, *We Might as Well Win* (Boston: Mariner Books, 2009), 30.

131   had no out-of-competition: Interview with Enrico Carpani,

spokesman for the International Cycling Union, 2012.

131 The difference between Bruyneel: Interview with Jonathan Vaughters, 2013; interview with Christian Vande Velde, 2013.

131 riders claimed that Bruyneel: Interviews with Jonathan Vaughters, David Zabriskie, Christian Vande Velde, 2013.

131 Bruyneel was obsessed: Bruyneel has denied the allegations that he helped riders dope, gave riders drugs or ever encouraged any use of banned drugs or methods on his teams. As of February 2014, he was involved in an arbitration with the USADA, in which he was fighting the lifetime ban the agency had given him in 2012. Bruyneel, through his lawyer, has denied requests for interviews for this book.

131 "You are doping": Interview with Jonathan Vaughters, 2013.

132 "The code word is butter": Ibid.; affidavit of Jonathan Vaughters in USADA case.

132 "Don't worry": Ibid.

133 "The whole team is ready": Ibid.

133 "You know, Emma": Affidavit of Emma O'Reilly in USADA case.

133 she had seen a fellow: Ibid.

133 His real job: Ibid.

134 a drug courier: Ibid.

134 "they would have a riot": Affidavit of Emma O'Reilly in USADA case.

134 pick up a bottle: Ibid.

134 Just before the team's: Ibid.

135 "How do you like": Armstrong, with Jenkins, *It's Not About the Bike*, 243.

136 "They want me to crack": Associated Press, July 22, 1999.

136 she heard him: Ibid.

136 team owner Thomas Weisel: Susanne Craig, "Banker Behind Armstrong Says He Was Unaware of Doping," *New York Times*, January 17, 2013.

137 "This is a real problem": Matt Lawton, "She Was the Whistleblower Who Hauled Him Down, Lance Armstrong Was the Drug Cheat,

So What Happened When They Were Brought Together Again by MailOnline?" *Daily Mail*, November 18, 2013.

137 "It's a bullshit story": Ben Rumsby, "Lance Armstrong 'has an agenda, has made my life a misery,'" *Telegraph*, December 17, 2013.

138 "mostly clean": Robin Nicholl, "Tour de France: Tour Has Test for New Drug," *Independent*, July 17, 1999.

138 nearly all of the nine: Interview with Jonathan Vaughters, 2013.

138 "This has got to stop!": James Startt, "Bassons: 'People Now See I Wasn't Lying,'" *Bicycling*, October 16, 2012.

138 a salary that would: Ibid.

139 "What are you, another": Affidavit of Jonathan Vaughters.

139 "What you are saying": Startt, "Bassons: 'People Now See I Wasn't Lying.'"

139 "If I made a mistake": Ibid.

140 "died at the stake": Alexander Wolff, "My Sportsman: Christophe Bassons," *Sports Illustrated*, November 12, 2012.

140 a Frenchman named Philippe: Affidavit of Tyler Hamilton.

140 Maire supposedly would follow the Tour: Ibid.

141 the A team could inject: USADA reasoned decision, 33.

141 shove the syringes: Affidavit of Tyler Hamilton.

141 The "B" team received: Affidavit of Frankie Andreu; interview with Frankie Andreu, 2013.

141 the whole team was taking: Interviews with Jonathan Vaughters and Christian Vande Velde, 2013.

143 "What can I do": "Grace Under Pressure: Armstrong Feels Stress of Yellow Jersey, Drug Accusations," Associated Press, July 19, 1999.

143 "I can emphatically": Poststage interview with Armstrong after Stage 14, posted on YouTube.

143 "Monsieur Le Monde": Jenny E. Heller, "Armstrong Makes His Position in Race—and on Drugs—Clear," *Los Angeles Times*, July 22, 1999.

144 "They say stress causes": Samuel Abt, "Armstrong Is Engulfed by Frenzy Over Salve," *New York Times*, July 22, 1999.

144   "He's understandably upset": Sal Ruibal, "Armstrong Rises Above Tour's Shame," *USA Today*, July 22, 1999.

144   "its healer after last": Christopher K. Hepp, "Tour de France Finds Its Healer After Last Year's Drug Scandal," *Philadelphia Inquirer*, July 17, 1999.

144   "doing his best to ignore": John Niyo, "Armstrong an Inspiration: Besides Overcoming Cancer, He's on a Roll in the Tour de France," *Detroit News*, July 16, 1999.

144   "a cancer survivor and": Anne Swardson, "Armstrong Rides Tour to the Top," *Washington Post*, July 15, 1999.

144   "an outspoken opponent": Samuel Abt, "Armstrong's Tour de France Tour de Force Rolls on Uphill," *New York Times*, July 14, 1999.

145   "This guy is so clean-living": "Armstrong's Spirit Fuels Comeback," Associated Press, July 14, 1999.

145   "It's like a miracle": William Fotheringham, "Armstrong Rebuffs Drugs Slur," *Guardian* (London), July 16, 1999.

145   "cutting-edge techniques:" Ruibal, "Armstrong Rises Above Tour's Shame."

145   "more revolutions:" Rachel Alexander, "Tour de Lance Is the Toast of France; Inspirational Armstrong: Cancer Survivor to Race Leader," *Washington Post*, July 22, 1999.

146   "Oh my God": Interview with Betsy Andreu, 2006.

147   "Who'd I end": Ibid.

148   "Did she say anything": Deposition of Frankie Andreu in *Armstrong v. SCA Promotions, Inc*, 2005.

148   "I'm in shock": Suzanne Halliburton, "American in Paris Wins It All: Armstrong's Tour Victory Emotional," Cox News Service, July 26, 1999.

148   "We can return to what": Jocelyn Noveck, "Vive La Lance! Armstrong Completes a Grand Tour," Associated Press, July 25, 1999.

149   "Fifty percent of this": Christopher K. Hepp, "Armstrong Triumphs," *Philadelphia Inquirer*, July 26, 1999.

149   "We're so proud": Bill Sullivan, "Lone Star Makes Texas Governor proud," *Houston Chronicle*, July 26, 1999.

149   "If Hollywood makes a movie": Alexander, "Tour de Lance Is the Toast of France."

149   "petty slander": Bernie Lincicome, "Hot Times This Summer for American Athletes," *Chicago Tribune*, July 26, 1999.

150   One shop owner: Beatriz Terrazas, "Going Postal," *Dallas Morning News*, July 31, 1999.

150   General Mills said: Bruce Horovitz, "Armstrong Rides to Market Gold," *USA Today*, May 4, 2000.

150   "millions and millions": Ibid.

150   "all-American": Ibid.

150   "He's the kind of guy": Ibid.

151   "And we haven't even": Halliburton, "Vive la Lance!"

151   Bristol-Myers Squibb: Ibid.

151   For the year 2000: Frank Litsky, "Hectic, but Armstrong Spins Along," *New York Times*, August 22, 1999.

152   "a business entity": Armstrong, with Jenkins, *Every Second Counts* (New York: Broadway Books, 2003), 9.

152   "If you ever get": Philip Hersh, "Cyclist Rides to a Miracle," *Chicago Tribune*, July 26, 1999.

CHAPTER 11

153   flew by private jet: Affidavit of Tyler Hamilton.

153   in a deserted luxury beach hotel: Tyler Hamilton and Daniel Coyle, *The Secret Race* (New York: Bantam Books, 2012), 122–125.

154   "Frankenstein-ish": Ibid., 120.

154   In the media room: Suzanne Halliburton, "Lance Says Hello to Yellow," *Austin American-Statesman*, July 11, 2000.

155   "The substances on people's": Erica Bulman, "IOC Bans Product at the Center of Armstrong Controversy," Associated Press, December 12, 2000.

155   "Everything I had": Armstrong, with Jenkins, *Every Second Counts*, 93.

155   the team had kept Actovegin: Ibid., 79.

155   Gorski insisted: "Armstrong Team Assures Tour de France Champ Will Return," Associated Press, December 17, 2000.

157   Tyler would later allege: Hamilton and Coyle, *The Secret Race*, 166–167.

157   who fought constantly: Interview with Christian Vande Velde, 2013.

157   "It's just so hard!": Interview with Alisa Schmidt (formerly Alisa Vaughters), 2013.

158   "I'm not surprised": Interview with Betsy Andreu, 2006.

158   Armstrong, Hamilton: Affidavit of Frankie Andreu.

158   "I don't want to": Interview with Betsy Andreu, 2006.

159   "Wow": Ibid.

159   "Liquid gold": Interview with Betsy Andreu, 2006; Betsy Andreu testimony in the SCA Promotions case, 2005.

159   "It's so the fucking press": Ibid.

159   "My numbers are great": Ibid.

159   Armstrong told Frankie: Ibid.

160   "get serious": Interview with Frankie Andreu, 2009.

161   duplicity and secrecy: Affidavit of Tyler Hamilton; Hamilton and Coyle, *The Secret Race*.

161   "None of your business": Interview with Jonathan Vaughters, 2013.

162   He told them the drug: Interview with Christian Vande Velde, 2013.

162   Ferrari also had advised: Hamilton and Coyle, *The Secret Race*, 139.

163   They weren't properly: World Anti-Doping Agency Independent Observers report, 2003.

163   When drug testers: Affidavit of Jonathan Vaughters.

163   Armstrong had just taken: Interview with George Hincapie, 2013; affidavit of George Hincapie.

163   Other times: Affidavit of Jonathan Vaughters and David Zabriskie; interviews with Jonathan Vaughters and David Zabriskie, 2013.

163   Haven Hamilton allegedly knew: Hamilton and Coyle, *The Secret Race*, 137.

164   "You won't": Ibid., 148–149.

164   Armstrong allegedly also told: Affidavit of Floyd Landis.

164   "You will never, ever": Ben Rumsby, "Lance Armstrong 'has an agenda, has made my life a misery,'" says former UCI President Hein Verbruggen, *Telegraph*, December 17, 2013.

164   The EPO test was so new: Interview with Martíal Saugy, 2013.

164   About a year later: Ibid.

165   The UCI set up: Ibid.

165   Saugy explained: Ibid.

166   "Do you realize that": Ibid.

166   a story by David: David Walsh, "Saddled with Suspicion," *Sunday Times*, July 8, 2001.

167   "has had a questionable": Samuel Abt, "Armstrong Says Doctor Never Talked About Drugs," *New York Times*, July 10, 2001.

167   "on dieting": Ibid.

167   "knows physiology": Ibid.

167   "proud" and "on a limited basis": Associated Press, July 10, 2001.

168   "People are not": Associated Press, July 23, 2001.

168   "If Lance is clean": David Walsh, "Paradise Lost on Tour," *Sunday Times*, July 29, 2001.

CHAPTER 12

171   An Italian criminal investigation: Affidavit of Renzo Ferrante, a law-enforcement agent with the Italian Carabinieri SAS, USADA reasoned decision.

171   "not gonna get": Hamilton and Coyle, *The Secret Race*, 132.

172   In less than two years: Dave Philipps, "Questions Remain About Doping Ties to Armstrong's Coach," *Gazette* (Colorado Springs, Colorado), January 20, 2013.

172   He said he woke up one night: Interview with Chris Carmichael, 2006.

173   In November or December 1999: J.T. Neal audiotapes; interview with Frances Neal, 2013.

173 many people in: J.T. Neal audiotapes; interviews with Lance Armstrong, John Korioth and a person with knowledge of the situation.

173 One wire transfer: USADA reasoned decision, 107.

174 In 1999, her company: J.T. Neal audiotapes.

174 Kristin Armstrong allegedly urged: Ibid.

174 Now he wouldn't even: Ibid.

175 To his wife's dismay: Ibid.

176 "Always have loved you": Armstrong Kelly, with Rodgers, *No Mountain High Enough*, 255.

177 "one of the few people": Ibid., 255.

177 she called Armstrong: Ibid., 256–257.

177 "He's out swinging": Ibid., 257.

178 "looked shell-shocked": Ibid., 257.

CHAPTER 13

181 "Yes, you will": Interview with David Zabriskie, 2013.

183 selling marijuana and cocaine: Ibid.; interview with Sheree Hamik (formerly Sheree Zabriskie), David Zabriskie's mother, 2013; records from Salt Lake City police department.

184 "Look, some guy's": Interview with David Zabriskie, 2013.

188 "Oh man, it's bad": Ibid.; interview with Matt DeCanio, 2013.

190 "tons of human growth": Interview with David Zabriskie, 2013.

191 injections came from: Ibid. Affidavit of Michael Barry, 2013.

193 "You are a pussy": Interview with David Zabriskie, 2013.

194 "Look, Dave": Ibid.

194 "No, it's not": Ibid.

194 "It's just how it is": Ibid.

194 "Don't you trust": Affidavit of Michael Barry; interview with Michael Barry, 2012.

194 he had found: Interview with Michael Barry, 2012.

194 Hincapie, who became close: Affidavit of Michael Barry.

195 Bruyneel and del Moral: Ibid.; interviews with David Zabriskie, 2013, and Michael Barry, 2012; affidavit of David Zabriskie.

195 "Be careful when you": Ibid.; interview with Michael Barry, 2012; Michael Barry affidavit.

195 As the administrator: Interview with David Zabriskie, 2013; interview with Michael Barry, 2012.

CHAPTER 14

198 he might drink: Interview with George Hincapie, 2013.

198 Landis battled: Interviews with many Postal Service riders, including David Zabriskie and Jonathan Vaughters. Many didn't want their names used because they didn't want to get entangled in the Armstrong doping scandal. Interview with Allen Lim, 2013.

198 he had popped: Interviews with David Zabriskie, 2013, and Allen Lim, 2013.

198 "His fucking money": Interview with David Zabriskie, 2013.

198 he wanted to "end it all": Ibid.

200 "Such an aggressive": Exhibit A, affidavit of Floyd Landis.

200 Armstrong told Landis: Floyd Landis affidavit in USADA case.

200 "Look, Floyd": Paul Kimmage, complete transcript of his interview of Floyd Landis, *VeloNews*, February 1, 2011.

200 For his first nineteen: Floyd Landis, with Loren Mooney, *Postitively False: The Real Story of How I Won the Tour de France* (New York: Simon Spotlight Entertainment, 2007), 3.

201 "Why is it that half": Ibid.

201 lay on the opposite side: Affidavit of Floyd Landis in USADA case.

202 to inject themselves: Interviews with Christian Vande Velde and George Hincapie, 2013.

202 "was remade": Samuel Abt, "Over the Years, the World According to Lance," *New York Times*, July 26, 2005.

202 "It's the organization": Ibid.

202 "France's motto": *Washington Times*, July 29, 2002.

202 "We have a sponsor": Samuel Abt, "Getting Things Right, So No One Can Follow," *New York Times*, July 29, 2002.

203 "Luke's name is Armstrong": Armstrong, with Jenkins, *Every Second Counts*, 93–94.

203 The two were on a beach: Interview with Mike Anderson, Armstrong's former bike mechanic/personal assistant, 2013.

203 Kristin had signed: Lawyers involved with Armstrong's legal cases, 2012 and 2013.

204 In 2004, Anderson: Mike Anderson, "My Life with Lance Armstrong," *Outside Online*, August 31, 2012.

205 Livingston—in his: Interview with Jonathan Vaughters, 2013.

210 The specific timing was contrived: Interviews with several people involved in the project. They didn't want to give their names because they don't want to be seen as damaging Livestrong or its mission.

210 Together with his foundation: Ibid.

211 "worst journalist": Claire Cozens, "Top Cyclist to Sue Sunday Times Over Doping Claims," *Guardian*, June 15, 2004.

212 "inappropriate": Suzanne Halliburton, "Discovery Channel to Back Team," *Austin American-Statesman*, June 16, 2004.

212 "If we're fucking lying": Daniel Coyle, *Lance Armstrong's War* (New York: Harper, 2004), 186.

213 A second after Betsy: Betsy Andreu affidavit in USADA case.

214 "To go around": Exhibit in the *Armstrong v. SCA Promotions, Inc.* case.

214 "You know your wife": Ibid.

215 Wilcockson told Walsh: David Walsh, *Seven Deadly Sins: My Pursuit of Lance Armstrong* (London: Simon & Schuster, 2012), 281–282.

216 the team bus came: Affidavit of Floyd Landis, 2013; interview with George Hincapie, 2013.

217 "You made a mistake": Affidavit of Filippo Simeoni.

218 "was protecting": Justin Davis, "Armstrong Settles Score with Simeoni," Agence France-Presse, July 23, 2004.

218 "I was surprised by what": Samuel Abt, "Armstrong Takes Time to Satisfy a Grudge," *New York Times*, July 24, 2004.

219 "I thought he was": Matt Lawton, "She Was the Whistleblower Who Hauled Him Down, Lance Armstrong Was the Drug Cheat, So What Happened When They Were Brought Together Again by MailOnline?" *Daily Mail*, November 18, 2013.

219 "I cannot understand": Exhibit in the *Armstrong v. SCA Promotions, Inc.* case.

219 and had even introduced: Interviews with George Hincapie and Frankie Andreu, 2013.

221 he told Johnson: Interview with David Zabriskie, 2013.

221 Johnson later said to me: Interview with Steve Johnson, 2013.

222 he had deposited: Testimony of Tyler Hamilton in the *Operación Puerto* doping ring case in Spain, 2012.

222 "a horror movie": Hamilton and Coyle, *The Secret Race*, 214.

222 "It felt like my skull": Ibid.

CHAPTER 15

232 "whether they're paying": Interview with Richard Young, partner at Bryan Cave law firm in Colorado Springs, former partner at Holme Roberts & Owen and an outside counsel for USADA.

235 "This is bullshit": Interview with Travis Tygart, 2013.

CHAPTER 16

239 flew to Belgium to: *United States of America ex. rel. Floyd Landis v. Tailwind Sports Corporation, Tailwind Sports, LLC, Montgomery Sports, Inc., Capital Sports & Entertainment, Thomas Weisel, Lance Armstrong, Johan Bruyneel, William Stapleton and Barton Knaggs*, filed in the United States District Court for the District of Columbia, 2010.

239 bikes-for-cash deal: Affidavit of Floyd Landis in USADA case; Reed

Albergotti and Vanessa O'Connell, "The Case of the Missing Bikes," *Wall Street Journal*, July 3, 2010.

240   When he called Trek: *Wall Street Journal*, July 3, 2010.

240   Bruyneel allegedly was furious: Ibid.

240   dumped one of Landis's: Ibid.; interviews with Jonathan Vaughters and David Zabriskie, 2013.

241   "Fuck, dude": Interview with Allen Lim, 2013.

242   "Good, dude": Ibid.

242   "You don't have to suffer": Interview with David Zabriskie, 2013.

243   "There's a system": Interview with Allen Lim, 2013.

244   Landis admitted that: Ibid. Affidavit of Levi Leipheimer in USADA case.

244   his father-in-law: Bonnie D. Ford, "ESPN.com's Q&A with Floyd Landis," *ESPN.com*, May 24, 2010.

245   "Sometimes to beat the devil": Interview with Allen Lim, 2013.

246   "Hey, Al, you're not": Ibid.

247   "That's the stupidest": Ibid.

248   "No, stay": Ibid.

248   "If you leave": Ibid.

250   He would help Leipheimer: Ibid.; interview with David Zabriskie, 2013; affidavit of Levi Leipheimer in USADA case.

253   Landis surmised: Interviews with Allen Lim, Jonathan Vaughters and David Zabriskie, 2013, affidavit of Levi Leipheimer in USADA case.

253   "Holy shit, remember": Interview with Allen Lim, 2013.

254   It began a string: Exhibit to the affidavit of Jonathan Vaughters in USADA case.

256   Leipheimer, who had transfused: Interview with Allen Lim, 2013.

257   "People say, I see": Kim Horner, "Banded Together Worldwide Army of Supporters Is United by Goal," *Dallas Morning News*, July 5, 2005.

257   Stores were requesting: Two people who work for Nike who do not want their names used because they are not authorized to speak publicly about company business.

259   The number of riders: Statistics provided by USA Cycling.

260   "If not for Lance": Richard Sandomir, "Stages in the Global Branding of the Tour de Lance Are About to Begin," *New York Times*, July 26, 2005.

CHAPTER 17

262   SCA balked after Hamman: Interviews with Bob Hamman, Chris Hamman and Jeff Tillotson, 2006 and 2013.

263   First, he hammered at Hamman's: Capital Sports and Entertainment advertisement, *Sports Business Journal*, September 2004.

264   Stapleton frequently made trips: Interviews with a person close to Stapleton who did not want to be identified for fear of retribution, and two people who worked at the UCI who also did not want to be identified because they fear for their job security.

265   McQuaid said that in 2002: Stephen Farrand, "McQuaid Reveals Armstrong Made Two Donations to the UCI," *Cyclingnews*, July 10, 2010.

265   part of Verbruggen's: Reed Albergotti and Vanessa O'Connell, "New Twist in Armstrong Saga," *Wall Street Journal*, January 17, 2013.

265   "stink to high heaven": Ibid.

266   "I'm so embarrassed": Interview with Jeff Tillotson, 2013.

267   "preposterous": Jim Vertuno, "Armstrong Gets Strong Backing from USA Cycling," Associated Press, August 26, 2005.

268   "Kafkaesque": Interview with Dick Pound, 2012.

268   "proven scientific facts": John Rawling, "Nasty Postscript to Hero's Tale," *Guardian*, August 29, 2005.

268   "He owes explanations": Ibid.

272   "How's it going to look": Interview with Frankie Andreu, 2013.

274   he perjured himself: Interviews with Stephen Swart, Lance Armstrong and George Hincapie, 2013.

275   First, they announced: Indiana University, News Release, October 27, 2005.

275   Nichols said he: Affidavit of Craig Nichols.

276   "I was in the room": Audiotape of the voice message Stephanie Mc-
      Ilvain left for Betsy Andreu.

CHAPTER 18

278   Even before the press: Interview with Jeff Tillotson, 2013.
279   "In no way will": Toby Sterling, "Dutch Lawyer Vows Independent
      Investigation into Armstrong Doping Allegations," Associated Press,
      October 10, 2005.
280   "he may have been right": Arthur Max, "Report Clears Armstrong
      of Doping in 1999 Tour de France," Associated Press, June 1,
      2006.
280   "Sweet Vindication": Fort Worth *Star-Telegram*, "Sweet Vindica-
      tion," June 5, 2006.
281   "so lacking in professionalism": Associated Press, June 2, 2006.
281   "Somebody send the photos": "Armstrong Picks Up Honorary De-
      gree," Associated Press, May 22, 2006.
288   The story ran: Juliet Macur, "2 Ex-Teammates of Cycling Star Ad-
      mit Drug Use," *New York Times*, September 12, 2006.
288   "a hatchet job": Jim Litke, "Armstrong Says Report Teammates
      Used EPO Was 'Hatchet Job,'" Associated Press, September 12,
      2006.
289   "a severe lack": Sal Ruibal, "Armstrong Chops Back at 'Hatchet
      Job,'" *USA Today*, September 13, 2006.
289   "Well, that's what we've": Interview with Betsy Andreu, 2006.
290   He had doped with: Interview with David Zabriskie, 2013.
290   Both men felt pressure: Ibid.
291   Witt was his source: In a Q&A between Landis and Bonnie D. Ford
      published on May 24, 2010, on ESPN.com, Landis said Witt "was
      involved, and he helped" with Landis's doping.
291   doping to Steve Johnson: Johnson denies ever being aware of any
      doping on the Postal Service team before Floyd Landis's allegations
      surfaced in the spring of 2010.

291   "If you ever do drugs": Interview with David Zabriskie, 2013.

292   "Shit, well, I guess": Interview with Allen Lim, 2013.

CHAPTER 19

293   Speaking for an hour: Chuck Salter, "Livestrong Leverage: How the $50 Million Foundation Helped Texas Win $3 Billion in Cancer Funding," *Fast Company*, November 3, 2010.

293   "It's only fun": Ibid.

293   "a regular 365-days-a-year": Douglas Brinkley, "Lance Armstrong Rides Again," *Vanity Fair*, September 9, 2008.

294   "The Tour was a bit": John Wilcockson, *Lance: The Making of the World's Greatest Champion* (New York: Da Capo Press, 2009), 6.

295   "Athletes still get away": Brian Alexander, "The Awful Truth About Drugs in Sports," *Outside*, July 1, 2005.

296   "You don't have the": Interview with Doug Ellis, 2012.

296   "You're spending": Ibid.

297   Pierre Bordry, the head: Interviews with several antidoping scientists who worked with Bordry. They didn't want their names used because their conversation with Bordry was supposed to remain confidential.

298   He and Armstrong had talked: Interview with Lance Armstrong, 2013; interview with Jonathan Vaughters, 2013.

300   "Us former riders generally": Agence France-Presse, "Cycling: Why Are You Coming Back, Lance? Asks Leblanc," September 30, 2008.

303   "did more in five minutes": Suzanne Halliburton, "Wait Till Next Year," *Austin American-Statesman*, July 27, 2009.

303   he had threatened: Interviews with Lance Armstrong, 2012 and 2013; interview with Johan Bruyneel, 2010.

303   he began threatening other: Ibid.; interviews with George Hincapie, Jonathan Vaughters, and David Zabriskie, 2013.

304   Williams felt bad: Interview with a close friend of Williams's who doesn't want to be identified for fear of betraying Williams's trust, 2013.

304 paid $200,000: Reed Albergotti and Vanessa O'Connell, "For Cycling's Big Backers, Joy Ride Ends in Grief," *Wall Street Journal*, December 18, 2010.

305 "To be honest": Albergotti and O'Connell, "For Cycling's Big Backers, Joy Ride Ends in Grief."

305 informing Williams that: Interview with Lance Armsttrong, 2013.

305 Williams was supposedly livid and vowed: Interview with a close friend of Williams's who doesn't want to be identified for fear of betraying Williams's trust, 2013.

305 Williams allegedly told a friend: Ibid.

306 "No, I'm sorry, man": Interview with David Zabriskie, 2013.

306 Landis felt safe: Ibid.; Interview with Jonathan Vaughters, 2013.

307 He allegedly could exact: Interview with a close friend of Williams's who doesn't want to be identified for fear of betraying Williams's trust, 2013.

307 Williams had previously denied: Albergotti and O'Connell, "For Cycling's Big Backers, Joy Ride Ends in Grief."

CHAPTER 20

308 Armstrong had eavesdropped: Affidavit of David Zabriskie; interview with David Zabriskie, 2013.

308 On Friday, April 30: Affidavit of Floyd Landis in USADA case, Exhibit B.

309 Landis claimed that: Ibid.

310 Stapleton, the agent who'd: Affidavit of Floyd Landis.

311 "I used performance-enhancing drugs": Interview with Andrew Messick, 2012.

311 Landis said he spent: Sara Corbett, "The Outcast," *New York Times Play Magazine*, August 19, 2007.

311 including at least $478,354: United States Attorney's Office, Southern District of California, Press Release: "Former Pro Cyclist Floyd

Landis Admits Defrauding Donors and Agrees to Pay Hundreds of Thousands of Dollars in Restitution," August 24, 2012.

311   "When you're in the Mafia": Interview with Andrew Messick, 2012.

312   later admitted: Jacquelin Magnay, "Spanish Cyclist Jesús Manzano Says He Was Given Dog, Cattle and Horse Medications by Eufemiano Fuentes," *Telegraph*, February 13, 2013.

313   "If I'm willing to come forward": Interview with Travis Tygart, 2012.

313   "We were all doing it": Ibid.

313   "the guys that want to": Ibid.

314   Landis recalled: Ibid.; interviews with law enforcement agents involved in the case, who are not authorized to speak publicly about the matters they've worked on.

315   "See all these security": Interview with George Hincapie, 2013; interview with Christian Vande Velde, 2013; interview with David Zabriskie, 2013.

315   Thanks in part: Interview with a close friend of Williams's and a colleague of Williams's who don't want to be identified for fear of betraying Williams's trust, 2013.

319   "What an idiot!": Interview with a person on the RadioShack team, who was not authorized to speak about any private conversations on the team bus, 2013.

319   "I can't believe it": *Los Angeles Daily News*, "Cyclists: Doping Charges Outlandish," May 22, 2010.

320   "They're going to": Interview with David Zabriskie, 2013.

320   "Why don't you just deny": Interview with George Hincapie, 2013.

320   Armstrong stared: Ibid.

320   "How do you feel?": YouTube video of Armstrong taken from the RadioShack team car, *Bicycling*, published on the Web on May 14, 2012. www.youtube.com/watch?v=kLor65LUslg.

CHAPTER 21

328   Danielson, once dubbed: Affidavit of Tom Danielson.

328   "Lance called the shots": Affidavit of Christian Vande Velde.

329   "I want to clear my": Bonnie D. Ford, "Landis Admits Doping, Accuses Lance," *ESPN.com*, May 21, 2010.

329   "If I don't say something": Ibid.

332   Landis, would do it all: Paul Kimmage, "Complete Transcript: Paul Kimmage's Interview of Floyd Landis," *VeloNews*, February 1, 2011.

332   "feel guilty at all": Ford, "Landis Admits Doping, Accuses Lance."

333   "You know, don't tell": Interview with David Zabriskie, 2013.

334   They wanted George Hincapie: Interviews with several investigators with knowledge of the case. They didn't want their names used because they aren't authorized to speak publicly about their cases.

334   He served him with a subpoena: Interview with Chris Manderson, Hamilton's lawyer, 2013.

335   Landis's claims that: Reed Albergotti and Vanessa O'Connell, "The Case of the Missing Bikes," *Wall Street Journal*, July 3, 2010.

336   a story in the *New Yorker*: Michael Specter, "The Long Ride," the *New Yorker*, July 15, 2002.

338   "You're the first person": Interview with Chris Manderson, 2013.

339   "I might be distracted": Neal Rogers, "Lance Armstrong: Crashes Not Result of Distraction by Federal Inquiry," *VeloNews*, July 18, 2010.

341   Doug Miller, the main: Interviews with several people involved in the case who are not authorized to talk publicly about the matter, 2012 and 2013.

343   Herman would pay: Reed Albergotti, "Armstrong Lobbying Targeted Investigator," *Wall Street Journal*, February 19, 2013.

343 First, he told Armstrong: Interview with two people with knowledge of Fabiani's conversation with Armstrong. Those people wanted to remain anonymous so as not to be seen as breaching Armstrong's trust.

348 "You are not a rat": Interview with Chris Manderson, 2013.

349 "How much are they": Hamilton and Coyle, *The Secret Race*, 258–259.

349 "Run don't walk": Affidavit of Levi Leipheimer.

350 Within a week of taking Armstrong on: Interview with two lawyers present at the meeting, who are not authorized to talk publicly about it, April 2013.

350 "You're going to have a hard time prosecuting": Ibid.

350 "You know you guys are going to": Ibid.

350 They were 99 percent sure: Interviews with two people with direct knowledge of the investigation who aren't authorized to speak publicly about the case, 2013.

351 Birotte told one investigator: Interview with the investigator who spoke to Birotte, 2013. He didn't want his name published because he was not authorized to speak publicly about the investigation or its outcome.

351 The Justice Department had received: Letter from the Justice Department regarding a Freedom of Information Act request.

CHAPTER 23

356 whose services Hincapie: Interview with a close friend of Williams's who doesn't want to be identified for fear of betraying Williams's trust, and with two people with knowledge of the situation who aren't authorized to speak about it, 2013.

357 "Can you believe all this": Interviews with Christian Vande Velde, February 2013, and George Hincapie, July 2013.

361 The ever-stubborn Gunderson: Interview with Micki Rawlings, Gunderson's sister, 2013.

361 "I can't assure you": Ibid.

362 Ulman chatted with Senator Kay Bailey: Pete Yost, "Influence Game: Armstrong's Lobbying Circle," Associated Press, July 17, 2012.

362 Among his next several stops: Interviews with staff members, including Philip Schmidt, of Representative Serrano's office.

363 "substantially if not all": Ibid.

363 "Livestrong was supposed": Ibid.

364 Stapleton supposedly asked USOC officials: Interview with two USOC officials and two USADA officials who didn't want to be named because they are not authorized to speak publicly on behalf of their organization, 2013.

365 Upon advice from Washington lawyer: Interview with Lance Armstrong, 2013; interview with a person on Armstrong's legal team who was not authorized to speak about the case.

CHAPTER 24

367 Fabiani, the spokesman, blamed: Interviews with several people with direct knowledge of the reaction to the USADA report's going online, 2013. Those people didn't want their names published for fear of losing Armstrong's trust.

370 Armstrong and his team were banking: Ibid.

372 Just before 2 p.m.: Interview with Annie Skinner, spokeswoman for USADA, 2013.

373 Armstrong clicked: Interviews with several people with direct knowledge of the reaction to the USADA report's going online, 2013. Those people didn't want their names published for fear of losing Armstrong's trust.

CHAPTER 25

377   though he was the person: Interview with Lance Armstrong, 2013.

378   foundation board members who had formed: Interview with Mark McKinnon, 2013.

378   "If Lance doesn't leave": Ibid.

382   Ungerleider helped broker: Interviews with two people involved in the meeting and several people briefed on the meeting, 2013. They didn't want their names used because they are not authorized to speak publicly about the meeting.

383   Even USADA: Ibid.

383   "Travis, you're a": Ibid.

384   Tygart said he could: Ibid.

385   "At the end of the day": Ibid.

386   "I can't get up in the": Ibid.

388   He was sick of: Interview with Lance Armstrong, 2013.

388   "So-and-so said this": Interview with Adam Wilk, 2013.

388   "I'm sorry for everything": Interview with Doug Ulman, Livestrong CEO, June 2013.

392   He offered them $1 million: Interviews with Bob Hamman and Jeff Tillotson, April 2013.

392   "We're all suckers": CBS News, July 19, 2013.

393   First, he offered the government: Interviews with two people involved in the case, 2013. They didn't want to be interviewed because the case is ongoing.

EPILOGUE

399   He'd shoot me an e-mail: Lance Armstrong e-mail message to author, October 10, 2006.

SELECTED BIBLIOGRAPHY

Allison, Scott T., and George R. Goethals. *Heroes: What They Do and Why We Need Them*. New York: Oxford University Press, 2011.

Armstrong, Lance, with Sally Jenkins. *It's Not About the Bike: My Journey Back to Life*. New York: Berkley Books, 2000.

Armstrong, Lance, with Sally Jenkins. *Every Second Counts*. New York: Broadway Books, 2003.

Armstrong Kelly, Linda, with Joni Rodgers. *No Mountain High Enough: Raising Lance, Raising Me*. New York: Broadway Books, 2005.

Ballester, Pierre, and David Walsh. *L.A. Confidentiel: Les secrets de Lance Armstrong*. Paris: La Martinière, 2006.

Bruyneel, Johan. *We Might as Well Win*. Boston: Mariner Books, 2009.

Campbell, Joseph. *The Hero with a Thousand Faces*. Novato, Calif.: New World Library, 2008.

Carlyle, Thomas. *On Heroes, Hero-Worship, and the Heroic in History*. Lexington, Ky.: 2013.

Coyle, Daniel. *Lance Armstrong's War*. New York: HarperCollins, 2005.

Hamilton, Tyler, and Daniel Coyle. *The Secret Race: Inside the Hidden World of the Tour de France: Doping, Cover-ups, and Winning at All Costs*. New York: Bantam Books, 2012.

Hatton, Caroline. *The Night Olympic Team: Fighting to Keep Drugs out of the Games*. Honesdale, Pa.: Boyds Mills Press, 2008.

Kimmage, Paul. *Rough Ride: Behind the Wheel with a Pro Cyclist*. London: Stanley Paul, 1990.

Landis, Floyd, with Loren Mooney. *Positively False: The Real Story of How I Won the Tour de France*. New York: Simon Spotlight Entertainment, 2007.

McGann, Bill, and Carol McGann. *The Story of the Tour de France*. Vol. 1, 1903–1964. Indianapolis: Dog Ear Publishing, 2006.

——— *The Story of the Tour de France*. Vol. 2, 1965–2007. Indianapolis: Dog Ear Publishing, 2008.

Millar, David. *Racing Through the Dark*. London: Orion Books, 2011.

Parisotto, Robin. *Blood Sports: The Inside Dope on Drugs in Sport*. Richmond, Australia: Hardie Grant Books, 2006.

Parkin, Joe. *A Dog in a Hat: An American Bike Racer's Story of Mud, Drugs, Blood, Betrayal, and Beauty in Belgium*. Boulder, Colo.: VeloPress, 2008.

Sharp, Kathleen. *Blood Medicine: Blowing the Whistle on One of the Deadliest Prescription Drugs Ever*. New York: Plume, 2012.

Thompson, Christopher S. *The Tour de France: A Cultural History*. Berkeley, Los Angeles and London: University of California Press, 2006.

Walsh, David. *From Lance to Landis: Inside the American Doping Controversy at the Tour de France*. New York: Ballantine Books, 2007.

Walsh, David. *Seven Deadly Sins: My Pursuit of Lance Armstrong*. London: Simon & Schuster, 2012.

Whittle, Jeremy. *Bad Blood: The Secret Life of the Tour de France*. London: Yellow Jersey Press, 2008.

Wilcockson, John. *Lance: The Making of the World's Greatest Champion*. New York: Da Capo Press, 2009.

World Anti-Doping Agency. *World Anti-Doping Code*, 2009.

INDEX